T0386622

The Ethics of Group Psychotherapy

The Ethics of Group Psychotherapy provides group psychotherapists with the ethical and legal foundation needed to engage in effective decision-making in their everyday group practices.

This text provides readers with a framework for understanding ethical dilemmas through a review of major models of ethical thinking, including principlism, feminism and the ethics of care, and virtue ethics. The authors use this foundation to explore those problems emerging most routinely in group practice, among which are safeguarding members' personal information, protecting members' autonomy, and helping members to process differences—particularly those related to privilege and oppression—in a way that furthers interpersonal relations and social justice. Throughout the text, practical tools such as using assessments to aid in member selection and tracking progress and outcome through measurement-based care are offered that bolster the group psychotherapist's effectiveness in ethical decision-making.

Featuring questions for discussion and items to assess the reader's master of the material, this text will be a valuable tool in classroom and small-group learning.

Virginia Brabender, PhD, ABPP, is a professor in Widener University's Institute for Graduate Clinical Psychology. She has written five prior books on group psychotherapy and numerous articles.

Rebecca MacNair-Semands, PhD, is a co-chair of the Science to Service Task Force for the AGPA Board of Directors. She authored the first edition of the *Ethics of Group Psychotherapy*.

AGPA Group Therapy Training and Practice Series
Series Editors: Les Greene and Rebecca MacNair-Semands

The American Group Psychotherapy Association (AGPA) is the foremost professional association dedicated to the field of group psychotherapy, operating through a tri-partite structure: AGPA, a professional and educational organization; the Group Foundation for Advancing Mental Health, its philanthropic arm; and the International Board for Certification of Group Psychotherapists, a standard setting and certifying body. This multidisciplinary association has approximately 3,000 members, including psychiatrists, psychologists, social workers, nurses, clinical mental health counselors, marriage and family therapists, pastoral counselors, occupational therapists, and creative arts therapists, many of whom have been recognized as specialists through the Certified Group Psychotherapist credential. The association has 26 local and regional societies located across the country. Its members are experienced mental health professionals who lead psychotherapy groups and various non-clinical groups. Many are organizational specialists who work with businesses, not-for-profit organizations, communities, and other "natural" groups to help them improve their functioning.

The goal of the AGPA Group Therapy Training and Practice Series is to produce the highest quality publications to aid the practitioner and student in updating and improving his/her knowledge, professional competence, and skills with current and new developments in methods, practice, theory, and research in the group psychotherapy field. Books in this series are the only curriculum guide and resource for a variety of courses credentialed by the International Board for Certification of Group Psychotherapists. While this is the series' original and primary purpose, the texts are also useful in a variety of other settings including as a resource for students and clinicians interested in learning more about group psychotherapy, as a text in academic courses, or as part of a training curriculum in a practicum or internship training experience.

Books in this Series:

Core Principles of Group Psychotherapy: An Integrated Theory, Research, and Practice Training Manual, *Edited by Francis J. Kaklauskas, Les R. Greene*

The Ethics of Group Psychotherapy: Principles and Practical Strategies, *by Virginia Brabender and Rebecca MacNair-Semands*

For more information about this series, please visit https://www.routledge.com/AGPA-Group-Therapy-Training-and-Practice-Series/book-series/AGPA.

The Ethics of Group Psychotherapy

Principles and Practical Strategies

**Virginia Brabender and
Rebecca MacNair-Semands**

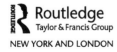

Routledge
Taylor & Francis Group

NEW YORK AND LONDON

First published 2022
by Routledge
605 Third Avenue, New York, NY 10158

and by Routledge
4 Park Square, Milton Park, Abingdon, Oxon, OX14 4RN

Routledge is an imprint of the Taylor & Francis Group, an informa business

Library of Congress Cataloguing-in-Publication Data
Names: Brabender, Virginia, author. | MacNair-Semands, Rebecca, author.
Title: The ethics of group psychotherapy : principles and practical strategies / Virginia Brabender and Rebecca MacNair-Semands.
Description: New York, NY : Routledge, 2022. | Includes bibliographical references and index. |
Identifiers: LCCN 2021050379 (print) | LCCN 2021050380 (ebook) |
ISBN 9780367615628 (hardback) | ISBN 9780367615611 (paperback) |
ISBN 9781003105527 (ebook)
Subjects: LCSH: Group psychotherapy–Moral and ethical aspects. | Group psychotherapists.
Classification: LCC RC488 .B73 2022 (print) | LCC RC488 (ebook) |
DDC 616.89/152–dc23/eng/20211112
LC record available at https://lccn.loc.gov/2021050379
LC ebook record available at https://lccn.loc.gov/2021050380

ISBN: 978-0-367-61562-8 (hbk)
ISBN: 978-0-367-61561-1 (pbk)
ISBN: 978-1-003-10552-7 (ebk)

DOI: 10.4324/9781003105527

Typeset in Times New Roman
by MPS Limited, Dehradun

Virginia dedicates this book to two beautiful souls, the late Dr. Patricia Bricklin and her daughter Carol Bricklin.

Rebecca dedicates this book to Nancy MacNair and the late Dr. Ray MacNair, kind and wise parents and models of social justice.

Contents

About the Authors   x
Preface   xi
Acknowledgments   xiv

1 Ethical, Legal, and Professional Fundamentals   1

2 Privacy, Confidentiality, and Privilege   26

3 Ethical Issues Related to the Role of Therapist/Leader   42

4 Selection, Preparation, and Norm Development among Members   67

5 Informed Consent   99

6 Supervision   119

7 The Group Psychotherapist as Ethical Decision-Maker: Process
   and Product   132

Afterword   171
Index   173

About the Authors

Virginia Brabender, Ph.D., ABPP (Cl), is a professor in Widener University's Institute for Graduate Clinical Psychology. She has been teaching group psychotherapy for four decades. She has co-authored with April Fallon the following texts in group psychotherapy: *Models of inpatient group psychotherapy*, *Essentials of group therapy*, *Group development in practice: Guidance for clinicians and researchers on stages and dynamics of change* and *Group psychotherapy in inpatient, partial hospital, and residential care settings.* She has also written *Introduction to Group Therapy.* She edited a two-part series on ethics, which appeared in the *International Journal of Group Psychotherapy* (2006–2007). She serves on the editorial board of the *International Journal of Group Psychotherapy* and is a fellow of the American Group Psychotherapy Association and division 49 of the American Psychological Association.

Rebecca MacNair-Semands, Ph.D., CGP, FAGPA, is currently in her ninth year as a co-chair of the Science to Service Task Force for the AGPA Board of Directors. She recently retired as the senior associate director of the UNC Charlotte Counseling and Psychological Services Center, where she was employed for over 25 years. In addition to coordinating the clinical and group services for the center, she delivered over 40 national and international professional presentations. She has published 30 articles and book chapters, as well as the first edition of the *Ethics of Group Psychotherapy.* In 2017, Dr. MacNair-Semands was named Group Psychologist of the Year by the American Psychological Association (APA)'s Society of Group Psychology and Group Psychotherapy. She is a fellow of the American Group Psychotherapy Association and division 49 of the APA.

Preface

Most group psychotherapists have had a course in professional ethics. Trainees will have such a course at some point during graduate training. What, then, is the purpose of this book? This text is necessary because group psychotherapy presents unique challenges, which are not likely to be covered in a general ethics course. A primary reason for the unique ethical concerns of this modality is the structure of the treatment, the fact that it almost always involves individuals who are strangers to one another (Brabender, 2021). This aspect distinguishes it from individual therapy in which only a single person (other than the therapist) participates in the treatment. It is also distinct from family therapy in which participants have a high level of familiarity with one another and access to a shared pool of information prior to the treatment. In group psychotherapy, it is only within the sessions that members learn about their co-members. This circumstance creates the condition for one of the most significant problems the group psychotherapist faces—how to ensure that each member retains control over one's personal information or as the popular slogan states, "What happens in Vegas stays in Vegas." The confidentiality problem is just an example of a challenge that faces group psychotherapists.

Another problem specific to group psychotherapy concerns responses to diverse identities. Members in the group are likely to encounter individuals very different from themselves. Any given group might be composed of members who differ in terms of race, culture, gender, gender identity, sexual orientation, socio-economic status, political beliefs, and so on. Such differences can be a fertile bed for conflict, evoking behaviors in members such as bullying and coercion that are at odds with therapeutic goals and also could be harmful. How does the therapist ensure that the harmful dynamics that exist in society at large, dynamics leading to the marginalization of some groups (MacNair-Semands, 2007), are not merely mirrored in the psychotherapy group? Teaching members to use supportive language means the leader must be aware of appropriate terms to use as they emerge and shift. Leaders often feel fearful when hurtful comments are made and may freeze rather than respond quickly due to this anxiety. Instead, the leader can learn to establish and maintain a group in such a way that differences among members serve as stimuli for positive change.

Group psychotherapy is distinctive in that the interests of multiple primary stakeholders must be considered in ethical decision-making. In individual therapy, the therapist must take into account how any given ethical or legal solution to a problem affects a single person—the patient. Although other stakeholders' interests can be weighed, those of the client are primary. The complexity that the presence of multiple primary stakeholders creates is that what might be beneficial to one group member could be detrimental to another. This circumstance often requires all of the thought and care that a group leader can muster. Having a solid knowledge base of common ethical problems and strategies for their solution—such as what this text provides—helps the group leader to contend with this complexity.

In addition to the uniqueness of group psychotherapy and the ethical problems related to this modality, it is also true that ever-emerging events and movements present new ethical challenges. Much has happened since the first edition of this text was published in 2005! The first edition had less emphasis on technology, diversity, and measurement-based care. In 2005, it was more common to hug clients or to allow members to hug each other without the developed thoughtful discussions about boundaries around touch and permission. As we write this book, we are amid a global pandemic. COVID-19 required clinicians to find new ways of delivering services other than in-person meetings. Many group psychotherapists moved their groups to online formats, introducing a host of new ethical and legal problems. For example, how does the group psychotherapist ensure that the group members' communications are confidential? This text also integrates recent empirical findings germane to the delivery of group treatment. For example, group psychotherapists have an ethical obligation to ensure that members are deriving benefit from participation in a particular group. This text describes how advances in routine outcome management help the therapist to meet this obligation.

In exploring the ethical issues we identify in this text, we draw upon a myriad of sources including the ethical literature, professional codes of practice, and our own experiences. Each of us has an extensive background in conducting and supervising group psychotherapy. Virginia's experience has been in inpatient and private practice settings. She has supervised and provided consultation to students in a great range of settings including residential treatment centers, public middle schools and high schools, and addiction treatment settings. Rebecca's experience has primarily been in various roles at a university counseling center, while also engaging in research on group therapy and developing measures specific to groups. She trained other agencies and administrators about starting and expanding group programs with an ethical approach; she also served as an administrator overseeing all clinical services, including developing policies and best practice guidelines. Both of us have conducted workshops on ethics and learned about the many ethical dilemmas that have affected our workshop participants in their group work.

In reading this book, you will be aided by a grasp of the overall structure. Chapter 1 provides the basic information about ethical and legal issues that the authors will draw upon throughout this text. This chapter begins with a discussion of broad theoretical systems that aid the group psychotherapist in framing ethical problems. An adequate analysis of ethical problems must include a consideration of the law and professional codes, which are also considered in Chapter 1. With these resources in tow, the reader is well-positioned to approach the next topic: the stages in solving an ethical problem. Ethical problems are complex—particularly in group psychotherapy with its multiple stakeholders—and the practitioner benefits from having an organized approach to addressing their multiple facets. Ethical problems also generate anxiety, which in turn can lead to quick, haphazard, and ill-considered solutions. An internalized set of problem-solving steps is an antidote to those hastily formed solutions that are largely designed to rid the practitioner of the problem rather than solve it most effectively. In Chapter 2, we address the critical issue of safeguarding member information and do so through an exploration of the topics of privacy, confidentiality, and privilege.

Chapters 3 and 4 focus on the roles of the leader and the roles of members respectively. Chapter 3 discusses competence in conducting groups as an ethical requirement of the therapist. It outlines many of the core tasks of the group psychotherapists and the various experiences that contribute to mastering these tasks. Two therapist tasks we explore in some depth because they are both associated with ethical problems. They are managing boundaries and differences in the group, particularly differences related to identity dimensions such as race, sexual orientation, and so on. This latter area has achieved increased importance as group psychotherapists consider how group treatment might advance social justice ends by enhancing individual members' abilities to respond to differences constructively. Chapter 4 focuses on selection, preparation, and relationships among members. Here, we address some of the complicated and even controversial issues that group leaders must address such as whether socialization among members outside the group will be permitted.

Chapter 5 is concentrated on informed consent, a topic that merits its own chapter because this agreement is the ethical and legal foundation of the group's work. The informed consent articulates risks and benefits of group participation and also performs the important function of delineating member responsibilities. Considering topics such as raising one's fee in a fair manner or setting norms around the members' use of social media about group psychotherapy are explored with a modern lens so clients understand the norms, risks, and benefits. The informed consent implications of online therapy groups are discussed.

Chapter 6 is devoted to supervision. Many group psychotherapists are thrust into supervisory positions without having had specific preparation for this role during their training. The task of developing strong ethical-mindedness in the supervisee is also one for which many new supervisors are unprepared. This chapter seeks to address this deficit through its delineating of many of the common challenges and ways to meet them. Included in this chapter is a consideration of the experiential training group and its ethical aspects.

In Chapter 7, we focus on how the group psychotherapist makes decisions when faced with ethical problems. We consider the array of factors—both rational and irrational—that can impinge upon the therapist approaching an ethical quandary. The outcome of the operation of these factors is the decision itself and how this decision will be judged by others and the professional community is our next topic, Standard of Care. Often, the circumstances that give rise to ethically fraught decisions carry a high level of risk. In this chapter, we provide the reader with guidelines on risk management. We offer them with the proviso that group psychotherapists also need to be knowledgeable about the laws in their state and jurisdiction of practice to respond competently in high-risk situations. Some risks can be averted if the therapist is aware of how members are faring in their group. Although the therapists' in-session observations play a critical role in making this assessment, they can be enriched greatly by measurement-based care, a topic into which we delve at the end of the chapter.

Because our text is intended to be used in training situations, we have included a variety of resources to aid the instructor or supervisor and learner. Following each chapter is a set of discussion questions, many of which place the trainee in a circumstance with an ethical or legal problem and invite the trainee to proceed through the process of forging a solution. These questions are ideal fodder for a group of trainees' considerations. Inevitably, participants will learn that others see aspects of the problem that they missed, a realization encouraging the learner to gather information about ethical problems emerging in group treatment in more comprehensive, flexible ways. We also include items that test the trainee's mastery of the material presented in the chapter. Finally, we have provided a series of vignettes corresponding to the content of each chapter. Role-playing the vignettes can be a powerful source of learning and can be evocative of some of the emotions that are likely to emerge as members confront ethical problems in their everyday practice. Enjoy the process of understanding the feelings that emerge and how they affect ethical and legal problem-solving!

Acknowledgments

We would like to express our great gratitude to the American Group Psychotherapy Association and Marsha Block for extending to us the invitation to write this second edition of *Ethics and Group Psychotherapy*. To have the opportunity to think and write about a topic in which we each have been passionately interested for many years has been quite a privilege. We wish to thank Angela Stephens for her support of this project from start to finish. Contributing immensely to this project have been the comments and recommendations of our three reviewers: Les R. Greene, Ph.D., CGP, DLFAGPA; Anthony S. Joyce, Ph.D., R.Psych; and Linda K. Knauss, Ph.D., ABPP. We also would like to thank Widener University for the Faculty Development grant that supported this work. Ariana Hays served as our graduate assistant on this project and did exceptional, painstaking work. From Routledge, we would like to acknowledge the competent efforts of Amanda Devine, Grace McDonnell, and Kris Siosyte. We wish to thank all of the students, supervisees, group members, and co-therapists with whom we have worked over a combined total of six decades.

Abundant thanks go to our wonderful families who provided the supportive, loving environments making creativity possible. Specifically, we thank our spouses, Arthur (VB) and Steve (RMS) and our children Jacob, Gabi, and Natasha (VB) and Allison (RMS). We are so appreciative of all the various ways you cheered us on!

Note: Neither the American Group Psychotherapy Association nor the authors of this text provide legal advice. Readers seeking legal advice should consult with an attorney with the appropriate expertise.

1 Ethical, Legal, and Professional Fundamentals

This chapter provides the basic tools that we, as group therapists, need to recognize, understand, and solve ethical problems that emerge in the practice of group psychotherapy, as well as evaluate the success of our solutions. This array of tasks entails our possession of two types of tools: (1) the basic definitions that help us to communicate with one another about ethical problems; and (2) the major models that illuminate different dimensions of any given ethical problem and help to identify courses of action to resolve these problems. Often, in facing a sticky, complex ethical problem, a group psychotherapist can feel very alone in the process. What this chapter points out to the reader is that a variety of resources—including human resources—are available to assist the practitioner. These forms of assistance do not alleviate the sense of aloneness altogether. After all, ultimately, the therapist or co-therapy team must make a final decision. However, having used all that is available, having proceeded through a comprehensive and thoughtful process of evaluating aspects of the situation and various solutions, the practitioner is far more likely to proceed with confidence.

Ethical Paradigms

When ethical problems emerge, they tend to evoke anxiety in psychotherapists, including the group psychotherapist, who wants to do right and avoid the negative consequences of ethical mistakes. This anxiety motivates practitioners to look for rules or laws that will unambiguously identify a correct course of conduct. In this search, as Acuff et al. (1999) note, the practitioner is likely to be disappointed:

> No code of ethics, however well written, can anticipate all of the various situations in which psychologists may confront ethical dilemmas, and no code of ethics may be able to specify concrete actions for the psychologist to follow in all situations. Consequently, some of the possible ethical conflicts faced by psychologists have no clear solution and require psychologists to engage in an ethical decision process involving the balancing of competing ethical standards. (p. 565).

The quality of the solution the group psychotherapist generates is likely to be based on the extent to which the problem at hand is fully understood. Potentially elevating the group psychotherapist's understanding of the problem at hand is to make use of dominant ethical paradigms, frameworks in which ethical quandaries can be examined. Principlism (Beauchamp & Childress, 1979, 2013) is likely the most familiar to group psychotherapists, ensconced as it is in the ethical codes of most mental health disciplines. Indeed, this text emphasizes principlism. However, increasingly, we are seeing that other paradigms provide additional information and insight that are critical to doing justice to the complexity of the

DOI: 10.4324/9781003105527-1

ethical problems that can emerge in psychotherapy groups. The ethical problem-solver need not choose a particular framework any more than a botanist needs to choose one lens to examine plant cells.

Principlism

Principlism is an ethical framework, created by Beauchamp and Childress, and described in their classic text *Principles of Biomedical Ethics*, first published in 1979 and now in its 7th (2013) edition. This framework initially assisted medical professionals and eventually, human service professionals more broadly, in solving ethical problems that emerge in everyday practice. Beauchamp and Childress identified five principles that they saw as having universal significance, that is, principles that can reasonably be applied to all clinical situations: Respect for Autonomy, Beneficence and Non-maleficence, Justice, and Fidelity:

- Respect for Autonomy means avoiding actions that would deprive or limit individuals' control over their own lives and, conversely, engaging in actions that would expand their autonomy. This principle is implicated in such clinical activity as providing informed consent when recruiting members for a group (Brabender, 2006). When patients are given all relevant information about the group they are considering entering, their autonomy (i.e., making a well-informed decision) is preserved.
- Beneficence refers to those clinical actions that aim to promote the welfare of the client. Specific Beneficence is directed at a particular party, typically the client, but also, perhaps, the client's family. General Beneficence has a non-specific referent. When practitioners strive to deliver services competently to contribute to the creation of a more just society, they are serving General Beneficence. Non-maleficence reflects the value of avoiding action that would harm a group member. For example, this principle would dictate that a group psychotherapist would avoid the use of a technique that, while having some potential to benefit a group member, could also damage the member in another respect.
- Justice entails that the therapist adopts an inclusive attitude toward the provision of services, offering members "...fair, equitable, and appropriate treatment in light of what is due or owed to persons" (Beauchamp & Childress, 2009, p. 241). For example, a therapist who conducts the group in a venue that is accessible to individuals with ambulatory challenges is acting in accordance with the principle of Justice. Justice is also served when a therapist is vigilant during the sessions to ensure that individuals who have been silenced or marginalized in society at large do not experience similar events in the group.
- Fidelity, or loyalty, is the practitioner's responsibility to place the patient's interest before self-interest. Adherence to Fidelity is seen in the behavior of the therapist who encourages an unimproved member to seek alternate treatment even though this recommendation might be at odds with the therapist's financial interests. At times, practitioners' relationships with third parties can threaten the observance of Fidelity (Beauchamp & Childress, 2009). For example, a group psychotherapist might allow a colleague to solicit group members for participation in a study. Even though creating this opportunity for the colleague might hold no advantage for members, the therapist might do so to enhance the collegial relationship. Fidelity does not demand that the therapist subordinate all self-interests to member interests. For example, a therapist might decide to move the group because the rent for the current office has risen dramatically. Even though the new location of the group might be somewhat less convenient for some members, the action is defensible because the therapist has a right

to contain costs. Where Fidelity is most critically considered is where the therapist's consideration of self-interest can hinder the member in deriving benefit from the group.

From the standpoint of principlism, ethical quandaries can arise because following one of these four core principles could entail compromising another. For example, if a group psychotherapist describes in detail all the risks associated with being a member of a psychotherapy group (thereby complying with Respect for Autonomy), the therapist might in effect be discouraging that prospective member's willingness to be in the group (thereby compromising Beneficence). Oftentimes, ethical problems entail a conflict between Respect for Autonomy and Beneficence because what a professional believes might be in a patient's or group's interest might not be freely accepted by that individual or group. For example, an individual therapist might strongly believe that a patient would benefit from group treatment. The therapist might know the group experience would evoke uncomfortable feelings in the patient. Were this professional to soft-pedal the likely negative reactions to obtain the member's receptivity to the group, that professional would be placing Beneficence ahead of Respect for Autonomy. However, within individualistic cultures, Respect for Autonomy is broadly viewed as having precedence over Beneficence. That is, individuals should be free to make bad decisions. Still, in more collectivist cultures in which individuals, particularly family members, assume a high level of responsibility for one another, Respect for Autonomy does not occupy the same privileged position (Elliott, 2001). Even in individualistic societies, professionals are called upon to emphasize Beneficence over Respect for Autonomy at times. For example, the group psychotherapist might need to sacrifice Respect for Autonomy to protect a suicidal member.

Table 1.1 lists the principles, their definitions, and one or more examples of each.

Although it is sometimes necessary to place one principle ahead of another, doing so should not entail abandoning those ethical principles that were not given the greatest

Table 1.1 Core Ethical Principles as Applied to Group Psychotherapy

Principle	Definition	Example of Behaviors Consistent with Principle
Non-maleficence	The group psychotherapist will avoid actions that lead to harm for group members or other entities such as the therapist's profession or society at large.	The group psychotherapist avoids using techniques that have been shown to be harmful to members.
Beneficence	The group psychotherapist will engage in actions that lead to positive outcomes for members.	The group psychotherapist develops a strong therapeutic alliance with members.
Respect for Autonomy	The group psychotherapist honors members' right to self-determination.	The group psychotherapist alerts the prospective member of the risks of group treatment.
Justice	The group psychotherapist strives to provide equitable and fair treatment.	The group psychotherapist works in a physical environment that is accessible to individuals with varying physical abilities.
Fidelity	The group psychotherapist gives priority to the members' interests over self-interest.	A group psychotherapist, rather than abandoning group members, makes provisions for them in case the therapist needs to terminate the group.

weight. The group psychotherapist should find solutions that, while giving deference to a particular principle, allow other principles to be honored as much as possible. In our example of the individual therapist attempting to encourage a member to pursue group treatment, it would behoove the therapist to acquaint the member with the likely benefits of the group and to provide the individual with tools for managing any negative feelings that group treatment would evoke. In this way, the clinician would be at once observing the principle of Respect for Autonomy (by giving the member information about possible uncomfortable experiences) while heeding Beneficence (by diminishing the likelihood that worry about negative feelings will control the member's decision-making). Box 1.1 describes a training circumstance involving a conflict between ethical principles.

Feminist Ethics and the Ethics of Care

Feminist ethics and the ethics of care are frameworks that focus on the relationship between patient and caregiver, see caregiving activities as inherently of value, and encourage avoidance of harmful power dynamics in the caregiving relationship, particularly those based on race, gender, or class (Gilligan, 1982). Feminist ethics recognizes that many human societies are organized into patriarchal structures wherein women suffer oppression while men retain power and privilege. Feminism sees the structures as built specifically to perpetuate the power imbalance between men and women (Lindemann, 2019). Although the feminist perspective initially was centered on gender inequities, it expanded to other identity facets such as those related to race, culture, and sexual orientation, and explores how these identities intersect to deepen patterns of oppression (Layton & Leavy-Sperounis, 2020; Lindemann, 2019). Psychotherapy bears the character of the society in which it is conducted. Differences in power and privilege are seen between therapists and group members, and among group members with different identities. At times, interactions among members can strengthen inequalities and work to the detriment of members in the group. To the extent that any psychotherapy group perpetuates the subjugation of individuals, it creates psychic pain and saps the potential of group psychotherapy to liberate members from binding forces such as symptoms, constricted interpersonal patterns, and toxic relationships. It instead reinforces role rigidity and undermines authenticity, as members feel compelled to operate under the sway of cultural prescriptions.

Feminism recognizes that power asymmetries cannot be altogether absent in professional relationships, given the distinctive responsibilities of each party. However, from a feminist perspective, the ethical practice requires that the therapist do whatever possible to prevent the power differential from affecting the treatment in malignant ways. One way in which the therapist attends to power dynamics is to acknowledge them. As simple as such a step might seem to be, it is actually profound in that it opens up power in the relationship as an acceptable topic of conversation. This openness encourages all parties to address power dynamics that might be harmful to participants. Consider the following situation:

> A group psychotherapist contacted a member's psychiatrist to say he thought the psychiatrist should consider adjusting the medication based on changes the group psychotherapist was seeing. The member came to a session expressing anger toward the therapist, saying that the therapist should have informed her that he was going to take this step. Instead of responding that the member had given him consent to speak with the psychiatrist, which was true, the psychotherapist acknowledged that this was a breach, apologized to the member in the group session, and indicated that he would respond differently in the future.

The therapist in the vignette realized that he used the power of his position beyond what was necessary, thereby disempowering the group member. For example, were the member to disagree with the group psychotherapist's judgment, she might wish to contact the psychiatrist and share her view. Although on the sound legal ground to engage in his peremptory action, the therapist was not on the strong ethical ground from a feminist perspective. More importantly, though, the therapist's receptiveness to the group member's perspective is relationship-building and revealing of a strong ethical sensibility. It also supports the group member's willingness to advocate for themselves rather than reflexively submit to power. This action on the part of the therapist was consistent with both principlism ethics and feminist ethics. In recognizing that he had overstepped in not informing the member of the extramural communication, he underscored the importance of the member's autonomy.

The feminist perspective on ethical practice places emphasis on the practitioner's attending to societal context without which the practitioner cannot appreciate how a group member's reaction to power is shaped by other experiences, both historical and present. Suppose a group member, a person of color, is given feedback by other members on the limitations of their passive stance. That feedback is likely to have lessened potency in the absence of an acknowledgment that the passivity has been self-protective in the face of a society that often interprets self-assertion by racial minorities as aggressive. Therefore, to understand the group member fully, the therapist needs to view the person not merely from a clinical perspective but also in terms of broader social dynamics.

The feminist viewpoint also requires that cultural considerations factor into the therapist's decisions about establishing boundaries. Whereas a traditional clinical perspective might have dictated that the therapist avoids any crossing of a boundary to avoid the slippery slope leading to boundary violations, the therapist operating from a feminist position acknowledges that failing to recognize culture can lead to experiences of shaming and humiliation (Vasquez, 2007). Consider the following example:

> Alicia had had a breakthrough session in which she opened up about some experiences in which she suffered abuse at the hands of a relative. Alicia had been a reticent member, but her level of openness was unprecedented in this session. In the following session, she brought in a dessert for members to share. She described her feelings of gratitude and told members that this cake was a special one in that it was one her mother baked for the family on special occasions. The therapist had always encouraged members to avoid eating and drinking during the group. Therefore, she felt herself to be in a quandary about Alicia's offering. Still, she decided to allow members to partake because she knew it would be crushing to Alicia to have her offering rejected. She emphasized to members the specialness of the occasion so that they would realize that the norm she established would continue to be in place despite its relaxation in this one session. She also fostered a discussion about gratitude and the diverse ways members can express this feeling.

A therapist need not be operating from a feminist position to allow members to eat the cake. It was the rationale for the decision that was consistent with a feminist posture. The therapist considered the possibility that a gift refusal would shame Alicia and convey that her expression of gratitude was not worthy of the group's reception. It could also be a negation of the cultural ties associated with the cake. As Brown (1994) noted in her classic article, when therapists establish rules and apply them rigidly, they are likely to run roughshod over the person's highly unique experience and prevent the therapist from fashioning an optimal response to the client. The therapist's attention to how members might perceive this relaxation in the rule as creating a demand for others to express gratitude in material ways is also consistent with a feminist position, which holds that therapists should be sensitive to forms of coercion in the therapeutic situation at all degrees of subtlety.

The ethics of care is tied to feminist ethics in its recognition of inherent imbalances of power existing in particular relationships such as those between child and parent, healthcare professional and patient, and teacher and student (Held, 2006). From this perspective, where care is provided lovingly and sensitively, morality resides. That is, to the extent that we provide care to those particular individuals for whom we have a responsibility, we are moral beings. The ethics of care is rooted in a conceptual view of the human being as essentially relational rather than autonomous and independent (Held, 2006). All human beings begin their lives in a state of dependency and throughout their lives satisfy their needs and accomplish their goals through interdependency with others.

One important link between the ethics of care and feminism is the recognition that women in many societies are often the care providers. Cultures that do not recognize the significance of care fail to acknowledge the importance of women's contributions by, for example, remunerating women's work in caregiving to children or elders, and often tolerate the exploitation of women (Parton, 2003). They also neglect to hold men as bearing responsibility for care provision. In a culture in which ethics of care prevails, caring responsibilities would be more equitably distributed.

Of relevance to the ethics of care to psychotherapy practice is the role of emotions. Although other ethical frameworks allow for the role of emotions, in no other theory do they have the centrality and salience that the ethics of care accords them. As we will discuss in Chapter 6, emotions can be an impediment to sound decision-making. However, the ethics of care holds that emotions can also lead to ethically sound behavior, that is, feelings of compassion, concern, and empathy can spur positive action on another's behalf.

A therapist who embraces an ethics of care position might view particular situations differently than a therapist employing an alternate ethical theory such as principlism (Elsner & Rampton, 2020). For the group therapist embracing principlism, the autonomy of the client is paramount. Treatment is monitored continually to ensure that it does not foster the client's dependency, for example, by keeping the client in treatment longer than necessary. The ethics of care, with its greater emphasis on interdependency, would not ask, "Could the group member function adequately on an independent basis?" but rather, "Does the group context support the individual's well-being?"

Virtue Ethics

Virtue ethics are rooted in the writings of the Greek philosopher Aristotle and the Medieval scholar Thomas Aquinas, both of whom saw character traits as of great consequence in a person's capacity for ethical action (Proctor, 2018). Virtues are features of a person that are long-standing dispositions rather than momentary states or specific behaviors (van Zyl, 2019). They are rooted in a deep-seated longing of human beings for goodness, the intention to be good. Although such traits can have their origins in inborn tendencies, they require development through life experiences. Aristotle's idea of *practical wisdom*, the overarching quality of the virtuous person, captures this concept (van Zyl, 2019). Practical wisdom requires very good judgment. It is achieved through experience, which leads to the formation of virtuous habits (Haidt & Joseph, 2008). Through experience, the individual learns how to respond to his or her highly unique and everchanging context in a way that promotes in self and others a state of well-being or happiness. However, the capacity to learn from experiences in this way requires an intent to be virtuous. Without this intent, the individual is not virtuous even if the person engages in behaviors consistent with virtuousness. For example, a therapist who is diligent about responding to group members in crisis is virtuous if the behavior is primarily rooted in a wish to be helpful rather than a fear of negative consequences.

A virtue approach to professional ethics shines a light on the *character* of the professional (Johnson, 2007; Laney & Brenner, 2020), with character corresponding to those traits that underlie good practice. The emphasis in virtue ethics is not on avoiding wrongdoing or observing rules but rather striving to fulfill the highest professional ideals (Jordan & Meara, 1990; van Zyl, 2019). Group psychotherapists practicing within a virtue ethics framework would establish as an explicit goal-achieving moral excellence in group work, constantly examining the consequences of their decision-making as well as the adequacy of the process itself. Supporting this quest would be the group psychotherapist's possession of particular virtues. For example, humility enables the therapist to recognize imperfections in decision-making. Self-acceptance creates a capacity to look at shortcomings without demoralization or even despair. Aristotle writes about having a capacity to avoid extremes and achieve the golden mean (Mizzoni, 2017), a quality involved in such processes as boundary regulation, therapist self-disclosure, and affect activation. The virtuous group psychotherapist knows how to titrate emotional exploration and expression and uses experience to do it even more effectively.

Recall our prior vignette about the group psychotherapist who shared his professional opinion about a member with a psychiatrist without apprising that group member of his intent to do so. The fact that the group psychotherapist did not break any law or professional standard would not be regarded by the virtue ethicist. The virtue ethicist would also not emphasize the fact that the consequence of the therapist's actions was negative (i.e., the group member was unhappy). What is important within this framework is the character trait that gave rise to the therapist's action. The virtue ethicist would observe that the action the group psychotherapist was taking was that of a shortcut. Even though he might have been motivated by his concern for the member's well-being, his manner of doing it privileged efficiency over the member's wish to be informed of vital information concerning her own person. On the other hand, in taking the member's reaction to heart, the therapist demonstrated a virtue of openness that would support the development of other important virtues. For example, it might foster a lessened tendency to take shortcuts out of increased empathy for the member's valuation of being notified versus being kept in the dark. Note that the virtue ethicist's primary focus is not on behaviors but on the character traits that behaviors reflect, not on the therapist's current moral status, but on the status to which the therapist aspires. It is an aspiration approach in that it aims to encourage the highest level of ethical functioning rather than specifying what is merely mandatory.

Box 1.1 Applying the Principles

Lettice was a second-year student in a doctoral program in clinical psychology. Lettice's academic advisor, who had her in a case conference that semester, noticed that she participated rarely. Lettice disclosed that she had always felt discomfort in group situations and frequently was passive. She expressed frustration over this longstanding reticence. The advisor recommended a particular private-practice outpatient group, which Lettice did join. Six months later, when the advisor met with her, he made a comment about an event in her family that she had mentioned in a group session and to a few close friends in the program. Lettice believed it was far more likely that he received information from the former rather than the latter source. She confronted him, saying it was evident to her that some communication had occurred between the therapist and advisor. She went on to say that both had acted unethically, and she intended to discontinue with the group. The advisor said that he had had a few conversations with the therapist and that it was to her benefit that some coordination occurs between her program and her treatment. Who was right?

Faculty in mental health training programs commonly refer students for psychotherapy (Elman & Forrest, 2004), and when interpersonal difficulties arise, group psychotherapy is one option proposed. Although many ethically fraught situations are not clear-cut, this one is. Unless Lettice had given her consent that communication occurs between the group therapist and the faculty member, any that did occur would constitute a violation of confidentiality. In giving consent, if she gave it, Lettice would need to know how the faculty member receiving the information would use it. Would it inform the program's evaluation of her and thereby affect her standing in the program? The ethical principles engaged in this situation are those of Beneficence and Non-maleficence. The supervisor saw himself as doing good for the student, and possibly the profession itself, in maintaining lines of communication with the therapist. Whether he was correct in this assumption is, of course, a matter for further inquiry. However, at least in his expressed intent, he was trying to achieve a good. The ethical situation also involves Respect for Autonomy insofar as Lettice's exercise of autonomy demanded both information and consent. In the absence of consent, confidentiality would be required of the therapist. Generally, Respect for Autonomy is regarded as having greater standing than Beneficence, given that violating an individual's autonomy deprives that person of a basic human right. One can imagine a world in which a professional—thinking he or she is doing good for another—could exert myriad types of control. Moreover, in this situation, any good that could come from the student's group participation could be undone by the student's loss of trust. Certainly, the fact that the student's contemplation of leaving the group because of the damaged trust makes this point even clearer.

In this circumstance, the faculty member was making a suggestion that he saw as helpful. Lettice was not required to pursue group psychotherapy as part of a remediation plan in her training program. When therapy is mandated by a remediation plan, frequently, the program will solicit certain information from the therapist such as whether the person fulfilled the requirement to attend sessions. The therapist might even be asked to state whether the individual participated in the sessions (i.e., communicated with the other members), derived benefit from participation, or both. Even though involvement is stipulated by the plan, the therapist can share information only if the student has consented to the release. Elman and Forrest (2004) make a number of useful recommendations about the inclusion of psychotherapy as part of a student remediation plan including the development of policies describing the use of psychotherapy as part of remediation plans, policies that are made available to incoming students, so they know about them in advance of their implementation.

Comment on Ethical Models

All of the models presented here offer a special perspective on any ethical situation and can be used in concert with one another. How the instructor or supervisor approaches the exploration of ethical situations is as important as the conceptual framework or frameworks the trainer employs. Knapp et al. (2018) distinguish between the positive and floor approaches to professional ethics. According to these authors,

> a positive approach would guard against an over emphasis on punishment and disciplinary mechanisms and highlight professional and personal values that motivate behavior. It would also guard against a tendency to do the minimum necessary to meet professional standards and encourage psychologists [and other professionals] to strive to do their best work. (p. 196)

In contrast, the floor approach entails teaching students what not to do—how to avoid what is clearly wrong. It emphasizes learning rules and laws and exercising care not to violate them to escape sanctions. The floor approach has a variety of disadvantages. It denies group psychotherapists the opportunity to strive for their ideals and to enjoy the satisfaction to be had in moving closer to them. This approach arouses anxiety in that the emphasis is upon the perils that attend making mistakes. Such anxiety can easily cloud judgment. It also leaves the practitioner stranded when no rule or law applies to a situation that is clearly ethically problematic. All of these disadvantages translate into the advantages of a positive approach. Although the positive approach does not regard rules and laws as unimportant, it places them within a larger framework in which group psychotherapists behave in a fashion that accords with both their personal values and those of the professionals. As Knapp and colleagues note, it prizes intrinsic motivation—engaging in a behavior because it is right—rather than extrinsic motivation (e.g., engaging in a behavior merely to avoid punishment). It also emphasizes process as much as a product. That is, it seeks to examine the decision-making process itself, an area that is often neglected in the training of professionals (Harding, 2007). That is, it looks at the various stages *en route* to solving a problem, ascertaining what internal processes and external behaviors along the way enable the clinician to make the best possible solution to an ethical dilemma.

Although ethical models are extremely important in ethical decision-making, they are insufficient to permit the therapist to find a legal and ethical solution to an ethical problem. The group psychotherapist also needs knowledge of the corpus of material that has been generated by professional organizations and legal entities in relation to what constitutes ethical and legal practice. Following the presentation of codes and standards, we then move on to see how ethical models are integrated with codes and standards to enable a group psychotherapist to reach an ethical and legal decision.

Codes of Ethics and Standards of Practice

All professions have codes of ethics (Welfel, 2015). Professions recognize that the work of its members affects the lives of clients in powerful ways (Pope & Vasquez, 2011). The professions of psychology, psychiatry, social work, and counseling share ethical foundations despite their unique identities and licensures (Rapin, 2011). In professional practice, the term *ethical* refers to codes that mandate or prohibit behavior; these documents are not all-inclusive of behaviors but do guide professionals through ethical decision-making according to various forms adopted by licensing boards.

Membership in professional associations requires adherence to formal ethical codes of conduct and standards of practice. Among others, the following organizations have been highlighted as regularly publishing or amending ethical codes or standards, with most having specific relevance for group therapy (Rapin, 2011):

American Counseling Association (ACA, 2005; ACA, 2014)

As a part of informed consent, includes social media use and cultural and/or language differences that may affect the delivery of services. The Association for Specialists in Group Work (ASGW), a division of the ACA, has also provided aspirational documents, including "Best Practice Guidelines" in 2007 that included addressing the integration of trends and technological changes (Thomas & Pender, 2008). ASGW also developed "Professional Standards for the Training of Group Workers," (ASGW, 2000), and "Multicultural and Social Justice Competence Principles for Group Workers" in 2012 (Singh et al., 2012).

American Group Psychotherapy Association (AGPA, 2002)

AGPA serves as an international resource and also provides significant training in group practice and certifications for those with more extensive and documented group training, with an earned credential entitled Certified Group Psychotherapist (CGP). AGPA put forth clinical practice guidelines for group psychotherapy inclusive of ethics as well as a core battery of measures that can be used for selection and tracking progress and outcome (Bernard et al., 2008; Burlingame et al., 2006). Both are currently being updated.

American Psychological Association (APA, 2002; See amendments in APA, 2010; and APA, 2017a on Avoiding Harm and Safeguarding Human Rights)

APA addresses roles in training groups and responsibilities for group educators, specifically directing programs to provide options for training in groups with unaffiliated leaders to the academic program. It also directs psychologists to describe the roles and responsibilities of all parties and the limits of confidentiality (code 10.03). In 2017, the organization's Council of Representatives adopted an updated set of ethical guidelines, "Multicultural Guidelines: An Ecological Approach to Context, Identity, and Intersectionality," which aimed to help psychologists understand and apply knowledge related to a person's cultural identities and background. APA has a specific division, The Society of Group Psychology and Group Psychotherapy, that also provides extensive training and education around group competencies and the group specialty practice. APA and the American Board for Group Psychology (ABPP) worked on intensive joint ventures over many years to establish procedures for the group specialty credential, by delineating these competencies unique to group practice (Barlow, 2012, 2013; Kaslow et al., 2009; Rapin, 2011). Group psychology and group psychotherapy garnered specialty status from ABPP in 1999; the APA Commission for the Recognition of Specialties and Proficiencies in Professional Psychology (CRSPPP) approved and identified Group Psychology and Group Psychotherapy as a specialty practice in 2018. As the APA has recognized group psychology and group psychotherapy as an evidence-based practice, this APA specialty status now qualifies academic doctoral, internship, post-doctoral, and post-licensure programs for accreditation. Under the domain entitled "Ethical and Legal Standards and Policies for Group," group leaders are expected to possess knowledge and skills of the ethical and legal standards by level of training. For example, graduate students must become *familiar* with the ethics code through both knowledge and applied efforts, but entry-level psychologists require even *more advanced levels of knowledge and applied competencies.*

National Association of Social Workers (NASW, 2008; NASW, 2017)

Before the revision in 2017, NASW's 2008 Code of Ethics specifically directed social workers to seek clarity and agreements regarding preserving confidentiality, but also to inform group members that they cannot guarantee that all members will honor confidentiality agreements and that confidentiality agreements are dependent on a state's statutes. The NASW Code of Ethics is the most accepted standard for social work ethical practice worldwide. NASW is also affiliated with the Canadian Association of Social Workers and endorses their companion documents (Canadian Association of Social Workers, 2005a; Canadian Association of Social Workers, 2005b). In 2015, the NASW National Committee on Racial and Ethnic Diversity developed "Standards and Indicators for Cultural Competence in Social Work Practice," which builds on the previous work and introduces new concepts (NASW, 2015).

American Psychiatric Association (APA, 2001, 2010, See amendments in 2013)

As the APA adheres to the American Medical Association's *Principles of Medical Ethics* and interprets these general guidelines in its annotations and published opinions, there are no specific guidelines for the practice of group therapy.

Other Professional Guidelines for Practice

Entry-level therapists engaging in group therapy are encouraged to focus on ethics. They should join group organizations and interest societies to develop an identity and build group skills through advanced knowledge and applied competencies. Membership and training within such organizations can have great influence and outcomes, such as encouraging the group professional to seek advanced credentialing, which in turn has implications for ethical competencies (Barlow, 2013). Some organizations and researchers have also intentionally put forth clinical guidelines and competencies for group psychotherapy that specifically address ethics and the use of evidence-based practice (Barlow, 2012, 2013; Barlow et al., 2015; Berman et al., 2017; Bernard et al., 2008; Burlingame et al., 2006; International Association for Group Psychotherapy and Group Processes, 2016; Leszcz & Kobos, 2008). Such ethical guidelines developed by professional associations are not designed to provide specific directives for all potential situations nor do they have regulatory influence, but they do provide important parameters to guide professional behavior around issues such as screening members, discussing confidentiality, and providing adequate informed consent. Because such documents are reflective of developing knowledge and are revised periodically, they might not anticipate emerging issues such as the use of social media or online technologies (MacNair-Semands, 2005; Woods & Ruzek, 2018).

In recent years, professional guidelines have been developed for specialty practices and for the use of telehealth in the delivery of mental health services. For example, the American Psychological Association (2013) adopted the Guidelines for the Practice of Telepsychology. The guidelines cover the areas of standards of care, informed consent, confidentiality, security and transmission of data, testing and assessment, and interjurisdictional practice. Likewise, the American Telemedicine Association (2013) has published Practice Guidelines for Video-based online mental health services. Although these various sets of guidelines provide therapists with a great deal of helpful information, they are not enforceable. Further information on telehealth can be found in Chapter 5.

See Rapin (2011) for a detailed history and comparison of the best group practice guidelines and the group training standards, with AGPA's CGP credential requiring the greatest number of documented hours of group experience of all the organizations. Rapin also observes that because membership in professional associations is optional, nonparticipating group counselors also may not be obligated to adhere to a specific code or standard in such documents.

Regulatory Bodies and the Law

Professions have effects on society, or segments of society, ranging from the highly beneficial to the highly detrimental, as well as all points in between. Accordingly, those governmental entities entrusted with protecting societal interests have a vested interest in ensuring, at minimum, that professional practices produce minimal harm. Regulation is the means by which the government protects society. Some regulations exist at a federal level and apply to healthcare broadly. For example, the Health Insurance Portability and Accountability Act is a set of regulations that seeks to guarantee the security, integrity, and availability of Personal Health Information (PHI). The HIPAA Journal provides a treasure trove of information about compliance and offers a useful compliance checklist. The regulations mandate how healthcare records should be maintained and stored, and what constitutes the official record. All healthcare professionals, including group psychotherapists, must abide by these federal requirements. Some federal regulations pertain to professionals who are working in specific systems such as the U.S. Department of Defense and the Department of Veterans Affairs. For example, while state law might not permit professionals to provide services across state borders, these federal regulations might allow professionals to do so within those systems. Group psychotherapists seeking to learn more about federal laws relevant to their practices can go to https://www.usa.gov/laws-and-regs.

When a state establishes a license in a given area, it also creates a board to administer that license. State licensing boards establish the minimum requirements for an individual to practice within a profession to prevent harm to the public; they are not created to promote the welfare of the professions themselves (Bricklin et al., 2003). As part of their mission to protect the public, licensing boards are entrusted with adjudicating complaints against professionals. In investigating and prosecuting complaints, a licensing board will apply a standard based on state law and possibly the ethics code of the national organization as well as the code of any overarching entity concerned with the regulation of a profession. For example, some psychology licensing boards use the ASPPB Code of Conduct of the Association of State and Provincial Psychology Boards (Association of the State and Provincial Psychology Boards, 2018; Knapp et al., 2013). Group psychotherapists licensed in one of the mental health professions must be knowledgeable about the standards of their state licensing board. For example, if engaging in telehealth, practitioners must be aware of and adhere to the laws in the state of the participating group member. Challenges can arise when the laws in different states dictate different actions. For example, some states such as California and Pennsylvania require that health providers report impaired driving to the Department of Motor Vehicles. Many states do not have this requirement. When conducting group psychotherapy with members in states with different requirements, the therapist must decide whether to have member-specific policies or group policies on such matters. In the latter case, the therapist would be obligated to establish the more stringent policy and make certain that it is fully spelled out in the informed consent. Group psychotherapists must be aware that they might be practicing side-by-side with other professionals governed by standards that, while undoubtedly similar in many ways, might also be different in some respects.

Therapy services are regulated by the state in which individuals are receiving the service. In some states, the therapist must be licensed in the state where the therapist is located and in the state where the client is located if they are in different states. This issue is important when delivering online services because the therapist might be in one state and the patient in another. Therefore, if a group leader is providing services in Pennsylvania but the client is located in Delaware, the leader must be licensed within Delaware. During exceptional circumstances such as the recent pandemic, states might waive the requirement that a practitioner is licensed within the client's state if the practitioner is licensed in the state in which the practitioner is located. The state might, though, require that the practitioner registers within the state prior to engaging in clinical activity. In ordinary circumstances, the therapist must obtain a license in each state in which a member is located during the group sessions. Licensing can be a time-consuming, complex process. However, some disciplines such as psychology have forged an interstate compact among participating states such that registry in the compact permits the practice of telepsychology and temporary, face-to-face treatment in those states. Compacts in Psychology, (the Psychology Interjurisdictional Compact [PsyPact]); nursing (the Nurse Licensure Compact; National Council of State Boards of Nursing, 2021), and Medicine (the Interstate Medical Licensure Compact administered by the Federation of State Medical Boards) currently exist.

For the most part, group psychotherapists need to concern themselves with federal and state laws and regulations. However, from time to time, the therapist's local jurisdiction is relevant. During the coronavirus pandemic, some state governors declared the stay-at-home order lifted whereas county elected officials in some cases kept the stay-at-home order in place. Given this order, unless the therapist were considered essential personnel, say, in a hospital setting, that therapist would be unable to hold his or her group meetings with members being physically proximate to one another.

Decision-Making Processes

In the prior section, we outline many of the elements that will enter into the group psychotherapist's considerations when responding to an ethical problem. Although the therapist's knowledge of these different elements is essential to good decision-making, it is not sufficient. Additionally, the therapist needs an approach to integrating these different elements. Fortunately, multiple decision-making models (Cottone & Claus, 2000) are available to the group psychotherapist. These models encourage a *systematic* process of decision-making. The use of a decision-making model has a number of potential benefits. A strategy can serve as an antidote to the anxiety that ethical problems often evoke. Guided by an orderly way of proceeding, the therapist is likely to have a can-do attitude in relation to the problem at hand. It can also bolster the therapist's confidence that important details germane to the present problem are recognized. The use of an organized process can facilitate communication with other professionals about various aspects of the problem about which more information is needed. When therapists document the various steps through which they proceed, they show that they have performed their due diligence, even if another party disagrees with the final decision. Although these systems have heuristic value, empirical support for one model over another is limited (Cottone & Claus, 2000).

Koocher and Keith-Spiegel Model Applied to Group Psychotherapy

The following offers a model of decision-making adapted from the work of Koocher and Keith-Spiegel (2016, 2019), Haas and Malouf (2005), and Cottone (2001). The model was first published in 1985 but has been recently updated in light of new research and emerging ethical problems. The model delineated ten stages of the decision-making process.

Stage 1 Defining the Problem

The first stage entails ensuring that the issue at hand has significant ethical implications. Often, when we dislike the actions of another professional, we are tempted to label them as unethical. The behavior (or lack of behavior) in question might be different from how we would proceed, clinically non-optimal, or violative of some other standard of human conduct such as politeness. Although unethical behavior can have these characteristics, any one of these elements can be mistaken as unethical behavior. Consider the following example:

> Two first-year psychiatry residents were conducting a psychotherapy group for the first time together. One therapist brought her phone to the sessions and on several occasions responded to text messages. On one occasion, she left a room to take the call and was absent for about 3 minutes. In the debriefing session, the therapist who had not been engaged with her phone confronted the other, saying that that the co-therapist's behavior was unethical. The therapist being confronted said she had an obligation to be available to all of her patients and was merely satisfying this obligation.

Many reasons exist why it is detrimental to a group's functioning for a therapist to have a competing engagement during the group and to shift attention away from the here-and-now of the group. In addition to interrupting the group's work, the therapist's behavior might be narcissistically bruising to group members. Although these consequences could be seen as violations of Non-maleficence, they are relatively minor and easily addressed. Framing them as "unethical" fosters defensiveness and could curtail a full processing of all the ramifications of this behavior (such as modeling unhelpful behaviors) for the group members, as well as interfere with the identification of potential solutions to the therapist's worry about being accessible to patients outside the group.

Koocher and Keith-Spiegel (2019) advise that one way to ascertain whether a given situation presents a true ethical concern is to question whether it engages one or more of the ethical principles. They point out that generally, if it does, it will also be reflected in a professional code of conduct, a law, or organizational policy. This assessment will likely help the questioner crystallize a formulation of the issue at hand.

Haas and Malouf (2005) observe that the complexity of clinical situations often means that multiple ethical problems can be associated with any one situation. Undoubtedly, the complexity increases as the range of recognized stakeholders expands. They counsel that clinical decision-making is well-served by the therapist's determination of which problems are more serious than others, thereby helping the therapists evaluate where to commence a process of decision-making.

Stage 2 What is Known and What Else Needs to be Known

The group psychotherapist should acquire all available information related to the problem. Rarely will the questioning individual at the outset of the process possess sufficient information to make an appropriate and defensible solution to the problem. Consider the following situation:

> A department head in a partial hospital called in one of the group psychotherapists, a relatively new employee, and informed the therapist that a group of visiting professionals wanted to observe a group session. The therapist became extremely anxious and said she believed that were she to allow these visitors to gain entry to her group, she would be committing an unethical act and could be reported to her professional group for disciplinary action. She rejected the request out of hand.

The emotional reaction of the group psychotherapist reflected a defensive reaction wherein she sought to remove herself from a situation that she saw as threatening. In fact, the therapist was correct in regarding this situation as one that should be taken seriously, not your everyday request by a supervisor. Bricklin (2001) noted that it is not unusual for healthcare professionals to be alerted to a problem initially through an emotional response, a sense of something feeling off or wrong about the situation. However, rather than cutting off the process of decision-making by offering a hasty "yes" or "no," the professional is better served to use that discomfort as a stimulus for clarification of the problem (Step 1) and for procurement of information related to the problem. Here is a sampling of the questions the concerned therapist might have posed to the department head:

- Did the informed consent signed by the patient upon admittance to the partial hospital program specify that professionals other than the on-site staff might observe therapeutic activities?
- Were the professionals required to sign a confidentiality statement in regard to content heard in the group?
- Would members be apprised of the visit prior to the session in which it occurred?
- Could the therapist accommodate members who might decide not to participate in the session?
- Would the visitors be invited to share their observations about the group, thereby providing members with the opportunity to receive something back from them?

Although a more extended conversation with the department head could have yielded valuable information, the therapist might also have consulted other group psychotherapists who had to respond to such requests in the past.

Stage 3 Explore Legal and Professional Standards

Once all the relevant information has been gathered, the decision-maker should then determine whether a standard exists that could direct the group psychotherapist's subsequent actions. Although every situation in all of its specificities is unique, most situations have been faced by other clinicians at least in a general way. Professional groups have used the corpus of experiences, seen through the lens of a profession's values, to develop the codes of conduct reviewed previously in this chapter. The therapist should consult these codes of conduct of their own or related professions for direction in relation to the present situation. Any laws relevant to the issue at hand should also be considered. For example, in our example of the group visitors, the therapist would benefit from examining those laws and sections of professional codes pertaining to informed consent. Haas and Malouf (2005) point out that it might be beneficial, at times, to obtain a consultation regarding the interpretation of what admittedly can be complicated material. A person highly familiar with a particular code can help the decision-maker to identify those sections that are relevant to the situation at hand.

Stage 4 Consider Personality and Cultural Influences

This step acknowledges that decision-making is more than a cognitive process. The decision-maker is a person with wishes, anxieties, affects, impulses, and biases. All of these elements can influence decision-making. Gans (1992) pointed out that the group psychotherapist's own self-interest must not unduly affect decision-making. For example, a therapist should not accept a member who is a poor fit for the group primarily because the member has an interesting background and the therapist wants to hear more about it. In Chapter 5, we will be discussing the ethics of self-referral further.

In considering all of the factors impinging on the decision-making process, Koocher and Keith-Spiegel (2019) argue that attention should also be paid to cultural factors. It is helpful for the group psychotherapist to recognize the group member's culturally derived worldview, beliefs, and values and how they differ from the therapist's. This awareness can affect not only the decision itself but how the decision should be communicated. For example, suppose the group psychotherapist receives a phone call from the parent of a 22-year-old client, seeking information on the member's progress in the group. Regardless of cultural factors, the therapist would not be able to provide information without the member's consent except in highly specific conditions (e.g., suicidality). However, noting that the parents operated within a cultural framework in which such communications are expected, the therapist could acknowledge the disparity between the parents' framework and the legal/ethical framework in which the group was operating as well as express empathy for their understandable confusion. This therapeutic stance could enable the therapist to interact with the parents positively while also upholding the therapist's legal obligation to the group member. Koocher and Keith-Spiegel provide the helpful reminder that heterogeneity exists within any cultural group and, therefore, the therapist should approach a member's connections with their cultural background with curiosity and not assumptions based on stereotypes.

Stage 5 Pursue Consultation

This stage involves seeking consultation from an individual who is qualified to address the therapist's ethical issue. Certainly, a situation that arises in relation to group psychotherapy requires a consultant who is knowledgeable about group psychotherapy. It is also important that the consultant have an ability to address the situation from a standpoint of neutrality. While it might be tempting to get the perspective of an individual who is generally sympathetic to the decision-maker's position, it would be preferable to solicit the view of someone capable of taking a contrasting position.

Stage 6 Identify all the Stakeholders

Koocher and Keith-Speigel underscore the import of recognizing all parties who are involved in the ethical situation and might be affected by the therapist's decision, and consider their "rights, responsibilities, and vulnerability…" (p. 20). In the initial appraisal of an ethically fraught situation, certain stakeholders will typically be more salient. However, if the decision-maker devises solutions to problems for these conspicuous stakeholders only, other parties might suffer adverse consequences. This potential exists particularly in group psychotherapy given a multiplicity of parties is inherent to the modality. When a group psychotherapist formulates a decision in relation to a single member, effects are likely to extend throughout the group.

Stage 7 Brainstorm Solutions

Next, the therapist should generate alternate solutions to the ethical problem. This process should be conducted in the spirit of brainstorming (see Furnham, 2000) in which solutions are not rejected out of hand due to impracticalities or other factors. This open attitude is much more conducive to creativity. It could lead to the refinement of the dominant solution or could lead the decision-making in a new direction altogether, one that enables the therapist to do justice to a greater array of the ethical principles. Steps 5 and 7 can occur in concert with one another if the consultant is able to suggest solutions that the therapist did not originally contemplate:

> A group psychotherapist obtained an informal consultation from a colleague about a referral she had received. The referred individual was potentially an excellent fit for her group except for one factor: He had mobility problems that would make it extremely difficult for him to get from his car to the group room. The group psychotherapist perceived the problem as insurmountable and lamented the client's possible exclusion based on ableness, seeing it at odds with her value of inclusion. Still, she focused on finding another group for him and hoped to obtain her colleague's help with this task. The colleague was puzzled why the group psychotherapist so quickly rejected the possibility of his inclusion in the group. The colleague suggested a variety of solutions. The group psychotherapist was surprised that she had not recognized these solutions that in retrospect seemed obvious.

The experience of this therapist is not unusual in that our own information-processing biases limit us in the range of solutions we contemplate for any problem (see Chapter 7 for further discussion of this problem). However, the therapist who makes a deliberate effort to broaden the range of solutions—especially with the aid of consultants—can gain access to a greater array of options. In some cases, the group members themselves can be enlisted to generate solutions to knotty problems.

Stage 8 Recognizing Consequences of Different Solutions

In the next step, the therapist revisits each identified solution generated in Stage 7 and identifies the various anticipated consequences of implementing each solution. It is at this point that our group psychotherapist in Step 7 would think about each alternative for accommodating the group member with mobility challenges. At this time, it would be useful to do a feasibility check of each of the different solutions. Koocher and Keith-Speigel advise us that documenting the advantages and disadvantages might be particularly useful should any question arise later about the ultimately chosen solution.

Stage 9 Making the Decision

The therapist, having collected all the requisite information, is now able to make the decision. Certainly, nothing could be more obvious than the fact that all of these steps must culminate in a decision. However, some therapists will detect in themselves a tendency to defer the decision indefinitely, perhaps employing the excuse that more information must be collected. Even a therapist who ordinarily is able to complete a decision-making process might avoid this step if it involves a difficult interaction. For example, a therapist functioning in a co-therapy pair might have detected alcohol on the co-therapist's breath on several occasions. Therapists have an obligation to address the subpar or unethical behaviors of colleagues (Haas & Malouf, 2005), and this obligation is particularly strong in a co-therapy situation because members have joint responsibility for the work performed. However, rather than deciding, a therapist might remain in an information-gathering mode to forestall the confrontation with the co-therapist. In any circumstance, more information could be collected but doing so should not be the therapist's means to escape from whatever unpleasantness attends making a decision.

Stage 10 Implementing the Decision

Once the decision is made, it must be implemented. As Koocher and Keith-Speigel note, this step often requires courage, especially when the therapist is likely to suffer some negative consequences when implementing the solution. For example, the therapist who confronts the co-worker about the latter's use of alcohol might well receive a range of negative reactions from the co-therapist. As Haas and Malouf (2005) observe, implementing the decision also involves, "...other (non-ethical) skills such as assertiveness, tenacity, the existence of a supportive network, and the ability to communicate one's chosen action in non-condescending and humane terms" (p. 17).

Critiques of Decision-Making Models

Any of the major ethical decision-making models have the potential to aid the group psychotherapist to make an ethically sound decision. Still, the application of a decision-making model does not guarantee that an ethical decision will be made. At any point, obstacles can emerge that hinder the therapist from using the model optimally, with many of these obstacles residing within the therapist. In Chapter 7, we identify some of the emotional factors and cognitive biases that interfere with good decision-making.

One limitation of ethical decision-making models is that they are conducive to use only *after* an ethical problem has emerged and forces the practitioner in a reactive position. With foresight and anticipation for treatment begins, many problems can be averted. Vergés (2010) urges practitioners to focus on the contexts in which they practice. Any given context has features that can lead to the emergence of a particular set of ethical problems. Therapists who recognize these features can take advantage of any opportunities to offset the operation of these factors. For example, in a fast-paced inpatient environment, little time might be available to provide an incoming member with an understanding of risks. The group psychotherapist realizing this challenge to an adequate informed consent might find alternate ways to prepare group members, such as through the provision of written material or an instructive video. Another advantage of a contextual analysis is that it can lead the practitioner to consider what might be an appropriate response where a particular type of problem emerges in a given setting. As such, it constitutes an antidote to therapist impulsivity that can lead to non-optimal therapist behavior (Vergés, 2010). In performing this contextual analysis, the group psychotherapist can be aided by the literature that addresses specific ethical problems in psychological healthcare practice with particular populations and specified settings. For example, Matusek and Wright (2010) identify ethical problems that frequently emerge in the treatment of eating disorder patients. Vergés notes that often a consultant, a professional knowledgeable about the context, is useful in this process. An optimal time to conduct a contextual analysis is in the early stage of a practitioner's work in that context.

Cottone (2004) argues that a limitation of many decision-making models is their emphasis on decision-making as a process in the mind of the decider. He observes that ethical problems are co-constructed. From an early emergence of an ethical problem to its full resolution, relational aspects are always present. For example, the group psychotherapist who was asked to allow observers into her group would be likely to receive the request differently if it was received from a highly trusted colleague versus one whose decision-making she has doubted in the past. The availability of different solutions will be affected by the presence of colleagues with whom a group psychotherapist can consult. In fact, Cottone et al. (1994) demonstrated that the more consultations counseling graduate students received in relation to ethical problems, the more frequently they were inclined to revisit their decisions in specific ethical situations. Cottone (2004) has developed a problem-solving model that captures the interpersonal aspect at each stage. Whether or not one adopts Cottone's model, the practitioner nonetheless should give due recognition to the profoundly interpersonal character of practitioner activity in ethically fraught situations. Cottone noted that a particular advantage of this perspective is that it invites the inclusion of multicultural data, noting that different perspectives based on different cultural backgrounds are inevitable in ethical decision-making situations.

Final Note

This chapter described the basic rudiments of ethical decision-making that every group psychotherapist should master. In the conduct of every practice, group psychotherapists benefit from knowing the basic terminology associated with professional ethics. Awareness of theories regarding ethical decision-making facilitates the therapist's recognition of different facets of any given ethical problem. Group psychotherapists operate within disciplines, each of which has its own Ethical Codes and Standards of Practice with which practitioners must be thoroughly familiar. In addition, group psychotherapists derive guidance from codes that have been developed by professional organizations such as the American Group Psychotherapy Association. Telehealth represents a recent expansion of group psychotherapy, and some disciplines have adopted practice guidelines that are useful to group psychotherapists moving into this realm. Group leaders are also accountable to regulatory bodies with a stake in protecting the public. As we discussed, group leaders need to be knowledgeable about the laws of their own jurisdiction and relevant case law. This chapter outlined a model of ethical decision-making, steps through which the group leader could proceed when ethical problems arise. An acknowledgment was made that any decision-making model will capture the process incompletely. The factors that are often not discussed in rational decision-making models are identified in Chapter 7.

CEU Questions

1. When group clients are also in individual therapy with a group leader, any information revealed in individual counseling may be disclosed in the group setting. (T/F)
2. When students in training must attend a therapy group as a course requirement, a program faculty member can lead the group even if they are giving a course grade as long as they do not base a grade on material revealed in the group. (T/F)
3. If a therapist is conducting an online group with members drawn from two different states, the therapist's duty to warn might take a different form from one member to another. (T/F)
4. Conscientiousness, which is defined as awareness and anticipation of how group processes may impact group members, is an example of virtue ethics. (T/F)
5. In recent writings about the principle of Justice, this concept often relates to a) stereotypes, b) majority identities, c) discrimination, d) privilege and equity, or e) all of the above.
6. Autonomy is often cited in *virtue* ethics, as it addresses group member independence and freedom to choose their own course of action. (T/F)
7. Standards of practice in professional associations hold more power than federal or state legal requirements. (T/F)
8. A group leader whose ethical decision-making considers broader societal goods is acting in accordance with General Beneficence. (T/F)

9. If individual treatment is offered as a replacement for group treatment, it is always permissible to exclude a member with a hearing impairment from a group. (T/F)

Answer key: 1. F; 2. F; 3. T; 4. T; 5. e; 6. F; 7. F; 8. T; 9. F

Discussion Questions

1. Name several moral principles that are at the root of your personal actions and discuss how they also influence your professional ethics and practice.
2. How are the tenets of the ethics of care consistent with your professional perspective?
3. How might Beneficence and Non-maleficence both be influencing factors when two members are in conflict?
4. How does your culture affect your values that may surface in your group responses?
5. How might the virtue ethics related to compassion and trustworthiness be communicated by the leaders, both directly and indirectly?
6. Aristotle held that a virtuous individual is likely to be a happy individual. Do you think that a virtuous group psychotherapist is more likely to be happier than one who is not?
7. What social and cultural themes in the last 20 years have contributed to a recent emphasis on professional codes of conduct?
8. What is the leader's responsibility around explicitly identifying moral issues in the group setting?
9. Do you see participation in group psychotherapy organizations key to maintaining competence as a group psychotherapist?

Vignettes/Role-Plays

1. The therapist interviewed a prospective member. He learned that the individual had insurance that the group therapist did not take. The therapist also knew that other reputable group psychotherapists in the area did take the insurance. Does the therapist have an ethical obligation to inform the prospective member of this fact?

    1. If you say "yes," what are the relevant principles?
    2. If you say "no," what are the relevant principles?
    3. Are there contextual features that would make a difference?

2. After a divisive election result was called the night before a group session, Daniella, who identifies as Latina, called the leader and asked to cancel her attendance. Daniella stated she was not willing to face the possibility that another member might discuss the outcome as positive when she felt emotionally devastated by this election.

    1. How might you balance the principles of Autonomy and Beneficence if you believe she might get more support than expected in group by attending?
    2. How might you address the norms around attendance?

3. A dominant male member came to the group session and stated he was upset because he had "an unfair test in a math class that totally *raped* me!" Two women in the group with histories of sexual assault looked stunned and upset but remained silent.

    1. How might the leaders balance the two aims of educating this member and processing the impact of his language? What constructive solution can be devised that considers the male member's potential shame issues?
    2. How would the principle of Justice apply to power dynamics in the room?
    3. How might leaders encourage other members to respond?

4. Leigh believes her co-leader Zach has been dressing in an unprofessional manner and uses inappropriate language as well as flirtatious behavior with group members.

    1. How might Leigh consider approaching these behaviors?
    2. What first steps might she consider if Zach is (a) responsive or (b) unresponsive?

5. As she begins to reveal herself in group, Leila discusses her past pregnancy and experience as a young single mother. Another group member, Emily, has just learned she is pregnant and is considering an abortion. Emily begins to question herself as several members in addition to Leila respond by stating that abortion is against their religious values. Leila lets the group know she feels unsupported, but members remain silent.

    1. How might the group leaders respond? Role-play different leader responses.
    2. How might the leaders address the values of other members as they encourage more emotional support for Emily?

6. A therapist notices that his intern co-therapist exhibits disapproval when members talk about certain issues such as divorce, abortion, and cohabitation. The therapist addresses these behaviors with the co-therapist. The latter responds matter-of-factly that these lifestyle issues are at odds with her religious principles. She says she realizes that others have different beliefs and she will try to control her facial expressions.

    1. Does this circumstance present the therapist with one or more ethical dilemmas and if so, what are they? How might different ethical frameworks see this situation differently?
    2. Role-play the conversation between the therapist and intern co-therapist. Identify the therapist's options following the role-play, given the co-therapist's stance.

References

Acuff, C., Bennett, B. E., Bricklin, P. M., Canter, M. B., Knapp, S. J., Moldawsky, S., & Phelps, R. (1999). Considerations for ethical practice in managed care. *Professional Psychology: Research and Practice, 30*(6), 563–575. 10.1037/0735-7028.30.6.563

Alder, S. (2018). *What is considered protected health information under HIPAA?* HIPAA Journal. https://www.hipaajournal.com/what-is-considered-protected-health-information-under-hipaa/

American Counseling Association. (2005). *ACA code of ethics.* https://www.counseling.org/docs/default-source/library-archives/archived-code-of-ethics/codeethics05.pdf

American Counseling Association. (2014). *2014 ACA code of ethics.* https://www.counseling.org/Resources/aca-code-of-ethics.pdf

American Group Psychotherapy Association. (2002). *AGPA and IBCGP guidelines for ethics.* http://ethics.iit.edu/codes/AGPA%202002.pdf

American Psychiatric Association. (2001). *Ethics primer of the American Psychiatric Association.* https://www.psychiatry.org/psychiatrists/practice/ethics

American Psychiatric Association. (2013). *The principles of medical ethics with annotations especially applicable to psychiatry* (2013 ed.). https://www.psychiatry.org/File%20Library/Psychiatrists/Practice/Ethics/principles-medical-ethics.pdf

American Psychological Association. (2002). Ethical principles of psychologists and code of conduct. *American Psychologist, 57*(12), 1060–1073. 10.1037/0003-066X.57.12.1060

American Psychological Association. (2010). Amending the ethics code. *American Psychological Association, 41*(4), 64. https://www.apa.org/monitor/2010/04/ethics

American Psychological Association. (2013). *Guidelines for the practice of telepsychology.* https://www.apa.org/practice/guidelines/telepsychology

American Psychological Association. (2017a). *Ethical principles of psychologists and code of conduct* (2002, amended effective June 1, 2010, and January 1, 2017). https://www.apa.org/ethics/code/index.aspx

American Psychological Association. (2017b). *Multicultural guidelines: An ecological approach to context, identity, and intersectionality.* http://www.apa.org/about/policy/multicultural-guidelines.pdf

American Telemedicine Association (2013). Practice guidelines for video-based mental health services. https://www.americantelemed.org/resources/practice-guidelines-for-video-based-online-mental-health-services-2/

Association for Specialists in Group Work. (2000). Professional standards for the training of group workers. *The Journal for Specialists in Group Work, 25*(4), 327–342. 10.1080/01933920008411677

Association for the Advancement of Social Work with Groups. (2005). *Standards for social work practice with* groups (2nd ed.). http://www.aaswg.org/files/AASWG_Standards_for_Social_Work_Practice_with_Groups.pdf

Association of the State and Provincial Psychology Boards. (2018). *ASPPB code of conduct.* https://cdn.ymaws.com/www.asppb.net/resource/resmgr/guidelines/code_of_conduct_2020_.pdf

Avci, E. (2017). A normative analysis to determine the goals of ethics education through utilizing three approaches: Rational moral education, ethical acculturation, and learning throughout life. *International Journal of Ethics Education, 2*(2), 125–145. 10.1007/s40889-017-0032-4

Barlow, S. H. (2012). An application of the competency model to group-specialty practice. *Professional Psychology: Research and Practice, 43*(5), 442–451. 10.1037/a0029090

Barlow, S. H. (2013). *Specialty competencies in group psychology.* Oxford University Press. 10.1093/med:psych/9780195388558.001.0001

Barlow, S., Burlingame, G. M., Greene, L. R., Joyce, A., Kaklauskas, F., Kinley, J., Klein, R. H., Kobos, J. C., Leszcz, M., MacNair-Semands, R., Paquin, J. D., Tasca, G. A., Whittingham, M., & Feirman, D. (2015). *Evidence-based practice in group psychotherapy.* American Group Psychotherapy. http://www.agpa.org/home/practice-resources/evidence-based-practice-in-group-psychotherapy

Bashe, A., Anderson, S. K., Handelsman, M. M., & Klevansky, R. (2007). An acculturation model for ethics training: The ethics autobiography and beyond. *Professional Psychology: Research and Practice, 38*(1), 60–67. https://doi.org/10.1093/occmed/kqu158

Beauchamp, T. L., & Childress, J. F. (1979). *Principles of biomedical ethics* (1st ed.). Oxford University Press.

Beauchamp, T. L., & Childress, J. F. (2009). *Principles of biomedical ethics* (6th ed.). Oxford University Press. 10.1093/occmed/kqu158

Beauchamp, T. L., & Childress, J. F. (2013). *Principles of biomedical ethics* (7th ed.). Oxford University Press. https://doi.org/10.1093/occmed/kqu158

Berman, M. I., Chapman, N., Nash, B., Kivlighan, D. M., & Paquin, J. D. (2017). Sharing wisdom: Challenges, benefits, and developmental path to becoming a successful therapist-researcher. *Counselling Psychology Quarterly, 30*(3), 234–254. 10.1080/09515070.2017.1293612

Bernard, H., Burlingame, G., Flores, P., Greene, L., Joyce, A., Kobos, J. C., Leszcz, M., MacNair-Semands, R. R., Piper, W. E., Slocum McEneaney, A. M., Feirman, D. (2008). Clinical practice guidelines for group psychotherapy. *International Journal of Group Psychotherapy, 58*(4), 455–542. 10.1521/ijgp.2008.58.4.455

Berry, J. W. (2003). Conceptual approaches to acculturation. In K. M. Chun, P. B. Organista, & G. Marín (Eds.). *Acculturation: Advances in theory, measurement and applied research* (pp. 17–37). American Psychological Association. 10.1037/10472-004

Brabender, V. (2006). The ethical group psychotherapist. *International Journal of Group Psychotherapy, 56,* 395–414. 10.1521/ijgp.2006.56.4.395

Brabender, V. M., & Fallon, A. (2009). Ethical hot spots of combined individual and group therapy: Applying four ethical systems. *International Journal of Group Psychotherapy, 59*(1), 127–147. 10.1521/ijgp.200.59.1.127

Bricklin, P. (2001). Being ethical: More than obeying the law and avoiding harm. *Journal of Personality Assessment, 77*(2), 195–202. 10.1207/S15327752JPA7702_03

Bricklin, P., Bennett, B., & Carroll, W. (2003). *Understanding licensing board disciplinary* procedures. American Psychological Association. https://www.apaservices.org/practice/ce/state/disciplinary-procedures.pdf

Brown, L. (1994). Boundaries in feminist therapy: A conceptual formulation. *Women & Therapy, 15*, 29–38. 10.1300/J015v15n01_04

Burlingame, G. M., Strauss, B., Joyce, A., MacNair-Semands, R., MacKenzie, K. R., Ogrodniczuk, J., & Taylor, S. (2006). *CORE battery—revised: An assessment tool kit for promoting optimal group selection, process and outcome.* American Group Psychotherapy Association.

Canadian Association of Social Workers. (2005a). *Code of ethics.* https://www.casw-acts.ca/files/documents/casw_code_of_ethics.pdf

Canadian Association of Social Workers. (2005b). *Guidelines for ethical practice.* https://www.casw-acts.ca/files/documents/casw_guidelines_for_ethical_practice.pdf

Cottone, R. R. (2001). A social constructivism model of ethical decision making in counseling. *Journal of Counseling & Development, 79*(1), 39–45. 10.1002/j.1556-6676.2001.tb01941.x

Cottone, R. R. (2004). Displacing the psychology of the individual in ethical decision-making: The social constructivist model. *Canadian Journal of Counseling and Psychotherapy, 38*(1). https://files.eric.ed.gov/fulltext/EJ719896.pdf

Cottone, R. R., & Claus, R. E. (2000). Ethical decision-making models: A review of the literature. *Journal of Counseling & Development, 78*(3), 275–283. 10.1002/j.1556-6676.2000.tb01908.x

Cottone, R. R., Tarvydas, V., & House, G. (1994). The effect of number and type consulted on the ethical decision making of graduate students in counseling. *Counseling and Values, 39*(1), 56–68. 10.1002/j.2161-007X.1994.tb01007.x

Elliott, A. C. (2001). Health care ethics: Cultural relativity of autonomy. *Journal of Transcultural Nursing, 12*(4), 326–330. 10.1177/104365960101200408

Elman, N. S., & Forrest, L. (2004). Psychotherapy in the remediation of psychology trainees: Exploratory interviews with training directors. *Professional Psychology: Research and Practice, 35*(2), 123–130. 10.1037/0735-7028.35.2.123

Elsner, A. M. & Rampton, V. (2020). Ethics of care approaches to psychotherapy. In M. Trachsel, J. Gaab, N. Biller-Andorno, S. Tekin, & J. Z. Sandler (Eds.), *The Oxford handbook of psychotherapy ethics.* Oxford University Press. 10.1093/oxfordhb/9780198817338.013.15

Furnham, A. (2000). The brainstorming myth. *Business Strategy Review, 11*(4), 21–28. 10.1111/1467-8616.00154

Gans, J. S. (1992). Money and psychodynamic group therapy. *International Journal of Group Psychotherapy, 41*(1), 133–152. 10.1080/00207284.1992.11732584

Gilligan, C. (1982). *In a different voice.* Harvard University Press.

Haas, L. J., & Malouf, J. L. (2005). *Keeping up the good work: A practitioner's guide to mental health ethics* (4th ed). Professional Resource Problem. https://books.google.com/books/about/Keeping_Up_the_Good_Work.html?id=LReYAAAACAAJ

Haidt, J., & Joseph, C. (2008). The moral mind: How five sets of innate intuitions guide the development of many culture-specific virtues, and perhaps even modules. In P. Carruthers, S. Laurence, & S. Stich (Eds.), *Evolution and cognition. The innate mind Vol. 3. Foundations and the future* (pp. 367–391). Oxford University Press. 10.1093/acprof:oso/9780195332834.003.0019

Handelsman, M. M., Gottlieb, M. C., & Knapp, S. (2005). Training ethical psychologists: An acculturation model. *Professional Psychology: Research and Practice, 36*(1), 59–65. 10.1037/0735-7028.36.1.59

Harding, T. (2007). Clinical decision-making: How prepared are we? *Training and Education in Professional Psychology, 1*(2), 95–104. 10.1037/1931-3918.1.2.95

Held, V. (2006). *The ethics of care: Personal, political, and global.* Oxford University Press. 10.1093/0195180992.001.0001

International Association for Group Psychotherapy and Group Processes. (2016). *Ethical guidelines and professional standards for group psychotherapy.* https://www.iagp.com/docs/Ethicalguidelines2009%20IAGP%20US%20V24.2.16.pdf

Johnson, W. D. (2007). The boundary waters are murky: A case for virtue. In Barnett, J. E., Lazarus, A. A., Vasquez, M. J. T., Moorehead-Slaughter, O., & Johnson, W. B. (Eds.), Boundary issues and multiple relationships: Fantasy and reality. *Professional Psychology: Research and Practice, 38*(4), 401–410. 10.1037/0735-7028.38.4.401

Jordan, A. E., & Meara, N. M. (1990). Ethics and the professional practice of psychologists: The rule of virtue and principles. *Professional Psychology: Research and Practice, 21*(2), 107–114. 10.1037/0735-7028.21.2.107

Kant, I. (1964). *Groundwork of the metaphysic of morals*, (H. J. Paton, Trans.). Harper and Row. (Original Work published 1785).

Kaslow, N. J., Grus, C. L., Campbell, L. F., Fouad, N. A., Hatcher, R. L., & Rodolfa, E. R. (2009). Competency assessment toolkit for professional psychology. *Training and Education in Professional Psychology, 3*(4, Suppl), S27–S45. 10.1037/a0015833

Keith-Spiegel, P., & Koocher, G. P. (1985). *Ethics in psychology: Professional standards and cases.* Crown Publishing Group/Random House.

Kimball, P. (2018). *When professional and personal values collide: A thematic analysis of counseling students' developmental journey through an ethics course.* [Unpublished doctoral dissertation]. Liberty University. https://digitalcommons.liberty.edu/doctoral/1847/

Knapp, S., Gottlieb, M. C., & Handelsman, M. M. (2018). The benefits of adopting a positive perspective in ethics education. *Training and Education in Professional Psychology, 12*(3), 196–202. 10.1037/tep0000195

Knapp, S., Handelsman, M. M., Gottlieb, M. C., & VandeCreek, L. D. (2013). The dark side of professional ethics. *Professional Psychology: Research and Practice, 44*(6), 371–377. 10.1037/a0035110

Koocher, G. P., & Keith-Spiegel, P. (2016). *Ethics in psychology and the mental health professionals: Standards and cases* (4th ed.). Oxford University Press. https://www.worldcat.org/title/ethics-in-psychology-and-the-mental-health-professions-standards-and-cases/oclc/910009481

Koocher, G. P., & Keith-Spiegel, P. (2019). "What should I do?" – Ethical risks, making decisions, and taking action. [Online course]. SocialWorkCoursesOnline. https://www.socialworkcoursesonline.com/active/courses/course050.php

Laney, M. & Brenner, A. (2020). Virtue ethics in psychotherapy. In M. Trachsel, J. Gaab, N. Biller-Andorno, S. Tekin, & J. Z. Sadler (Eds.), *The Oxford handbook of psychotherapy ethics.* Oxford University Press. 10.1093/oxfordhb/9780198817338.013.17

Layton, L., & Leavy-Sperounis, M. (2020). *Toward a social psychoanalysis: Culture, character, and normative unconscious processes.* Routledge. 10.4324/9781003023098

Lehnert, K., Park, Y. H., & Singh, N. (2015). Research note and review of the empirical ethical decision-making literature: Boundary conditions and extensions. *Journal of Business Ethics, 129*(1), 195–219. 10.1007/s10551-014-2147-2

Leszcz, M., & Kobos, J. C. (2008). Evidence based group psychotherapy: Using AGPA's practice guidelines to enhance clinical effectiveness. *Journal of Clinical Psychology, 64*(11), 1238–1260. 10.1002/jclp.20531

Lindemann, H. (2019). *An invitation to feminist ethics* (2nd ed.). Oxford University Press. https://global.oup.com/academic/product/an-invitation-to-feminist-ethics-9780190059316?cc=us&lang=en&

MacNair-Semands, R. R. (2005). *Ethics in group psychotherapy* (1st ed.). American Group Psychotherapy Association.

MacNair-Semands, R. R. (2007). Attending to the spirit of social justice as an ethical approach in group therapy. *International Journal of Group Psychotherapy, 57*(1), 61–66. 10.1521/ijgp.2007.57.1.61

Matusek, J. A., & Wright, M. O. D. (2010). Ethical dilemmas in treating clients with eating disorders: A review and application of an integrative ethical decision-making model. *European Eating Disorders Review, 18*(6), 434–452. 10.1002/erv.1036

Mizzoni, J. (2017). *Ethics: The basics* (2nd ed.). Wiley.

National Association of Social Workers. (2008). NASW *Code of ethics.* https://www.socialworkers.org/LinkClick. aspx?fileticket=KZmmbz15evc% 3D&portalid=0

National Association of Social Workers. (2015). *Standards and indicators of cultural competence in social work practice.* https://www.socialworkers.org/LinkClick. aspx?fileticket=7dVckZAYUmk% 3D&portalid=0

National Association of Social Workers. (2017). *Code of ethics of the National Association of Social Workers*. https://www.socialworkers.org/About/Ethics/Code-of-Ethics/Code-of-Ethics-English

National Council of State Boards of Nursing. (2021). *Nurse licensure compact (NLC)*. https://www.ncsbn.org/nurse- licensure-compact.htm

Parton, N. (2003). Rethinking professional practice: The contributions of social constructionism and the feminist' ethics of care. *British Journal of Social Work*, *33*(1), 1–16. 10.1093/bjsw/33.1.1

Pope, K. S., & Vasquez, M. J. T. (2011). *Ethics in psychotherapy and counseling: A practical guide* (4th ed.). Wiley. 10.1002/9781118001875

Proctor, C. (2018). Virtue ethics in psychotherapy: A systematic review of the literature. *International Journal of Existential Positive Psychology*, *8*(1), 1–22. http://journal.existentialpsychology.org/index.php/ExPsy/article/view/237

Psychology Interjurisdictional Compact. (n.d.). *Psypact.* https://psypact.site-ym.com/

Rapin, L. S. (2011). Ethics, best practices, and law in group counseling. In R. K. Conyne (Ed.). *The Oxford handbook of group counseling* (pp. 61–82). Oxford University Press. 10.1093/oxfordhb/9780195394450. 013.0005

Singh, A. A., Merchant, N., Skudrzyk, B., & Ingene, D. (2012). Association for specialists in group work: Multicultural and social justice competence principles for group workers. *The Journal for Specialists in Group Work*, *37*(4), 312–325. 10.1080/01933922.2012.721482

Sinnott-Armstrong, W. (2019). Consequentialism. In E. N. Zalta (Ed.), *The Stanford encyclopedia of philosophy archive*. Metaphysics Research Lab. https://plato.stanford.edu/archives/sum2019/entries/consequentialism/

Thomas, R. V. & Pender, D. A. (2008). Association for specialists in group work: Best practice guidelines 2007 revisions. *The Journal for Specialists in Group Work*, *33*(2), 111–117. 10.1080/01933920801971184

van Zyl, L. (2019). *Virtue ethics: A contemporary introduction*. Routledge.

Vasquez, M. J. T. (2007). Cultural difference and the therapeutic alliance: An evidence-based analysis. *American Psychologist*, *62*(8), 878–885. 10.1037/0003-066X.62.8.878

Vergés, A. (2010). Integrating contextual issues in ethical decision making. *Ethics & Behaviors*, *20*(6), 497–507. 10.1080/10508422.2010.521451

Welfel, E. R. (2015). *Ethics in counseling & psychotherapy: Standards, research, and emerging issues* (6th ed.). Cengage Learning. https://www.cengage.com/c/ethics- in-counseling-psychotherapy- 6e-welfel/9781305089723PF/

Woods, J. D., & Ruzek, N. A. (2018). Ethics in group psychotherapy. In M. D. Ribeiro, J. M. Gross, & M. M. Turner (Eds.), *The college counselor's guide to group psychotherapy* (pp. 83–100). Routledge. 10.4324/9781315545455

2   Privacy, Confidentiality, and Privilege

Group psychotherapy is predicated on trust. Group members enter the group with the expectation that they will make themselves known, and that doing so will be beneficial. Members expect that the therapist will create a culture in which their disclosures are safeguarded—not used for purposes of exploitation, not exported out of the group, not employed in any way to their detriment. The paradox is that, despite this act of trust, the therapist cannot strictly control what members are going to do with the information concerning other members. Despite this limitation, therapists can do a great deal to develop trust in them, the other members, and the group as a whole, as we will discuss.

Basic Terms

Privacy, confidentiality, and privileged communication are core terms that pertain to the treatment of client information. *Privacy* is freedom from unwanted intrusions of all sorts but the type of privacy most important for group psychotherapy is informational privacy—control over one's own personal information. The right to safeguard one's personal information is ensconced in the Bill of Rights of the United States Constitution (Haas & Malouf, 2005). This definition is to be distinguished from the use of "privacy" in a HIPAA context in which privacy is the ability of the individual to control the communication of Personal Health Information (PHI). Privacy is an overarching concept in which the concepts of Confidentiality and Privileged communication are embedded. In the 1996 legal case of Jaffee vs. Redman, the Supreme Court upheld the principle that trust could exist in the relationship between patient and therapist.

Consider the following examples in which issues pertaining to confidentiality and privileged communication arise:

> 15 minutes into a group session, Florence asked Ava why she appeared so anxious. Ava responded that she had a large favor to ask of members. She reminded group members that the prior week, she had told the members she had filed a restraining order against her spouse for punching her. He was now disputing her account. Ava wondered if the group members would be willing to testify in a court proceeding about what she had said. Reactions varied from enthusiastic willingness to outright refusal. The therapist felt at a loss. She worried that the court might be able to compel members' testimony whether they wish to render it or not. She also worried that if members did testify, they could share material that could be legally injurious to Ava and have long-term negative effects on trust in the group.

> A faculty member is on an admissions committee of a doctoral program in clinical psychology. He recognizes that an application has been submitted from an applicant

DOI: 10.4324/9781003105527-2

who had formerly been in his psychotherapy group. The faculty member noted that certain aspects of the application material differed significantly from what was learned in the course of therapy, posing questions about his obligation to the applicant, the program, and the public.

A patient was seeing a therapist in both individual and group psychotherapy. In her individual therapy sessions, she had shared her doubts and confusion about her sexual orientation. In the group, she began to note that every time another member talked about her own sexual orientation issues, the therapist would make eye contact with her and on several occasions pressed her to share her reactions to the other member's disclosures. She felt that the therapist was using her knowledge derived from the individual sessions to pressure her to make a disclosure she was not ready to make.

The reader might confront none of these situations but, undoubtedly, will be faced with dilemmas related to confidentiality and privileged communication because these challenges are inherent in a modality in which individuals who meet as a group of strangers acquire private information about one another.

Confidentiality is an understanding between a healthcare professional and a patient or client that the latter's information will remain within the treatment situation. When practitioners act to preserve confidentiality, they are observing important ethical principles. The first is Respect for Autonomy in that the group leader is striving to ensure that the individual is autonomous in determining with whom and how that individual's information is shared. The second might be less obvious: the group psychotherapist acts in accord with Non-maleficence by protecting the individual from any harm that could come from information exported from the group about a member without that member's consent (Lasky & Riva, 2006). In contrast, when members enjoy the experience of their confidences being honored, their well-being is likely to be enhanced—an outcome consistent with the principle of Beneficence (Lasky & Riva, 2006).

The distinction between confidentiality and privileged communication is important. According to Haas and Malouf, "...privilege is a legally guaranteed right of the patient, whereas confidentiality is an ethical obligation of the service provider" (2005, p., 33–34). *Privileged communication* rests on the fact that governmental entities regard open communication in particular types of relationships as so crucial for the well-being of society that it protects those communications. Examples of such relationships are the communications of one spouse to another, of penitent to confessor, or—most pertinently to our interests—patient to psychotherapist. Although the psychotherapist-patient privilege is derivative of the physician-patient privilege, it now has standing in its own right. Mueller et al. (2018) state,

> The justifications for a psychotherapist-patient privilege are viewed as stronger than those underlying the physician-patient privilege. A psychotherapist relies almost entirely on disclosures from the client, whereas the physician often treats injuries or illnesses that can be observed, diagnosed, and treated by procedures not dependent on patient communications. Matters disclosed in psychotherapy are often more personal and more likely to cause embarrassment (or potential civil or criminal liability) than matters disclosed to a physician, leading some to conclude that the privilege has a constitutional basis in the right to privacy (p. 2).

The protection afforded these communications is highly specific. Privileged communication means that the person who holds the privilege in a protected relationship can keep information shared in that relationship from entering a court proceeding. In the case of psychotherapy, the patient is the holder of the privilege, meaning that it is the client and not the psychotherapist who decides whether a communication within a session is shared with the court. For example, a patient might direct the therapist to share treatment notes with the patient's attorney for possible use in a court proceeding. However, the therapist would not be able to take this action independently except under highly specific circumstances.

Identifying and Managing the Challenges of Confidentiality and Privileged Communication

This section identifies the threats that can emerge to confidentiality and privilege and the ways in which therapists can eliminate or reduce these threats.

Confidentiality

Just as the challenges to the preservation of confidentiality are multiple, so too are the tools the therapist can deploy to address these challenges.

Challenges to Confidentiality

Imagine Damon entering a psychotherapy group, sharing with the group leader and other members sensitive information—perhaps information shared with few others—and learning that one or more of the members divulged that very information with someone in the outside community. We can expect that feelings of anger and betrayal would result from such a breach. But we can also anticipate the thought "If I had known that this would happen, I would not have joined the group." Indeed, members share personal material because they trust that such material will be held in confidence. Even though members expect confidentiality to be observed, confidentiality is a protection that neither the therapist nor the organizations sponsoring psychotherapy groups can guarantee.

Why would one member violate the confidentiality of another? In order for a group leader to implement measures to discourage violations, the leader must understand the reasons breaches occur. A violation of confidentiality is so objectionable, so undermining to the group's well-being, that it might be assumed to be an act of aggression—with this notion, the violator is thought to have intended to hurt the violated member (e.g., by shaming the member). Such a motive undoubtedly operates in some instances. However, other motives also exist.

> A group member, Autumn, discovered that her young adult son had had a summer job with another member in the group, Deke. Both young men worked at a well-known establishment and their knowing one another was likely, given the nature of the workplace. Autumn provided her son with a physical description of the member. The son then confirmed that he knew this individual. Autumn excitedly shared the news with the group—that Deke and her son worked together. She went on to say that because they shared many of the same difficulties, they ought to become friends. Deke became enraged, saying that he intended to leave the group immediately because Autumn had broken his trust. Autumn became quite tearful and said that she did not violate confidentiality because she did not say what difficulties Deke had—she had merely told her son that they were similar to his own.

The violation of confidentiality in this example is twofold. Autumn revealed Deke's status of being a group member, a piece of information that should be under Deke's control.

Second, even though Autumn did not discuss Deke's specific difficulties, she nonetheless gave her son information about Deke beyond the mere fact of his group membership. Again, Deke's concerns expressed in the group should be his to convey to outsiders. This example highlights that at times, violations in confidentiality occur because the member's construction of what confidentiality is differs from that of the therapist or other healthcare professionals. Autumn appeared to believe that violations of confidentiality are restricted to actual content shared by members. Additionally, it seemed that Autumn took pleasure in making the disclosure to her son. Human beings enjoy gossiping and observing confidentiality requires a denial of this pleasure (Klontz, 2004).

Violations of confidentiality can occur because a member lacks the cognitive resources to observe it. Members must have sufficient resources to remember the confidentiality agreement and to understand how it is applied. Some members may begin a group in possession of such resources only to have them deteriorate over time. In such cases, violations of confidentiality are unintentional. Another example of an unintentional breach is when a member is taken by surprise and impulsively discloses information about another member. For example, Wolf might encounter Nadine while Nadine is accompanied by others. If Wolf and Nadine greet one another, Nadine's companions might inquire how the two individuals know one another. Such a seemingly innocuous question could elicit a revelation that the individuals are attending group psychotherapy together. One of the most frequent confidentiality violations is members identifying one another as group members to others (Roback et al., 1992).

A multiplicity of motives might account for members' confidentiality violation—anger at the violated member, enjoyment at the sense of control over another's information, satisfaction in having interesting information to share, a thrill in violating a group rule, or a defense against some element within the violator's inner life, to name a few. The best way to foster confidentiality is through a multi-component plan with components addressing different potential factors that could induce a lapse. In this way, the group leader can create the conditions in which members will adhere to confidentiality even if the leader cannot, strictly speaking, guarantee that they will.

Consequences of Breaches in Confidentiality

Violations of confidentiality can produce harm in multiple ways. The most obvious negative effect is the set of feelings—hurt, anger, embarrassment, and humiliation-stimulated by the discovery of the breach. The transgressed-against member's commitment to the group is also jeopardized. Beyond these immediate and potentially long-term reactions, other types of tangible harm can come to group members. For example, an individual's social connections and employment could be endangered (Roback et al., 1996).

Violations also affect other group members. One way in which group psychotherapy works is that members identify with one another's experience (Brabender, 2002). When any member suffers a negative experience in the group, other members tend to place themselves in that member's shoes. When a member suffers a violation of a confidence, the other members privately conclude, "My confidences could be leaked also." In this way, breaches have a chilling effect upon self-disclosure in the group, which in turn can limit interpersonal learning (Farber, 2003). Violations also lead to anger toward the therapist, greater resistance, and precipitous terminations (Roback et al., 1992).

Violations of confidentiality also undermine the trust the public has in group psychotherapy. When individuals experience significant adverse events in group psychotherapy, especially if those events are treated in a lax or casual manner, they understandably share their disappointment beyond the confines of the group. Such negative reports can shape the attitudes of the recipients of these communications regarding this modality. Given the relative lack of familiarity that even mental health professionals have with group psychotherapy (Taylor et al., 2001), reports to other professionals providing services to the injured member can create doubt about the usefulness and safety of the modality.

Multi-component Plan to Foster Confidentiality

Given the range of possible negative consequences that can ensue from violations of confidentiality, group psychotherapists should think carefully about how they will protect the confidentiality of each group member. The therapist needs to consider not merely how to create the conditions in which confidentiality is upheld, but also, how to provide a constructive response when it is not.

An adequate plan for maintenance of confidentiality requires therapist activity at different junctures over the course of a member's group participation: (a) during screening and orientation for the group; (b) at regular defined intervals; (c) when evidence exists of violations; and (d) at termination.

PRE-GROUP MEETINGS AND PREPARATION

Members must learn about confidentiality before they participate in group sessions. Specifically, the therapist needs to instruct the entering member on what confidentiality is and what kinds of events would constitute infractions. As illustrated in the example of Autumn and Deke, prospective group members can have ideas about what confidentiality is that different from those of the therapist, often reflecting a concept with a narrower scope than that of the therapist. The therapist must ensure that the potential member's definition of confidentiality is in alignment with the therapist's. One way for the therapist to discern the prospective member's idea of confidentiality is to present hypothetical situations, for example, "What would you do if you saw a member on the street and you were accompanied by a friend who asked about the encounter?" Such a question delivers to members the critical message that seemingly ordinary behaviors such as greeting a member with that member's name can have significance for the protection of confidentiality. In this process, the therapist should take into account the new member's cultural background (Brabender, 2021). In some cultures, the notion of strict communication boundaries might be alien. The therapist should acknowledge the disparity between the client's expectations and the requirements of the group, and explain why in the group setting, it is so important that the member adheres to confidentiality requirements.

Another element that should be introduced at this time is the idea of communicating the harm that could arise from confidentiality violations. Almost always, it is a revelation to new members that long-term damage can be done to others when their confidentiality is compromised. It can also be noted that members often alter their behaviors in the group in an unhelpful direction by withdrawal or defensiveness when the group learns of a violation. Again, it is generally more effective if the therapist engages the incoming member in a dialogue that encourages the person to mentalize others' reactions, for example, asking "What effect would you imagine it would have for group members to learn that one member's confidentiality was violated?" In some specialty groups, disclosures can lead to particular types of harm, and members should be helped to anticipate what they might be. For example, individuals who are known to have HIV are frequently subjected to stigmatization (Vanable et al., 2006). Therefore, if an individual is identified as being a member of a group for individuals diagnosed with HIV, that person's disease status is also revealed.

A particularly important piece of information to convey is to specify the consequences of confidentiality violations. Group psychotherapists have varying sanctions that they impose, but common to all of them is a thorough exploration of the violation within the group. The violation must be labeled as such and the members' various reactions to the violation should be acknowledged. Some therapists hold open the option of removing the transgressing member from the group, particularly if reason exists to believe that the member will engage in future violations. Therapists sometimes consider the circumstances surrounding the violation to determine the level of the sanction. For example, violations that occurred because the violator was taken off-guard might be sanctioned less heavily than those occurring with forethought (see an example of unwitting disclosure in Brabender, 2021).

As the therapist works with the incoming member on matters of confidentiality, it is important for the therapist to be attuned to any cultural factors that might make the task of maintaining confidentiality difficult for the member. Some members come from a culture in which personal information is routinely shared with family members and close friends, a style likely to affect their group behavior (McRae & Short, 2010). In such instances, maintaining confidentiality might seem unnatural and burdensome. These reactions need to be acknowledged at the same time that the therapist affirms the necessity of observing confidentiality.

The therapist must also assure the incoming member that the therapist will be maintaining confidentiality. The therapist should identify any legally-mandated exceptions to confidentiality (Rapin, 2010) such as the need to protect a suicidal group member, the need to protect others from a member who intends to hurt one or more people, or the need to respond to a court order. If the therapist hopes to interact with other professionals working with the group member, the therapist will need to obtain consent for those communications in the context of this broader discussion. One study found that students in training to be healthcare and legal professionals exhibit an insufficient appreciation of confidentiality breaches and see them as less significant than they are once they are recognized (Elger & Harding, 2005). In another study, it was found that as experience accrues, health-care professionals become more skilled at recognizing confidentiality issues (Elger, 2009). Therefore, supervisors of new leaders should be attentive to this aspect of the supervisee's functioning. In some cases, the group psychotherapist might be seeing the member in combined individual and group psychotherapy. The therapist should share information obtained from the individual therapy only with the individual's permission and should avoid pressuring a member in the group session to disclose information obtained in individual therapy sessions. If the group psychotherapist sees a member in individual psychotherapy and wishes to share information gleaned there with the co-therapist, permission to share that information should be obtained first.

Generally, the conversation about confidentiality should be accompanied by a written document that captures the major points of the discussion, which the new member signs. However, the written document should not be used as a substitute for a thoroughgoing conversation about confidentiality.

OVER THE COURSE OF GROUP PARTICIPATION

Even with a full discussion of confidentiality during preparation, the therapist cannot count on every member remembering the specificities of confidentiality from the pre-group meetings over the course of the group. Moreover, at various junctures in the group process, members' motivation to violate confidentiality might intensify. For example, the events in the group could stimulate one member's sadistic impulse to damage another member. In some cases, members' original understanding of what constitutes confidentiality drifts back to their original conceptions:

During the pre-group meeting, the leader told Fabienne that she was not permitted to discuss the events of the group or the communications of other members with anyone outside the group. As time passes, Fabienne becomes less conscious of the rationale for and definition of confidentiality and begins to divulge material to her wife. Once the therapist recognizes this misunderstanding, it is corrected for not only her, but also, all of the group members.

Although Fabienne's loss of conscious attention to confidentiality might be cognitively based, her revised understanding might also have emotional underpinnings, that is, she might wish to share with her wife this information. Therefore, it is important for the therapist to keep the obligation of confidentiality active in members' awareness. One way this awareness can be cultivated is to introduce the topic of confidentiality at various intervals (Brabender, 2002).

Another way in which the therapist can maintain members' awareness of confidentiality is to explore with members any situations in which they encountered one another outside of the group sessions:

Paula said she was surprised to see Alexa at a food fair that was located quite remotely from where the group was held, and Alexa admitted that she had the same reaction. Adesh changed the topic, conveying his assumption that the exchange between Paula and Alexa had run its course. The therapist, Gloria, intervened saying, "Wait—I'd like to hear more about what was going through your minds, Paula and Alexa, during this surprise encounter." Alexa said [to Paula], "I wanted to say 'hello' to you, but you were with a group. I worried later that maybe I hurt your feelings." Paula responded, "Not at all! I knew you were protecting me." "Exactly," Alexa exclaimed, "But I'm relieved that you realized that." Stan noted, "Even if you did hurt her feelings, protecting everyone's privacy is even more important. Had you greeted her, folks might have been curious about how you know her."

A conversation such as this is extremely beneficial to the group because members could very well be placed in this circumstance in the future. If they can recognize in advance that the ordinary social customs should not hold sway among group members when they see each other outside of the group, they are less likely to engage, impulsively, in overlearned, socially expected responses.

A CONFIDENTIALITY VIOLATION

The most important occasion on which to return to the topic of confidentiality is when a violation has occurred. In some cases, the therapist might not be certain that the violation occurred and would need to explore. For example, a highly suspicious group member might say, "When I passed you on the street, I heard you talking about me to your companion." A denial by the other member will prevent the therapist from declaring a violation and imposing sanctions unless other evidence is present. However, even the possibility of a violation would justify a review of the confidentiality rule. At times in the life of a group, it can be clear that a violation has taken place such as in our prior example when Autumn revealed to the group the violation (without acknowledging it as such). In such instances, it is important for the therapist to explore with the violator the experiences that accompanied the violation. We discussed previously that Autumn's notion of a violation was too narrow. A recognition of this distortion would allow the group to help Autumn broaden and clarify the meaning of confidentiality for the group. Still, such a discussion does not go far enough. The other factors that operated to lead to the breach are important to identify. For example, exploration might reveal that Autumn felt she possessed information that would be highly interesting to her son and penetrate his dismissive attitude toward her. It is likely that Autumn's recognition that she at times needs to use information to achieve connection could protect her and the group members from further violations.

Above all, it is essential for the group to explore confidentiality violations or possible violations because such attention conveys to every member of the group that such events are very significant. As the group develops, members' sophistication in recognizing the implications of violations (see Box 2.1 for a relevant example). In these discussions, the violator undoubtedly experiences discomfort. Members' observation of this adverse consequence

---

Box 2.1 The Group Processes a Confidentiality-Related Incident

Edwina got on the elevator with Rex to go to the floor on which the group session took place. Another person was on the elevator. Edwina said to Rex, "I hope you-know-who doesn't monopolize the group." Rex stared back at her. When the session began, Rex said, "I have an issue I feel I must bring up. Edwina spoke about another member in the elevator. She didn't mention anything the member said, and she didn't even give the member's name. But I feel we're on a slippery slope if we talk about particular members outside the group." Another member said, "I think that's a violation of confidentiality." Still another member said, "To me, this discussion is over-the-top. If the other person on the elevator didn't know who it was or what the person said, how can there be any harm?" Rex said, "Maybe the harm is that it makes me feel not quite as safe in here."

Questions for Discussion

a. As the therapist, would you see Edwina's comment as a violation of confidentiality?
b. Members have a differing understanding of the group's confidentiality rule. How would you foster a process to help clarify the rule?
c. As the therapist, would you make a statement about whether Edwina had violated confidentiality?
d. If you say "yes," is any further discussion necessary? If you say "no," is any further discussion necessary?
e. What does this vignette suggest about members' open communication in the group?

No group psychotherapist will be able to anticipate all of the challenges to confidentiality and therefore cannot craft a rule for all situations. The benefit of this likely reality is that opportunities to talk about the application of the confidentiality rule will emerge. Discussions such as the ones in which the members in the vignette participated enable clarification and refinement of this rule. One question that the therapist must answer is whether the group can decide what boundary crossings represent violations. In any decision about members' decision-making latitude, the therapist should factor in the developmental maturity of the group. As members' experiences with one another build, they acquire a greater ability to engage in a mature decision-making process characterized by a consideration of various aspects of a problem (Brabender & Fallon, 2009). The reader might identify other group-level factors that the group leader should consider when deciding whether the group has an adequate capacity to engage in ethical decision-making within the group.

serves as a deterrent. Additionally, it must be recognized that a violation in confidentiality typically creates a rupture in their alliance with the therapist and one another and can interfere with members' capacity to progress toward their therapeutic goals. Some members might directly express their displeasure whereas other members might manifest their discontent behaviorally, for example, by missing sessions, coming late, or remaining passive throughout the session (Marmarosh, 2021). The task of the therapist is to help the group repair the rupture by first acknowledging its presence and members' diverse ways of experiencing the rupture. For example, the member who committed the violation might withdraw from relationships in the group because of an extreme level of shame. The member whose confidentiality was violated might feel angry at the therapist who did not prevent the violation. The therapist can foster repair by facilitating a thorough exploration of these reactions. Therapists themselves are likely to have powerful reactions to confidentiality violations. Emotions such as anger toward the violator are important for the therapist to recognize and explore lest they hinder the therapist from doing the work of repair most effectively.

AT TERMINATION

Members might believe that the rules of the group remain operative only as long as they are in the group. This belief applies to many other life circumstances: When one leaves a system, one is no longer subject to the requirements of the system. Reciprocally, without direction otherwise, remaining members might imagine that it is acceptable to talk about the departed member with others outside the group. However, members can do as much damage to one another after they leave the group as when they are in it. Therefore, it is important at the time of termination that the therapist makes clear that the protections that have been accorded the members should continue to be provided. That is, the member who departs should not violate the confidentiality of remaining members, and vice versa.

In a time-limited group, the leaders should give specific attention to the progression of time over the course of the group and the disbanding of the group. The termination phase of a group is a unique period with its own processes and purposes, involving a review and reinforcement of the changes in each of the members. The leaders serve the principle of Beneficence by establishing a structure and procedures that help group members to resolve any remaining conflicted relationships with one another and the leaders. With particular attention to diversity and differences in identities, leaders can instill a social justice mindset for equity, inclusion, and acceptance in future relationships. One way in which this mindset is cultivated is through the acknowledgment of what members have contributed to one another across their varied identities. The awareness of differences in privilege can surface as members recognize contrasting opportunities—in therapy and other realms—following the ending of the group. Working on authority issues is also crucial. Losing the therapist, the members, and the group as a whole can activate feelings of helplessness and dependency, the exploration of which provides an opportunity for members to redress conflicts related to loss and dependency (Piper et al., 2011).

A successful leaving from a group should be a beneficial learning experience for all members. Making the ending complete means leaving relationships as *transparent* as possible, with past conflicts and supportive dynamics as highlighted learnings. Leaders with an ethical stance guide group members to predict potential stressors and practice the coping skills which have been developed in the group and can be applied in the future. Therapists who stop leading groups through a change in practice setting, retirement, or medical status have an ethical responsibility to help the members find a new treatment modality when needed. A reminder in the last group that the confidentiality agreement is everlasting respects the members' autonomy in controlling their personal information.

Privileged Communication Challenges and Strategies

One of the most significant challenges for the group leader is to know whether privileged communication exists in the relationship between the group psychotherapist and members, and among members. Group psychotherapists need to be aware of the privileged communication law in their jurisdictions, although not all do (Lasky, 2005). Such information can typically be accessed through state psychological associations. When therapists conduct online groups, the added complexity is often present: Therapists must be aware of the privileged communication law in the jurisdictions of their group members, jurisdictions that can vary from member to member (Prabhakar, 2013).

A complication exists in the relationship between group psychotherapy and privileged communication in that the model on which privileged communication rests is a one-to-one model: one communicator and one recipient of the disclosure. When an additional party is brought into the communication, it is typically regarded as an implicit waiver of the privilege. Making a disclosure to a third-party is tantamount to making it to the world (Slovenko, 2009), thereby giving the court a right to the information. By definition, group psychotherapy is a circumstance that involves multiple parties, and therefore could be regarded as failing to satisfy the conditions for privileged communications. The argument that could and would be advanced to the court is that the multiplicity of parties is inherent to group psychotherapy. Because the multiplicity is integral to the modality, communications made within the group are not those made to third parties extraneous to the treatment. This argument was made to the Minnesota Supreme Court in the case of State vs. Andring and was found to be compelling, that is, privilege was upheld. Whether this argument would hold sway with other courts is uncertain.

Even though privilege is not guaranteed, the therapist's actions can make it more or less likely that a member's material will enter a judicial proceeding in the absence of the member's authorization. First, in the informed consent, the therapist should make it clear to the incoming member that privilege is not guaranteed. That is, the therapist might be obligated to disclose information about the member to the court that the member does not wish to be disclosed. The therapist must assess the client's understanding of the concept of privilege, and if a full understanding is lacking, explain it clearly. The therapist must also cultivate the member's recognition of how a privilege issue might arise in the group. It is useful to have some examples at the ready (e.g., if a member were to be involved in a custody dispute, records might be sought on the member's report of parenting difficulties in the group). The therapist should also indicate what the therapist would do in the event of a request by an attorney or a court for information. The inclusion of information about privileged communication in the informed consent entails the therapist's respect for the member's autonomy in that the therapist is educating the member regarding potential consequences of disclosing particular types of information in the group.

A second way to protect member confidentiality is by keeping individual records on group members and avoiding the creation of records in which other members are mentioned. Recall the scenario presented at the beginning of this chapter where Ava sought to have other members testify on her behalf in court. In writing other members' notes, were the therapist to refer to what Ava shared, the material would have greater evidentiary value to Ava's case. Even the use of first names of other members should be avoided in note-writing. In this way, the therapist with proper authorization can submit records about a given group member without compromising the privacy of other group members (Knauss, 2006; Knauss & Knauss, 2012).

Third, once the member enters the group, the group leader should make every effort to keep the member's information confidential. At times, the therapist's aim to keep member information confidential might be at odds with the court's aim to collect information relevant to a court decision. The more relevant information is to a judicial decision at hand, that is, the greater the evidentiary value of the information, the more invested the court will be in obtaining the information (Brabender, 2002). At outset, the group leader must determine whether the communication is a subpoena or a court order. A *subpoena* is a device to discover information, typically from an attorney or court clerk, seeking evidence (testimony or documentation). On the other hand, a *court order* is a written command issued by a judge, and it requires that the therapist submit written material or provide testimony.

Responding to a Subpoena

Consider the following situation:

> A group psychotherapist who had been in practice for five years received a subpoena for the records of one of her group member's records. The anxiety the subpoena evoked in her led her to respond quickly. She copied the requested records and submitted them. Having done so, she felt she satisfied her obligation.

The therapist's anxiety is not unusual and makes the therapist vulnerable to precipitous action. The therapist was right about one matter: A valid subpoena requires a response; ignoring it could open the therapist to legal sanctions. However, *responding to the subpoena does not mean that the therapist must provide the requested privileged information.* Among the factors that dictate whether the therapist is required to yield the information are the following:

- Is the subpoena valid? For example, a valid subpoena allows sufficient time for the therapist to respond.
- Has the group member or the group member's attorney requested that the therapist submit the privileged information? Because the group member holds the privilege, the group member can waive it.
- Does the group member realize the possible consequences of release of information? The therapist should help the client to understand the implications of waiving privilege. This is particularly important if a record has information (e.g., material on substance abuse or sexual or family experiences) that could harm the client. Before the therapist releases the material, written authorization from the client should be obtained.

In deciding how to respond to a subpoena, the therapist should not only involve the client and the client's attorney early in the process but also an attorney who represents the therapist. Often such a person will be provided by the therapist's professional liability company (Felton & Polowy, 2015) who, in advising the therapist, will attend to a variety of factors including the specific laws governing subpoenas in the therapist's jurisdiction of practice. Whereas the client's attorney keeps in mind the client's best interest, the therapist's attorney serves the therapist's interests. As our analysis suggests, a therapist who receives a subpoena should respond, unlike the therapist in our vignette, with thoughtfulness, deliberation, and consultation.

Responding to a Court Order

If the therapist receives a court order, a writ from the judge presiding over a case, the therapist must comply. Although it is not impossible to challenge a court order, the therapist should do so rarely and generally obtain appropriate legal consultation before doing so (Knapp et al., 2013). In some cases, the judge might be willing to examine client records *in camera*, that is, in the judge's chamber in order to ascertain which documents have real evidentiary value to the current case. In this way, the group member's exposure within a larger forum can be limited.

Final Note

This chapter focused on the all-important topic of privacy, individuals' right to the protection of their information. The leaders' careful and proper handling of information will contribute to members' trust in the therapist and readiness to disclose in the group. Privacy relates to the topics of confidentiality and privilege. Adhering to confidentiality entails avoiding the transmission of material the client shared within the group outside of the group. Both the therapist and members must observe confidentiality although in particular well-defined circumstances, the therapist is required to breach confidentiality. Members should be informed of the requirement group membership confers upon them to observe confidentiality, the possible consequences of their failure to do so, and the harm that could result to other members from any violations. The member, too, should be apprised of the limitations of confidentiality. Privilege is the statutory and federal right of the client to control information from entering a judicial proceeding. Because group psychotherapy is a multi-person modality, members' right to privilege is not guaranteed, a fact that should be explicated as part of the informed consent.

CEU Questions

1. In the legal case of Jaffee vs. Redman, privacy concerns were upheld by the Supreme Court so that trust could exist in the relationship between patient and therapist. (T/F)
2. State laws specify circumstances in which a group therapist must breach confidentiality. (T/F)
3. Leaders can guarantee group member confidentiality, as long as each member signs a written contract and is informed of the limits of confidentiality. (T/F)
4. The greatest harm that can result from a violation of confidentiality is shame and embarrassment. (T/F).
5. When individuals with particular illnesses such as HIV enter a group, their identification as a member outside of the group can lead to their stigmatization. (T/F)
6. In hospitals and prisons, decisions about responding to a subpoena are often made by the institution's attorney. (T/F)
7. The most common breaches of confidentiality by group members involve another member's criminal behavior. (T/F)
8. The client has the right to be informed at the start of group treatment about the limitations of confidentiality. (T/F)
9. Not all states in the United States have established therapist-patient privilege. (T/F)
10. Identify three strategies the therapist can employ to encourage members to observe confidentiality.

Answer Key: 1. T; 2. T; 3. F; 4. F; 5. T; 6. T; 7. F; 8. T; 9. F; 10. Emphasize confidentiality during the informed consent; establish consequences for violations; process any member contacts outside of the group; model confidentiality.

Vignettes/Role-Plays

1. Fanny comes to the group and confesses that she had seen co-member Linette's posting on the FB page of one of her friends. Fanny revealed further that she used this posting to go to Linette's page and get a great deal of additional information about her, information that was unknown to other group members. Fanny perceived her own action as impulsive and wondered if it constituted a type of confidentiality violation. The therapist felt confused about whether it was a violation and how to best focus the group's discussion. The leader was also aware that Linette appeared very distressed. Questions:

    1. What ethical principles are at play in this situation?
    2. Who are the stakeholders?
    3. What solutions might the therapist devise and what are the advantages and disadvantages of each?

2. Gina reported at the beginning of the session that she had run into another member, Joy. Gina was with a number of her friends and was distressed that Joy greeted her in a conspicuous way and as they passed each other said, "See you Thursday night." Gina said Joy placed a burden of explanation upon her, which she resented. Joy said that had she not acknowledged Gina, she thought Gina would feel rejected by her. Different members ally with each of the members.
    Questions:

    a. Identify steps that might have been taken in the group prior to the encounter that might have diminished the likelihood of Joy and Gina having different understandings of appropriate behaviors when encountering one another outside of sessions.
    b. What steps should the therapist take now?
    c. How would the therapist know if the interventions were successful?

3. Terrence reported to his group that after his terminally ill wife had months of pain and no quality of life left, he ended her life at her request by giving her more morphine than allowed. Another member wants the leader to report this to the police because it violates her religious values.

    a. Is the leader legally mandated to report Terrence to legal authorities?
    b. How might you respond as a leader to both members, and the group as a whole?

4. Vanessa and Sheila were both aware that a group norm prohibited the use of social media to connect with other members, but Vanessa reached out to Sheila via Instagram. It later was revealed in group comments that they had been communicating and sharing photos. Several other members stated that the social media did not bother them and that they didn't agree with the norm anyway. How might this impact the inclusion dynamics of the other members, or the pair on Instagram, and how might the leaders consider responding?

5. David has been a group member for several months when Renita accuses him of telling a non-member that she is in a counseling group. Renita feels her confidentiality has been broken and wants to address it in group. Renita also asked the group leaders to prohibit David from returning to group.

6. Terri is extremely angry and rageful about her ex-wife, who has a lawyer and is trying to take the children away. She threatens to hurt her ex-wife at her house and tells the group she plans to do this tonight.

7. Susan, a shy person and newer member of the group, is feeling pressure to talk about her abusive childhood before she is ready to do so in the group. After asking the group to give her space, one member continues to push her. What is the leader's responsibility regarding coercion, sharing of information, and privacy?

Discussion Questions

1. In an inpatient setting, group members encounter one another outside of the group both informally and in other activities. How does this extra-group contact constitute a threat to maintaining confidentiality? How can the therapist work to counteract this threat?
2. Rufus gets caught having violated the confidentiality of another member. When asked by another member about his motive, he shrugs and says, "I did it for the fun of it." As the therapist, how would you work with Rufus's response?
3. How might you address confidentiality issues with group members whose disciplinary practices with children conflict with legal statutes? How might you include exploration of one's cultural/religious values in relation to confidentiality?
4. How do you approach conflicts around confidentiality issues with respect to other healthcare providers or administrators who might have less stringent standards?
5. What might be an ethical approach for addressing breaches of the confidentiality agreement by a co-leader or supervisee?
6. How can confidentiality breaches be repaired within a group?
7. What are some of the negative and positive treatment factors for your group members as you follow the laws and ethics around privacy and information control in your practice?
8. Bayley needs to miss an online session. She requests that the therapist record it so that she can view it later. She promises to erase the video as soon as she has viewed it.

    1. What ethical hazards are present in this situation?
    2. If ethical problems were not present, would clinical problems remain?

References

Brabender, V. (2002). *Introduction to group therapy*. Wiley. https://www.wiley.com/en-us/Introduction+to+Group+Therapy-p-9780471378891

Brabender, V. (2021). Identifying and resolving ethical dilemmas in group psychotherapy. In M. Trachsel, J. Gaabs, N. Biller-Andorno, S. Tekin & J. Z. Sadler, (Eds.), *The Oxford handbook of psychotherapy ethics* (pp. 625–641). Oxford University Press. 10.1093/oxfordhb/9780198817338.001.0001

Brabender, V., & Fallon, A. (2009). *Group development in practice: Guidance for clinicians and researchers on stages and dynamics of change*. American Psychological Association.

Committee on Legal Issues (2016). Strategies for private practitioners coping with subpoenas or compelled testimony for client/patient records or test data or test material. *Professional Psychology: Research and Practice*, *47*(1), 1–11. 10.1037/pro0000063

Elger, B. S. (2009). Factors influencing attitudes towards medical confidentiality among Swiss physicians. *Journal of Medical Ethics*, *35*(8), 517–524. 10.1136/jme.2009.029546

Elger, B. S., & Harding, T. W. (2005). Avoidable breaches of confidentiality: A study among students of medicine and of law. *Medical Education*, *39*(3), 333–337. 10.1111/j.1365-2929.2005.02097.x

Farber, B. A. (2003). Patient self-disclosure: A review of the research. *Journal of Clinical Psychology*, *59*(5), 589–600. 10.1002/jclp.10161

Felton, E. M., & Polowy, C. I. (2015). Quick reference guide for responding to a subpoena. https://naswcanews.org/quick-reference-guide-for-responding-to-a-subpoena/

Fisher, M. A. (2008). Privileged communication statutes in Virginia compared to other states. Retrieved from https://centerforethicalpractice.org/ethical-legal-resources/virginia-legal-information/legal-position-papers/privileged-communications-statutes-in-virginia-compared-to-other-states/

Glosoff, H. L., Herlihy, B., & Spence, E. B. (2000). Privileged communication in the counselor-client relationship. *Journal of Counseling & Development*, 78(4), 454–462. 10.1002/j.1556-6676.2000.tb01929.x

Haas, L. J., & Malouf, J. L. (2005). *Keeping up the good work: A practitioner's guide to mental health ethics* (4th ed.). Sarasota, Fl: Professional Resource Press.

Jaffee v. Redmond (1996). 518 U.S. 1. (United States Supreme Court).

Klontz, B. T. (2004). Ethical Practice of group experiential psychotherapy. *Psychotherapy: Theory, Research, Practice, Training*, 41(2), 172–179. 10.1037/0033-3204.41.2.172

Knapp, S., Yonggren, J. N., VandeCreek, L., Harris, E., & Martin, J. N. (2013). *Assessing and Managing Risk in Psychological Practice: An Individualized Approach*. (2nd ed.). The Trust.

Knauss, L. K. (2006). Ethical issues in recordkeeping in group psychotherapy. *International Journal of Group Psychotherapy*, 56(4), 415–430. 10.1521/ijgp.2006.56.4.415

Knauss, L. K., & Knauss, J. W. (2012). Ethical issues in multiperson therapy. In S. J. Knapp. (Ed.), *APA Handbook of Ethics in Psychology, Vol. 2*. (pp. 29–44). American Psychological Association.

Lasky, G.B. (2005). Confidentiality in groups: Rate of violations, the consent process, and group leader level of experience. Unpublished doctoral dissertation, University of Denver, Colorado.

Lasky, G. B., & Riva, M. T. (2006). Confidentiality and privileged communication in group psychotherapy. *International Journal of Group Psychotherapy*, 56(4), 455–476. 10.1521/ijgp.2006.56.4.455

Marmarosh, C. L. (2021). Ruptures and repairs in group psychotherapy: Introduction to the special issue. *Group Dynamics: Theory, Research, and Practice*, 25(1), 1–12. 10.1037/gdn0000150

McRae, M. B., & Short, E. L. (2010). *Racial and cultural dynamics in group and organizational life: Crossing boundaries*. Sage.

Mueller, C., Kirkpatrick, L. C., & Richter, L. (2018). Psychotherapist-Patient Privilege. Evidence §5.35 (6th ed. Wolters Kluwer 2018); GWU Law School Public Law Research Paper No. 2018-68; GWU Legal Studies Research Paper No. 2018-68. Available at SSRN: https://ssrn.com/abstract=3277054 Retrieved from https://scholarship.law.gwu.edu/cgi/viewcontent.cgi?article=2649&context=faculty_publications

Pepper, R. S. (2015). Is group psychotherapy inherently unethical? *Group*, 39(2), 159–160. 10.13186/group.39.2.0159

Piper, W. E., Ogrodniczuk, J. S., Joyce, A. S., & Weideman, R. (2011). *Short-Term Group Therapies for Complicated Grief: Two Research-Based Models*. American Psychological Association.

Prabhakar, E. (2013). E-therapy: Ethical considerations of a changing healthcare communication environment. *Pastoral Psychology*, 62(2), 211–218. 10.1007/s11089-012-0434-3

Rapin, L. (2010). Group development. In Conyne, R. K. (Ed.). *The Oxford Handbook of Group Counseling*. (pp. 61–82). Oxford.

Roback, H. B., Moore, R. F., Waterhouse, G. J., & Martin, P. R. (1996). Confidentiality dilemmas in group psychotherapy with substance-dependent physicians. *The American Journal of Psychiatry*, 153(10), 1250–1260. 10.1176/ajp.153.10.1250

Roback, H. B., Ochoa, E., Bloch, F., & Purdon, S. (1992). Guarding confidentiality in clinical groups: The therapist's dilemma. *International Journal of Group Psychotherapy*, 42, 81–103. 10.1080/00207284.1992.11732581

Rosen, D., Aronson, B., Litt, D. G., McAlinn, G. P., & Stern, J. P. (2017). *An introduction to American law* (3rd ed.). Carolina Academic Press.

Slovenko, R. (2008). *Psychotherapy and confidentiality: Testimonial privileged communication, breach of confidentiality, and reporting duties*. Charles C Thomas.

Slovenko, R. (2009). *Psychiatry in law/law in psychiatry* (2nd ed.). Taylor & Francis.

Smokowski, P. R., Rose, S. D., & Bacallao, M. L. (2001). Damaging experiences in therapeutic groups: How vulnerable consumers become group casualties. *Small Group Research*, 32(2), 223–251. 10.1177/104649640103200205

State v. Andring, 342 N. W.2d 128 (Minn. 1984).

Taylor, N. T., Burlingame, G. M., Kristensen, K. B., Fuhriman, A., Johansen, J., & Dahl, D. (2001). A survey of mental health care provider's and managed care organization attitudes toward, familiarity with, and use of group interventions. *International Journal of Group Psychotherapy, 51*(2), 243–263. 10.1521/ijgp.51.2.243.49848

Vanable, V. A., Carey, M. P., Blair, D. C., & Littlewood, R. A. (2006). Impact of HIV-related stigma on health behaviors and psychological adjustment among HIV-positive men and women. *AIDs and Behavior, 10* (5), 473–482. 10.1007/s10461-006-9099-1

3   Ethical Issues Related to the Role of Therapist/Leader

Ethical practice in group psychotherapy demands competence. However, becoming a competent group psychotherapist is no simple matter. Although group psychotherapy has been demonstrated to be an effective (Barkowski et al., 2020; Burlingame et al., 2020; Grenon et al., 2017) and efficient modality, it is typically given short shrift in graduate training (Marcus & King, 2003; Ohrt et al., 2014). The consequence of this training gap is that to achieve competence, the aspiring group psychotherapist must muster great initiative to pursue a self-directed learning program (Brabender, 2020). Specifically, developing group psychotherapists must ensure that they acquire the knowledge, skills, and attitudes (Kaslow, 2004) relevant to this modality. Many of the specific competencies are listed in Box 3.1 (see Barlow, 2012, for a more extensive discussion of group competencies). The mastery of the extensive set of competencies needed for group leadership requires multiple types of training experiences: Didactics, opportunities to observe senior group psychotherapists conducting groups, close supervision of group work, and exposure to groups in different contexts. Fortunately, professional organizations such as AGPA have filled the gap by providing students and professionals with group training.

Monitoring Competence

Ethical group leaders monitor their competence levels throughout their careers. Various factors can impinge upon competence with the following examples:

- Continuing Education—Does the therapist stay current with emerging research and theory as presented in the literature and workshops?
- Supervision and Consultation—Does the group psychotherapist know when supervision or consultation might be essential to competence performance as a group leader?
- Contextual Capability—Is the group psychotherapist qualified to work with a particular population, in a given context, employing a specific approach? Running a long-term outpatient group does not qualify a therapist to run short-term inpatient groups without additional training.
- Lack of Cognitive and Emotional Interferences—Does the group leader engage in appropriate self-care to regulate stress caused by personal events (e.g., births, illness, and death) and societal phenomena (e.g., pandemics and acts of terrorism) as well as internal vulnerabilities such as proneness to diminished self-esteem? Because certain stressful changes, in whole or in part, might be detrimental to the professional's functioning as a group psychotherapist, the therapist must monitor any alterations in the self as they affect group work and take actions to address them (Kaklauskas & Greene, 2020).

DOI: 10.4324/9781003105527-3

Box 3.1   Specific Competencies for Group Psychotherapy

- Selecting an Appropriate Theoretical Approach for the Population and Setting
- Engaging in Productive Self-Reflection
- Forming Working Alliances with Members
- Assessing and Selecting Members
- Preparing Members for Group Experiences
- Developing Cohesive Groups
- Managing Group Boundaries
- Understanding Group Dynamics
- Intervening at different levels (individual, dyadic, subgroup, and group as a whole)
- Demonstrating Multicultural Sensitivity and Humility
- Responding to microaggressions appropriately.
- Staying Abreast and Drawing upon Research
- Monitoring and Evaluating Outcomes
- Repairing Ruptures
- Engaging in Ethical and Legal Decision-making
- Developing a Pro-Group Environment in the Broader Treatment Context
- Managing Terminations and Transfer of Members

Leadership Challenges

Two tasks pose significant ethical challenges for the group leader: management of boundaries and management of differences among members.

Managing Boundaries

Group psychotherapists must be skilled in managing the boundaries or maintaining the framework of the group. Consistent, predictable boundaries - as in reinforcing the time and space boundaries of the group and defining the work roles of the members - are a source of safety for members, creating the conditions that members require to reveal themselves in the group and take the risks needed for their progress (Rutan et al., 2014).

Distinguishing among a rigid boundary, a boundary violation, and a boundary crossing is critical to ethical decision-making (Barnett, 2015; Gutheil & Gabbard, 1998). A *rigid boundary* is the maintenance of a particular boundary despite whatever events occur in the treatment. For example, a group psychotherapist might set the boundary that members cannot enter the session late and unswervingly maintain it. A *boundary violation* is an action that would exploit, oppress, or otherwise harm the client. A *boundary crossing* is ".... a benign variant where the ultimate effect of the deviation from the usual verbal behavior may be to advance the therapy in a constructive way that does not harm the patient" (Gutheil & Gabbard, 1998, p. 3). A variety of situations can lead the therapist to believe that a boundary should be crossed (Zur, 2004). For example, a change in the life of a therapist might do so, as is seen in the following example:

> Dean, a psychiatric resident leading the group, anticipated the birth of his first child in the next several weeks. His plan was to take a two-week sabbatical from the group

once his child was born. He decided to reveal to the group the reason for his upcoming absence. He reasoned that it would help them understand his inability to specify precisely when he would be absent as well as any more subtle differences in his demeanor in the group. Because this decision was at odds with his usual stance of low transparency about events in his personal life, he fostered a discussion with members of how they experienced his sharing a personal development.

What makes Dean's decision a boundary crossing is the fact that he did not customarily make this type of self-disclosure. However, he had a well-developed rationale for deviating from his customary way of relating. Moreover, he was open to members' reactions to relaxation of a boundary. Given that members' reactions to boundary alterations are not wholly predictable and might include some that are difficult for members to process on their own, this step is an important element of Dean's responsible decision-making. It would also be prudent for Dean to think about the possibility that this boundary crossing would open the door to other boundary crossings, for example, gift-giving in relation to the newborn given that major life events elicit gift-giving (Davies et al., 2010), and how the additional boundary crossings might be handled.

At times, boundary crossings will be necessitated by the particular issues with which a group member or the group as a whole is grappling:

> The group psychotherapist, Annie, was writing her notes after the conclusion of her group when Natalie appeared in her doorway. The session had concluded approximately 20 minutes prior, and Annie had assumed that all members had departed. Natalie explained that she had taken a long time in the ladies' room and now was frightened to take the elevator and walk to her car by herself. She wondered if the therapist would escort her to her car. Natalie previously had an abusive partner who continued to frighten her even though she had not encountered him in several years. Physical isolation such as walking through a desolated parking lot evoked intense anxiety. Annie was well-aware of Natalie's past and her fright in relation to certain situations in the present. She agreed to walk with Natalie to the exit and watch her until she safely got into her automobile. However, upon returning to her office she considered the possibility that Natalie might make this request on future occasions. Annie made a plan that if Natalie made a similar request in the future, she would explore with Natalie how she might feel safe travelling to her car without requiring the therapist's accompaniment.

Annie's decision entailed a boundary crossing in that her typical behavior did not include escorting a group member to her car. She decided to accede to Natalie's request because she knew Annie's distress was genuine and its continuation would serve no beneficial purpose. At the same time, she recognized that in doing so, she might be re-defining her relationship with the client in a way that could undermine Natalie's treatment. She therefore decided to develop a plan to mitigate any risks associated with the boundary crossing.

Good risk management requires that, whenever possible, consultation is obtained before deciding to cross a boundary, particularly if a crossing is significant. For example, if a member is extremely distressed at the end of a session, the therapist might decide to spend a few additional minutes speaking with that member. It would not be practical to obtain a consultation in this instance, and neither would it be necessary given that this type of boundary crossing is fairly routine. It is when boundary crossings are more significant and carry significant risks that consultation becomes essential. Consider the following:

Galen had been a group member for two years and had recently been experiencing elevated distress due to the dissolution of his marriage, which had taken him by surprise and involved infidelity on the part of his spouse. His work was sending him to a geographically remote area for six weeks. He petitioned the group and the therapist, Sheldon, to be able to attend the group virtually. Sheldon never had received such a request and never had done any work with virtual therapy. He found himself confronted with two sets of issues: (a) what were the advantages and disadvantages of on-line treatment, and how could he prepare himself to deliver it competently and ethically; and (b) what would be the ramifications of having a single member temporarily attend virtually while other members attended in-person?

This vignette highlights a circumstance in which a boundary crossing of potential significance could occur. Beyond investigating whether Sheldon practices in the jurisdiction in which Galen was located during those sessions, Sheldon would need to contemplate the ramifications of a manner of conducting the session that was quite different from the group's usual format. It would be important to consider how this variation would affect Galen but also the other group members. Before Sheldon committed to this temporary alteration, given the complexity of issues, it would be of utmost importance to get at least one consultation on the matter—the consultant might recognize aspects of the situation that Sheldon had missed. For example, had Sheldon agreed to the arrangement, he might not realize the need to get a new informed consent from Galen to cover the risks of tel-etherapy and any other stipulations the therapist might wish to set (e.g., the time limitation of the arrangement). The selection of an appropriate consultant is always an important issue. Sheldon should identify a professional who is competent in conducting psychotherapy groups and knowledgeable about ethical matters.

The circumstances raising potential for boundary crossings are limitless. However, three types of situations invite the therapist to engage in decision-making in relation to boundaries: therapist self-disclosure, gift-giving, and extra-group contact.

Therapist Self-Disclosure

Therapist self-disclosure in the psychotherapy group can take various forms. The disclosure could concern some past, present, or future aspects of the therapist's personal life outside the group. For example, a therapist might talk about a past struggle, a current experience, or an anticipated event. Another type of self-disclosure is when the therapist shares a here-and-now reaction stimulated by the group. Admitting to feeling torn between the competing needs of two members, expressing sadness over the termination of a member, or communicating regret over a therapeutic mistake are all examples of therapist emotional reactions pertaining to the group itself. Most therapists engage in self-disclosure at times (Edwards & Murdock, 1994). Even so, the topic of therapist self-disclosure remains controversial because of the awareness that this activity can have both positive and negative consequences for the group members. Among the benefits, therapist self-disclosure:

- Models the disclosure process for group members (Shechtman, 2002).
- Strengthens the real relationship wherein each party is experienced as genuine and real (Gelso, 2014)
- Increases the client's perception of the therapist as warm (Henretty & Levitt, 2010).
- Lessens the power differential between therapist and group member (Mahalik, et al., 2000).
- Conveys that member reactions are a natural part of human experience.

- Communicates that the therapist understands experiences associated with the client's minority status because the therapist shares that status (Guthrie, 2006).
- Establishes the humanity of the therapist (Lane & Hull, 1990).

Among the risks and potential disadvantages of therapist disclosure are the following:

- Creates a burden for group members if the therapist discloses personal difficulties (Dies, 1973).
- Reduces the space for the members to imagine aspects of the therapist and the therapist's life (Hanson, 2005).
- Lessens the client's perception of the therapist as an expert; reduces confidence in the therapist (Dies, 1973).

To decide what to reveal at any moment in the group, the group psychotherapist must think contextually, that is, hypothesizing what the likely positive and negative consequences will be of the disclosure in this particular group at this particular time. For one group, a given therapist disclosure might be anxiety-producing and for another, reassuring. Therapist disclosures that are unnerving early in the developmental life of the group might be beneficially absorbed when the group gains greater maturity. In any case, processing the effects of the disclosure is crucial. Group psychotherapists must also recognize that a particular disclosure might affect group members differently and be prepared to work through any unintended harm done.

Gifts and the Psychotherapy Group

At times, therapists will need to contend with members' efforts to provide gifts to the therapist or co-therapy team, or to one another (see Fallon & Brabender, 2018; Shapiro & Ginzberg, 2002; Smolar & Eichen, 2013). As is true for most categories of boundary crossings, group psychotherapists do well to consult professional codes and standards. The ethical guidelines of the American Counseling Association (2014) provide useful guidance on gift-giving and receiving:

> Counselors understand the challenges of accepting gifts from clients and recognize that in some cultures, small gifts are a token of respect and gratitude. When determining whether to accept a gift from clients, counselors take into account the therapeutic relationship, the monetary value of the gift, the client's motivation for giving the gift, and the counselor's motivation for wanting to accept or decline the gift.

This standard highlights the necessity of the therapist's response to accepting a gift being predicated upon a consideration of many factors. The meaning of gifts and gift-giving varies greatly from culture to culture (Davies et al., 2010), and with a diversity of members in a psychotherapy group, a diversity of beliefs and expectations about gift-giving will almost always be present and deserve exploration (Spandler et al., 2000). Relative to the individual therapist, the group psychotherapist has a more complicated task. Whereas the individual therapist's main focus is the individual client, the group psychotherapist must consider all of the members. For example, were a member to present a gift to the therapist, no matter how modest the gift might be, other members could well experience a pressure to emulate the gift-giver. Whatever stance the group psychotherapist makes in relation to the gift must be transparent and available for the entire group's exploration. Moreover, apart from the decision made, engaging the members in processing the gift-giving situation can provide valuable insights (Knox, 2008).

As in all matters, the therapist must weigh risks and benefits in decision-making. In refusing a gift, the therapist must recognize that feelings of hurt and humiliation are likely to be evoked. Where gift-giving is a natural part of a culture, the gift refusal could be seen as a nonacceptance of the member's identity (Knox, 2008). These reactions are especially likely if the therapist spurns the gift with little or no explanation. In some instances, the intensity of the member's reactions might lead that person to leave the group precipitously. However, the negative outcome might not end there in that the departed member might be disinclined to pursue further treatment. This is not to say that the therapist should always accept gifts to avoid eliciting uncomfortable feelings in the group member. Certain types of gifts (those beyond nominal value, those of a sexual nature, or those that set up a dual relationship such as a member offering babysitting services for the therapist's new baby) should always be refused, even though they precipitate negative feelings.

Acceptance of a gift and its exploration need not be at odds with one another, and it is important to understand that accepting the gift need not deprive the individual and the group of the opportunity of uncovering the meaning of the gift, the gift giver's intentions and what is going on in the group (cf. Smolar & Eichen, 2013).

In Box 3.2, a list of questions is raised for the therapist when a member seeks to offer a gift.

Extra-Group Contact

Although many types of boundary crossings can occur, one that is particularly common takes place when a member wishes to communicate with the therapist outside of sessions. Such requests represent a therapeutic challenge in that they can deprive the member of the opportunity to address a matter within a session. Consider the following example:

Box 3.2   Questions for Group Psychotherapists to Ask Themselves about Accepting a Gift

- What are the likely effects of the therapist's accepting or rejecting the gift including on the real relationship and the therapeutic alliance?
- What might the member have in mind (consciously or unconsciously) in exchange for the gift?
- When in the life of the member's participation in the group is the gift being offered (for example at the beginning, midpoint, termination)?
- How would the presentation of a gift be construed within a given member's culture?
- What is the likelihood that the exploration of the meaning of the gift will raise awareness of aspects of the member's intrapsychic or interpersonal life?
- What interpretation are other members likely to make of the therapist's acceptance or rejection of the gift?
- What is the expense of the gift?
- Particularly in the case of a gift made to the group, is it feasible or beneficial to have the group as a whole participate in the decision-making vis-à-vis accepting the gift?

Lucille called the group leader and said she had an urgent matter that she needed to discuss with the leader. She insisted that she had to make this communication in person. The leader suggested that she bring it up in the next group session, but she said she could not wait that long, and she truly needed to speak to the therapist privately but not on the phone. The therapist accommodated this request and scheduled a meeting for Lucille the next day. During the meeting, Lucille revealed that she was considering dropping out of the group because she felt that another member was looking at her in an amorous way. She found it to be distracting and frightening. She thought the member might make an advance upon her after she left the session. The therapist suggested that this might be an opportunity for her to learn about herself by addressing this matter in the group. She didn't take up this suggestion; while she returned to the group, she never raised her concern.

Many contextual factors might bear upon the therapist's decision, factors such as Lucille's fragility or even the length of the span until the next session. However, in making the decision about extra-group contact, the therapist's decision-making process would be strengthened by the recognition that a request for a private session likely means that the patient does not want to share something with the group. A group exploration of the ramifications of keeping the content private or secret between therapist and patient could be a useful forerunner to member's sharing the material with the group.

Another possibility for extra-group contract involves a member extending an invitation to the therapist to attend an event connected to the therapist:

As members were leaving a long-term group, Annabelle exclaimed to the leader, "I am going to play in a recital next month with my quartet. I'd love for you to attend. You've helped me so much with my anxiety about performing. I want you to see the fruits of your labor!" The leader asked Annabelle to bring it up in the next session, which she did. The members questioned Annabelle's awarding the therapist so much credit for her progress. They wondered why their own contributions were not recognized. Anabelle excitedly invited all of the members to the performance, saying that it simply had not occurred to her to invite them. She also encouraged everyone to remain for the reception after the concert. One member, Imogen, who tended to be reserved, began to ask questions about the number of people who would likely be at the concert. Upon hearing that it would be a relatively small audience, Imogen began to wonder whether it would be awkward for them to run into one another at this event. Should she introduce the other group members to her husband who would accompany her? As members processed the complexities of navigating this event, a consensus developed that the challenges of deftly handling one another's presence would be daunting. Annabelle remarked that knowing that members were apprehensive about seeing one another might compromise her confidence in herself and her pleasure in performing. One member suggested that the therapist could attend the concert and would represent the entire group. The therapist said she was amenable to this idea but wondered if it could introduce any other complexities. Annabelle then suggested that the therapist not attend the reception because it might create a pressure on Annabelle to explain the therapist's role in her life. Another member said a possible complication was that everyone would want the therapist to attend events, and briefly jested about the therapist having no life of her own, running as she would be from one event to the next. Several group members acknowledged that it would be unrealistic to expect the therapist to frequently attend members' events. However, they reasoned that this event was different from many other major events in members' lives in that

Anabelle's recital was closely tied to the work she did in the group. The group settled upon the notion that the group would talk about any invitation members wished to present to the therapist, offer a recommendation, but ultimately, the therapist would decide for herself whether she would attend.

In this session, the members themselves recognized some of the important considerations that should bear upon this type of boundary crossing decision. Mature groups are capable of engaging in this type of processing about therapy-related decisions, and often do so to their betterment (Agazarian & Peters, 1981). Moreover, group members offer a multiplicity of perspectives and can identify facets that might be hidden to the therapist. When allowing the group to weigh in on a decision, the therapist can be transparent with members about matters that affect them.

Managing Differences among Members

One of the most significant tasks for a group psychotherapists is to manage all of the types of differences that exist among members, differences due to identity, experiences, and positions in relation to basic psychological conflicts.

Multicultural Competence and Cultural Humility

Group psychotherapists have an ethical obligation to adhere to the principle of Justice, ensuring that their groups serve all individuals. Increasingly group psychotherapists' groups will be composed of members who have identities and backgrounds different from those of the therapist and different from one another. Multicultural competence is the ability to respond to these differences constructively, that is, in a way that strengthens the relationships among members and with the therapist, enabling members to accomplish more fully their therapeutic goals (Mbroh, et al., 2020). Group psychotherapists' multicultural competence contributes to a group environment that supports social justice in which oppression is avoided, biases are identified and challenged, and rights and responsibilities are equally distributed (MacNair-Semands, 2007; Sensoy & DiAngelo, 2017). In a psychotherapy group in which social justice is served, space is created for those who have been colonized (that is, had their culture and personal effects appropriated by another group) to understand their experiences of having been subjugated and move toward decolonization (Lewis et al., 2018). Presumably, members' experience of social justice within the micro-society of the group will enable them to work toward social justice in the society at large (Chen, 2013).

In this context, an individual's culture is seen as corresponding to the constellation of identities of a person and their intersection (Taloyo & Neal, 2020). These identities include, but are not limited to, race, ethnicity, sexual orientation, gender identity, religion and spirituality, immigration and citizen statuses, socio-economic level, language, and education (see Comas-Diaz, 2012; and Hays, 2008, for further discussion). Moreover, identities can be fluid across the life of an individual and might not fit into established categories, thereby requiring adaptability on the part of the therapist (Ribeiro, 2020). For example, the extent to which an immigrant identifies with the culture of the host country might change the longer the individual is in that country. Multicultural competence in the group psychotherapist requires knowledge of how a member's identities influence the individual's experience and behavior. Group leaders cannot be expected to have pre-existing knowledge of the backgrounds of all the members who enter their groups but, certainly, the willingness to acquire this knowledge once a particular member is accepted is necessary.

The concept of *cultural humility* introduced by Tervalon and Murray-Garcia (1998) is very helpful in conceptualizing this process. A danger of the notion of competence is its potential for being viewed as a fixed commodity—one becomes competent and thereafter enjoys this state. Cultural humility acknowledges that cultural learning is a lifelong quest, entailing continual openness to acquiring knowledge and self-reflection about the limits of one's current knowledge (Hook et al., 2017).

Both processes will support a group psychotherapist's expression of curiosity about an incoming member's culture, honesty in acknowledging missing or incomplete information, and recognition of the client's status as expert in this regard (Chung & Bemak, 2002). However, competence also frequently requires the therapist's conscientiousness in pursuing other sources of information about a member's culture. Some identities are associated with expectations about the ways in which others are likely to behave. For example, a particular cultural expectation might be, "When tension exists in a relationship, one must lessen it by taking responsibility for the creation of the tension." The therapist's appreciation of such cultural prescriptions provides a foundation for empathy when the member engages in interpersonal behaviors that appear to undermine that member's well-being.

For some group psychotherapists, cultural humility is a hard-wrought virtue. It requires the avoidance of two extremes, one being excessively confident in one's multicultural capabilities and the other, epistemic despair, the paralytic sense that one cannot know anything in the midst of so much complexity. The first position easily leads to stereotypic thinking about individuals' identities, i.e., "I know from my experience that cultural group 'x' responds in way 'y'...," thereby failing to recognize that members in a group do not respond in the same way in most areas. This therapist is prone to impose stereotypes on members that do not fit them. The second position leads to an effort to accommodate the member in the absence of any systematic attempt to learn about a member's cultural identity. This therapist is deprived of the guiding notions that would elucidate particular member behaviors. Supervisors play a seminal role in this process of helping the supervisee to develop more robust cultural humility. A skilled supervisor can identify the assumptions a supervisee holds about a member's identity status, recognize any ways of relating to members that might be rooted in bias, and can point out opportunities for cultural learning that the supervisee might have missed. Owen et al. (2016) found more favorable outcomes in groups led by culturally humble therapists, suggesting that this quality operates in the service of Beneficence. In our discussion of multiculturalism and the group psychotherapist, we use the term "competence," but think about it not as a static acquisition or a complete mastery, but as a lifelong effort on the part of the group psychotherapist consistent with the notion of cultural humility.

Power configurations are complex and changing and require the ethical group leader's attention. A key responsibility of the group psychotherapist is being cognizant of any identity statuses that are connected to stigmatization and marginalization, an awareness that should be shared by practitioners of all modalities. However, the group psychotherapist must be particularly sensitive to these phenomena because it is often in a group setting that they reveal themselves: Individuals are bullied in groups and shunned by groups. Psychotherapy groups are a place in which wounds can be re-opened or healed (Haen & Thomas, 2018). Group psychotherapists must recognize that members' real-life histories affect how they process the here-and-now events of the group. What might appear to be an overreaction to a social stimulus might be fully comprehensible given a member's history. The group psychotherapist knowing this history is likely better equipped to ensure that the member's interactions with others yield outcomes that are favorable rather than adverse, healing rather than harmful.

In pondering what constitutes a marginalized identity, the group psychotherapist might think of race, gender identity, sexual orientation, and other relatively stable features of a person's identity. However, the marginalization of a given identity can be fluid—a person might be subordinated in one context and not another. For example, a politically conservative student might study at a progressive college and be marginalized by classmates. International students might experience marginalization if they are not fluent in the language of the host country. Moreover, sociocultural events affect privilege. For example, during the COVID pandemic, the view that the virus originated in China led to the subordination of Chinese Americans. Hence, the therapist is best served by holding to broad notions of prejudice and privilege, appreciating that from context to context, who is marginalized can vary.

Thinking about a group member's marginalized status is not the only task for a group psychotherapist. It is also necessary for the group leader to be aware of the history, beliefs, values, and norms associated with the identities represented in a given psychotherapy group. Fortunately, the literature in this area is rapidly accruing. In Tables 3.1 (articles and chapters) and 3.2 (organizational guidelines), we list resources for the group psychotherapist attempting to increase multicultural competence in relation to a particular identity group. Our list is non-exhaustive, and we have given priority to more recent publications because their list of references will give the reader access to past contributions. A part of the therapist's multicultural competence is a mastery of terminology in relation to different identity statuses, a mastery that is consistent with the ethical principle of Justice, reflecting an inclusive attitude toward the fullness of group members' identities. For example, a respectful group psychotherapist knows and uses pronouns that correspond to individuals' gender identities while being mindful that group members might have individual preferences about terminology and these preferences should be revealed and honored. For example, Chen et al. (2020) point out that in a psychotherapy group composed of transgender group members, some members might prefer "he" or "she" and others, gender-neutral pronouns such as the singular "they" and "them," or "ze" and "hir."

As therapists strive to achieve multicultural competence and humility, they can be aided by exploration of their own racial and cultural identities (Platt, 2020). This process helps therapists to anticipate their own blind spots and recognize their own biases. In this effort, therapists might usefully consult racial identity theory as Helms (2008) proposed for White Identity theory and Cross et al. (2012) for Black Identity theory. Privilege attaches itself to different identities, and therapists who understand their own privilege in relation to that of group members will recognize a greater range of potential meanings of behavior within the group. For example, excessive deference toward the therapist might be readily construed as a manifestation of dependency. Alternatively, though, the member might be following an unspoken social rule demanding obsequiousness in relation to individuals with a particular privileged identity. In some instances, the therapist could possess less privilege than a member on some identity variable (see Fors, 2018), such as when a member might clearly occupy a high socioeconomic status. A therapist unaware of internalized subordination might be less responsive to this member's boundary crossings in such matters as paying fees than to other members engaging in the same behavior.

In managing boundaries competently, the group psychotherapist must attend to culture. Consider the following example:

> A group psychotherapist has an appointment with a 25-year-old woman, Isla, to evaluate her appropriateness for the group. The therapist steps into the waiting room and sees that three individuals are present rather than the single person he expected. The prospective member introduces these individuals as her parents. He proceeds to

Table 3.1 Resources for Multicultural Competence and Humility for Different Cultural Identity Groups: Articles and Chapters

Identities	Articles and Chapters
Ableness	• Freedman, W., Klein, L., & Kopp-Miller, K. (2020). Chronic health conditions/ability issues in group therapy. In M. D. Ribeiro (Ed.), *Examining social identities and diversity issues in group therapy: Knocking at the boundaries* (pp. 53–65). Routledge. https://www.taylorfrancis.com/chapters/chronic-health-conditions-ability-issues-group-wendy-freedman-leslie-klein-katheryne-kopp-miller/e/10.4324/9780429022364-4?context=ubx&refId=6be69e74-67a5-4a90-bf22-26fad1347515
Acculturation/Immigration	• Buchele, B. (2020). Immigration and implications for group work: Commentary on the works included in this Special Issue. *International Journal of Group Psychotherapy, 70*(2), 293–306. https://doi.org/10.1080/00207284.2020.1717881 • Klein, R. H. (2020). Introduction to the special issue on migration problems in the US and their implications for group work. *International Journal of Group Psychotherapy, 70*(2), (141–161). https://doi.org/10.1080/00207284.2020.1718503 • Leiderman, L. M. (2019). Psychodynamic group therapy with Hispanic migrants: Interpersonal, relational constructs in treating complex trauma, dissociation, and enactments. *International Journal of Group Psychotherapy, 70*(2), 162–182. https://doi.org/10.1080/00207284.2019.1686704 • Ponzer, K. A., Mastropolo, E. & Molina, L. S. (2020). Immigration law and its impact on the family: What group psychotherapists need to know. *International Journal of Group Psychotherapy, 70*(2), 183–211. https://doi.org/10.1080/00207284.2020.1719012 • Thomas, N. (2020). Immigration: The "illegal alien" problem. *International Journal of Group Psychotherapy, 70*(2), 270–292. https://doi.org/10.1080/00207284.2020.1718504
Age	• Giannone, Z. A., Cox, D. W., Kealy, D., & Ogrodniczuk, J. S. (2020). Identity-focused group interventions among emerging adults: A review. *North American Journal of Psychology, 22*(1), 41–62. • Mangione, L., & Forti, R. (2018). Beyond midlife and before retirement: A short-term women's group. *International Journal of Group Psychotherapy, 68*(3), 314–336. https://doi.org/10.1080/00207284.2018.1429927 • Shechtman, Z. (2017). *Group psychotherapy with children and adolescents: Theory, Research, and Practice.* Routledge. • Tavares, L. R., & Barbosa, M. R. (2018). Efficacy of group psychotherapy for geriatric depression: A systematic review. *Archives of Gerontology and Geriatrics, 78*, 71–80. https://doi.org/10.1016/j.archger.2018.06.001
Gender	• Moreno, J. K., Kramer, L., Scheidegger, C. M., & Weitzman, L. (2005). Gender and group psychotherapy: A review. *Group*, 351–371. • Paquin, J. D., Abegunde, C., Hahn, A., & Fassinger, R. E. (2020). A brief history of group therapy as a field and the representation of women in its development. *International Journal of Group Psychotherapy, 71*(1), 13–80. https://doi.org/10.1080/00207284.2020.1798176 • Pure, D. L. (2011). Single-gender or mixed-gender groups: Choosing a perspective. In J. L. Kleinberg (Ed.). *The Wiley-Blackwell Handbook of Group Psychotherapy* (pp. 381–396). Wiley-Blackwell. https://doi.org/10.1002/9781119950882.ch19

(Continued)

Table 3.1 (Continued)

Identities	Articles and Chapters
Gender Identity	• Heck, N. C. (2017). Group psychotherapy with transgender and gender nonconforming adults: Evidence-based practice applications. *Psychiatric Clinics of North America, 40*(1), 157–175. https://doi.org/10.1016/j.psc.2016.10.010 • LeFay, S. (2020). Gender identity in group. In M. D. Ribeiro (Ed.), *Examining social identities and diversity issues in group therapy: Knocking at the boundaries* (pp. 41–52). Routledge. https://doi.org/10.4324/9780429022364-3
Indigenous People	• Heilbron, C. L., & Guttman, M. A. J. (2000). Traditional healing methods with First Nations women in group counselling. *Canadian Journal of Counselling, 34*(1), 3–13. https://files.eric.ed.gov/fulltext/EJ603067.pdf
Race and Ethnicity	• Bemak, F., & Chung, R. C. Y. (2019). Race dialogues in group psychotherapy: Key issues in training and practice. *International Journal of Group Psychotherapy, 69*(2), 172–191. https://doi.org/10.1080/00207284.2018.1498743 • Bermudez, G. (2018). The social dreaming matrix as a container for the processing of implicit racial bias and collective racial trauma. *International Journal of Group Psychotherapy, 68*(4), 538–560. https://doi.org/10.1080/00207284.2018.1469957 • Haen, C., & Thomas, N. K. (2018). Holding history: Undoing racial unconsciousness in groups. *International Journal of Group Psychotherapy, 68*(4), 498–520. https://doi.org/10.1080/00207284.2018.1475238 • Kivlighan III, D. M., Owen, J., & Antle, B. F. (2020). Do racial/ethnic disparities differ between relationship education groups? Testing the cultural effectiveness of racially diverse relationship education groups. *Couple and Family Psychology: Research and Practice, 9*(1), 1–12. https://doi.org/10.1037/cfp0000130
Religion and Spirituality	• Abernathy, A. D. (2020). Spirituality as a resource in group psychotherapy. In M. D. Ribeiro (Ed.), *Examining social identities and diversity issues in group psychotherapy: Knocking at the boundaries* (pp. 149–160). Routledge. https://doi.org/10.4324/9780429022364
Sexual Orientation	• Bertsch, K. (2021). Inclusivity of multiple identities in sexual identity based therapy groups in university and college counseling. In M. D. Ribeiro (Ed.), *Examining social identities and diversity issues in group psychotherapy: Knocking at the boundaries* (pp. 66–77). Routledge. • Heilman, D. (2018). The potential role for group psychotherapy in the treatment of internalized homophobia in gay men. *International Journal of Group Psychotherapy, 68*(1), 56–68. https://doi.org/10.1080/00207284.2017.1315585 • Israel, T., Gorcheva, R., Burnes, T. R., & Walther, W. A. (2008). Helpful and unhelpful therapy experiences of LGBT clients. *Psychotherapy Research, 18*(3), 294–305. https://doi.org/10.1080/10503300701506920
Socio-economic Status	• Ziadeh, S. (2020). Group interpersonal psychotherapy in the context of poverty and gender: Toward a culturally sound adaptation of IPT-G to socioeconomically disadvantaged and depressed lebanese women. In M. D. Ribeiro (Ed.). *Examining social identities and diversity issues in group psychotherapy: Knocking at the boundaries* (pp. 204–222). Routledge. https://doi.org/10.4324/9780429022364

(*Continued*)

Table 3.1 (Continued)

Identities	Articles and Chapters
Veterans	• Lewis, M. (2020). Managing microaggressions within veterans' psychotherapy groups. In M. D. Ribeiro (Ed.), *Examining social identities and diversity issues in group therapy: Knocking at the boundaries* (pp. 119–133). Routledge. https://www.taylorfrancis. com/chapters/chronic-health-conditions-ability-issues-group-wendy-freedman-leslie-klein-katheryne-kopp-miller/e/10.4324/ 9780429022364-4?context=ubx&refId=6be69e74-67a5-4a90-bf22–26fad1347515

Table 3.2 Organizational Resources to Address Diverse Identities

Identities	Organizational Guidelines
Ableness	• American Psychological Association. (2012). Guidelines for assessment of and practice with persons with disabilities. *American Psychologist, 67*(1), 43–62. https://doi.org/10.1037/a0025892
Acculturation/ Immigration	• Pottie, K., Greenaway, C., Feightner, J., Welch, V., Swinkels, H., Rashid, M., Narasiah, L., Kirmayer, L. J., Ueffing, E., MacDonald, N. E., Hassan, G., McNally, M., Khan, K., Buhrmann, R., Dunn, S., Dominic, A., McCarthy, A. E., Gagnon, A. J., Rousseau, C., ... Zlotkin, S. (2011). Evidence-based clinical guidelines for immigrants and refugees. *CMAJ, 183*(12), E824-E925. https://doi.org/10.1503/cmaj. 090313
Age	• American Psychological Association. (2014). APA guidelines for psychological practice with older adults. *American Psychologist, 69*(1), 34–65. https://doi.org/10.1037/a0035063
Gender	• Girls and Women Guidelines Group. (2018). *APA guidelines for psychological practice with girls and women.* American Psychological Association. http://www.apa.org/about/policy/psychological-practice-girls-women.pdf • Boys and Men Guidelines Group (2018). *APA guidelines for psychological practice with boys and men.* American Psychological Association. http://www.apa.org/about/policy/psychological-practice-boys-men-guidelines.pdf
Gender Identity	• American Psychological Association. (2015). Guidelines for psychological practice with transgender and gender nonconforming people. *American Psychologist, 70*(9), 832–864. https://doi.org/10.1037/a0039906 • The World Professional Association for Transgender Health. (2012). *Standards of care for the health of transsexual, transgender, and gender nonconforming people* (7th version). https://www.wpath.org/ publications/soc • Association of Lesbian, Gay, Bisexual, and Transgender Issues in Counseling. (2009). *Competencies for counseling transgender clients.* https://www.counseling.org/docs/default-source/competencies/ algbtic_competencies.pdf?sfvrsn=d8d3732f_12
Indigenous People	• Rivera, E. T., Garrett, M. T., & Crutchfield, L. B. (2004). Multicultural interventions in groups: The use of indigenous methods. *Journal for Specialists in Group Work, 18(2)*, 86–93. https:// psycnet.apa.org/doi/10.4135/9781452229683.n21 • Roessel, M. H. (n.d). *Working with indigenous and native American peoples.* American Psychiatric Association. https://www.psychiatry.

(*Continued*)

Table 3.2 (Continued)

Identities	Organizational Guidelines
	org/psychiatrists/cultural-competency/education/best-practice-highlights/working-with-native-american-patients
Race and Ethnicity	• APA Task Force on Race and Ethnicity Guidelines in Psychology. (2019). *APA guidelines on race and ethnicity in psychology: Promoting responsiveness and equity.* American Psychological Association. https://www.apa.org/about/policy/guidelines-race-ethnicity.pdf
Religion and Spirituality	• Awaad, R. & Abbasi, F. (2019). *Stress & trauma toolkit for treating muslims in a changing political and social environment.* American Psychiatric Association. https://www.psychiatry.org/psychiatrists/cultural-competency/education/stress-and-trauma/muslims
Sexual Orientation	• American Psychological Association. (2012). Guidelines for psychological practice with lesbian, gay, and bisexual clients. *American Psychologist, 67*(1), 10–42. https://doi.org/10.1037/a0024659 • Cabaj, R. P. (2020). *Best practice highlights: Working with LGBTQ patients.* American Psychiatric Association. https://www.psychiatry.org/psychiatrists/cultural-competency/treating-diverse-patient-populations/working-with-lgbtq-patients
Socio-economic Status	• American Psychological Association. (2019). *APA guidelines for psychological practice for people with low-income and economic marginalization.* https://www.apa.org/about/policy/guidelines-low-income.pdf
Veterans	• The Management of Posttraumatic Stress Disorder Work Group (2017). *VA/DoD clinical practice guidelines for the management of posttraumatic stress disorder and acute stress disorder.* Department of Veteran Affairs and the Department of Defense. https://www.healthquality.va.gov/guidelines/MH/ptsd/VADoDPTSDCPGFinal012418.pdf

take Isla into his office where she explains abashedly that her parents wanted to "lay eyes" on him. She went on to say that she would greatly appreciate the therapist's explaining to her parents how group psychotherapy works. Upon detecting a look of puzzlement on the therapist's face, Isla explained that within her culture, it was not uncommon for parents—especially first-generation parents—to be aware of the involvements of their adult children. She stated her recognition that the therapist should not and could not be updating her parents on her progress. However, she felt that some explanation of the workings of group psychotherapy would reassure them and add to her own harmony with them. The therapist thought the request unusual and worried that acceding to this request could be at odds with the prospective member's long-term developmental needs. He demurred from offering them any specific information in relation to Isla. However, in deference to Isla's culturally-rooted request, he agreed to meet with the parents briefly to offer them introductory information about the modality.

Typically, in the case of an adult, the group psychotherapist would not be meeting with other parties in an incoming member's life. However, Isla made a special request based on the notion that what was typical for this therapist (and other therapists) was atypical for her culture. Indeed, first-generation Hispanic immigrants show relatively low utilization rates of mental health care (Vásquez et al., 2020), and it would not be surprising if this treatment were somewhat alien to Isla's parents. From the stance of cultural humility, the therapist was a learner about her culture and open to the possibility that it could enhance her well-being for her parents to learn about group psychotherapy. Another therapist, also exhibiting cultural humility, might have provided Isla with educational materials about group psychotherapy to share with her parents. Both solutions would be examples of factoring culture into clinical decision-making.

Identity Differences within the Microcosm

The group psychotherapist has an ethical obligation to ensure that differences among members do not emerge in a way that brings harm to members. Process-oriented psychotherapy groups are based on the notion that individuals bring their customary difficulties in relating to others in their everyday worlds to the relationships in the psychotherapy group. This concept combines with the construct of "microcosm"—the group is a little world with a range of personalities conducive to the emergence of interpersonal behaviors that could be observed in the member's life outside of the group (Yalom & Leszcz, 2020). The idea is that what is outside the group enters the group where it can be addressed. However, what can enter the group is broader than individuals' idiosyncratic behaviors. As a part of society, the group is likely to be permeated by the values, tensions, and struggles of the society in which it is embedded (Bemak & Chung, 2019). Most societies are afflicted by cultural oppression— the separation of society into castes of the privileged and the oppressed—based on such factors as race, ethnicity, gender, gender identity, sexual orientation, immigration status, and religion, to name some major factors. These societal forces of oppression and subjugation inevitably enter the group creating a circumstance wherein members who have been societally victimized can be subjected to this process again (Chang-Caffaro & Caffaro, 2018). However, the fact that the group provides an environment in which interactions are explored creates the potential for members to learn to interact in non-oppressive ways and for members who have been harmed by toxic societal forces to experience healing and understanding (Haen & Thomas, 2018). When group psychotherapists tap into this potential of groups, they are acting in consistency with the core ethical principle of Justice.

The psychotherapy group has not historically been seen as a resource for addressing societal problems of oppression, marginalization, and racism. Individuals' unique issues rooted in their own developmental histories have been regarded as the proper province of the group's attention. Group psychotherapists themselves as persons enjoying some measure of privilege likely had a vested interest in preserving the existing power structure. Recently, a societal shift has occurred—due in part to well-publicized and horrific evidence of racism—that has created a new openness to the dismantling of power structures. With this shift has come a greater appreciation of the group psychotherapy community of the need for group psychotherapists to work not merely for individual ends but also, for social justice ends. In fact, social justice ends are highly compatible with the goal of fostering healthy interpersonal change. The marginalization and oppression of groups have not contributed to interpersonal harmony but led to conflict and strife. Therefore, fostering individual social adjustment and social justice are complementary goals.

Although some manifestations of prejudice are blatant, more often they are subtle, taking the form of what has been popularly termed "microaggressions" (Sue et al., 2007; Sue, 2010). The "micro" aspect of the aggression pertains to its hidden aspect, not its impact (Platt, 2020). Certain forms of oppression such as racism are no longer socially condoned in most (but not all) sectors of society such that individuals expect to get sanctioned for direct expressions, and indeed, might sanction themselves for such manifestations. Yet, in any country in which racism has taken hold, a shift in public sentiment leads racism to go underground because it is based upon a power structure that those with privilege seek to perpetuate. Microaggressions serve to maintain the status quo of privilege and domination while obscuring this from others and often themselves ("I can be a good person and still have my privilege"). Examples of microaggressions are failing to acknowledge another's presence in the group, making barely discernible put-downs, and failing to show empathy for another's difficulties. Group leaders are also capable of microaggressions directed at members such as forgetting a member's name, making an ill-timed intervention, or missing an important issue present in the group (Rutan, 2021). Ignoring microaggressions violates the principle of Non-maleficence. Conversely, the therapist's willingness to acknowledge and repair these empathic lapses will contribute to members' openness to exploring microaggressions occurring in the group.

Beyond helping members to grapple with discrimination based on their identity statuses, the group psychotherapist must also help members to engage in appropriate acts of self-advocacy. The member who has minority status in the group by virtue of coming from a different culture or having some other distinguishing feature is at risk of succumbing to subtle pressure to submit to the norms established by other members (Fenster, 1996). We are not referring here to the norms that the therapist carefully cultivates that are necessary for members to reach their therapeutic goals such as attending sessions consistently. Rather, the norms we are referencing are those rules that are idiosyncratic to subgroups of members. For example, individuals from some cultural groups might be more prone to hesitate before speaking. Although the therapist and members might interpret this behavior as defensiveness, a cultural hypothesis might also be considered. The group psychotherapist can help members distinguish between goal-related versus identity-related norms and acquire the ability not to submit to the latter simply because they reflect the ways of the majority.

Competence in Managing Difficult or Antitherapeutic Member-to-Member Relations

The leader should disallow all forms of intimidation or verbal abuse and respond promptly to any fledgling manifestations to protect members. Group psychotherapy carries with it the risk for member-to-member relations that can affect one another adversely. As noted in the prior section, potentially harmful interactions can reflect discrimination based on facets of identity. However, other possibilities exist. For example, members can coerce a member into making a self-disclosure that the member would refrain from making in the absence of pressure. The therapist must possess the skill to recognize and disrupt group coercion (Greene & Kaklauskas, 2020) and be ready to seek prompt supervision or consultation if the therapist's efforts are unsuccessful. Therapists must also monitor their groups for the emergence of scapegoating. Scapegoating has been understood in various ways but is commonly understood to represent the projection of negative qualities members see within themselves onto a particular member whom they then marginalize. This dynamic places the scapegoat in peril because that individual must endure group-level rejection and ridicule along with the host of negative feelings scapegoating is likely to precipitate. Different theoretical models offer different strategies for doing so. For example, systems-centered theory recommends *functional subgrouping* by which members can join with others with similar positions as a method for repairing ruptures and avoiding group-level maneuvers that isolate and coerce members (Gantt, 2021). Moreno (2007) and Clark (2002) indicate that alongside group- or subgroup-level interventions, the therapist might help the scapegoated individual to learn about any social behaviors that might make the person vulnerable to such group activity. Whether a therapist embraces these strategies or some others, it is crucial that the therapist recognize and act upon the responsibility to protect all members from scapegoating.

In Chapter 7, we also discuss measures of racism and ethnicity-related stress and other measurement-based care systems (MBC). At times it is necessary to monitor specific aspects of the group process to track how they are functioning. One such area that we now discuss from the recent literature is *rupture and repair* in groups.

Using Measures to Address Rupture and Repair in Groups

Marmarosh (2021) reminds us that not addressing members' dissatisfactions and disappointments can have a deleterious effect on group therapy. However, when leaders are made aware of deterioration in the group relationships, we know that leaders can process them and enable repairs (Burlingame et al., 2018). Group therapists are directed to pay keen attention to conflict and disruptions in the group (Yalom & Leszcz, 2020), and recent literature identifies relational *rupture and repair* as processes that need more research and intentional training for leader understanding. It is our ethical responsibility to avoid rupture harms and provide repair and healing when they occur.

Rutan (2021) describes ruptures related to insensitivity to cultural diversity, equity, and inclusion; forgetting information about members; poor timing of interventions; countertransference; and insufficient boundary maintenance. Rutan examines how leader privilege or lack of awareness of microaggressions may lead to ruptures and reduced cohesion and outcome. We know that group members show up with different intersecting identities (Ribeiro, 2020). These identities impact how likely one will be involved in a rupture and how one may respond to a rupture.

To that end, Lefforge et al. (2020) created a training model and video programs to help leaders address microaggressions in group treatment. They portray the anxiety group members and leaders have when exploring these ruptures, using role plays and providing helpful guidance for leaders during pauses to consider responses. They recommend intentionally approaching ruptures and avoiding shaming the members who commit ruptures. Similarly, Gantt (2021) describes how systemic-level conflicts have the potential to lead to greater cohesion and personal change when using *functional subgrouping* to repair such ruptures. She provides examples of how System-Centered Theory directs group leaders to intervene by shifting member roles around weakness and power as they are repeated in the present group, encouraging a reparative action. More research would be useful to understand how these member factors and leader responses influence ruptures and the activity of repair.

A multitude of web-based systems have emerged to support MBC monitoring systems, which are now widely adopted in clinical practice (Wampold, 2015). The Group Questionnaire (GQ; Burlingame et al., 2017) was developed to assess relationship structures in group therapy and identify how and where ruptures tend to originate. It can be used as an outcome measure to monitor treatment progress in MBC systems or as a sole measure to assess the ruptures in the therapeutic relationship. The GQ is an evidence-based combination of the three structural relationships in group (member-to-therapist, member-to-group, and member-to-member) and four relational constructs (alliance, cohesion, empathy, and climate), gauging the overall relationship quality of the group. As a tool to potentially address ruptures, it measures (a) *what* is involved in the rupture—is the issue around the *tasks* or *goals* of therapy (positive work) or the relationship *bond* (positive bond and negative relationship); (b) *who* is involved (member-member, member-group, and member-leader); and (c) *when* ruptures originate in a group (Burlingame et al., 2021). Burlingame and colleagues (2021) explain that the GQ has two dimensions: The first assesses the quality of the therapeutic relationship with three subscales (positive bond, positive work, and negative relationships), and the second measures the three-relationship structures in group (member-member, member-group, and member-leader). The GQ uses two types of alerts, change alerts and status alerts. The recommendation is for group members to complete the GQ after each group session. Scores are only computed for the three GQ quality subscales, with two assessing *bonds* and a third assessing *tasks* and *goals*. The GQ *positive bond* subscale includes member-member (cohesion), member-group (climate), and member-leader (alliance) items. The goal of crossing positive bonds with relationship structures is to offer the group leader greater detail about what is contributing to the positive bond subscale score (see Burlingame et al. for more details).

Another MBC group measure that assesses *member relationships* is the Group Sessions Rating Scale (GSRS; Quirk et al., 2013). This visual analog measure has four items and assesses the cohesion a member experiences in the group. It was also developed to supplement an outcome measure, the Outcome Rating Scale (ORS; Miller et al., 2003; Miller et al., 2015). Results are interpreted immediately after the end of the group session relative to past scores on the analog. It is described as a quick and affordable way to assess cohesion and can provide both trainees and experienced leaders immediate feedback about sessions.

Scope of Responsibility for Therapist Competence

As the following example underscores, therapists' responsibility for competence extends beyond their own functioning:

> Darren and Ruby had been running a process group for several years and enjoyed an excellent working relationship. Several months prior, Darren had confided in Ruby that his marriage was deteriorating. Ruby had noticed that during the last several sessions, Darren was less active in the group, appeared tired, and yawned frequently. In fact, one member had commented that Darren appeared to be exhausted. On recent occasions, she detected a smell of alcohol on his breath during the post-group processing. She decided to schedule a meeting with him during which she confronted him with her observation. He responded with anger, agreeing that he had been experiencing and possibly expressing fatigue but denying any consumption of alcohol before the group sessions. He speculated that Ruby might have been smelling the alcohol in his mouthwash. Ruby, feeling unsatisfied with his explanation, told Darren that she wanted to think about what he was saying. In fact, Ruby wanted to obtain a consultation from a former supervisor about her concern about Darren. However, the following day, Darren called her and acknowledged that he had indeed been medicating himself with alcohol. He planned to take a sabbatical from the group and obtain help for both his marital difficulties and recent dependence on alcohol.

According to Guideline 3 of the AGPA and the IBCGP Guidelines for Ethics (American Group Psychotherapy Association, 2002), "The group psychotherapist acts to safeguard the patient/client and the public from the incompetent, unethical, and illegal practice of any group psychotherapist." Ruby was acting in compliance with this guideline in confronting Darren's behavior in the group, likely compromised by alcohol and the press of his marital difficulties. From a virtue ethics standpoint, she was exhibiting courage in entering into a difficult conversation. Ruby's responsibility to monitor this problem would continue as Darren re-entered the group following his sabbatical.

Final Note

Achieving and maintaining competence is an ethical requirement for group psychotherapists. Among the knowledge bases and skills, the therapist must master is the ability to work through ethical problems. Two common tasks performed by the group leader have particular ethical significance. The first is the management of boundaries. Boundary violations are never acceptable. However, because any given boundary crossing might be useful or not, the therapist's discernment is required. Areas in which group psychotherapists are commonly called upon to exercise good judgment about boundaries are those of therapist self-disclosure, gift-giving, and extra-group contact between therapist and members. The second area is the management of differences among members, particularly in relation to members' identity statuses. Ethical group therapists recognize the potential for members to respond to differences with bias and prejudice in a fashion mirroring society at large. Therapist multicultural competence and cultural humility contribute to a group environment that supports social justice outcomes in which biases are challenged and group members can develop into better members of society. In addition to fostering constructive processes, ethical group therapists safeguard members from toxic processes such as coercion and scapegoating that can occur in any group. The competent group therapist realizes that ruptures with the therapist and between and among members are a natural part of group life and takes care to repair them. In addition to taking responsibility for their own conduct, such therapists promote the competence of other group psychotherapists to serve the welfare of the group members and the public.

CEU Questions

1. Therapists can improve their ethical decision-making by enlisting the opinions of the members about the issues at hand. (T/F)
2. It is unethical for either leaders or members to use intense pressure to keep members in the group who may be considering leaving, even if they are at risk for deteriorating. (T/F)
3. The initial approach when dealing with a colleague who seems to be practicing in a manner that you deem unethical should be to report them to their supervisor or administrator. (T/F)
4. Helping members to become better members of society honors *General Beneficence*. (T/F)
5. Identify three potential benefits of therapist self-disclosure (essay).
6. All boundary crossings are unethical. (T/F)
7. The GQ looks at three types of relationships: member-member; member-leader; member-group. (T/F)
8. Why is it important to detect rupture through measurement activities?

Answer Key: 1. T; 2. T; 3. F; 4. T; 5. For example: strengthens the real relationship, conveys that client reactions are a natural part of the human experience; models self-disclosure for the group; 6. F; 7. T 8. To create the possibility for repair.

Discussion Questions

1. In what ways do you see communication norms in groups being influenced by Western or White values that might discourage storytelling or providing cultural context?
2. What benefits may be gained from exploring cultural and social issues that impact our members and our group practice?
3. You realize that you have been calling one female Black member by another female Black member's name during a particular session. You notice that both members look dejected and you suspect a rupture has occurred between you and them. How do you establish that a rupture occurred and if so, how do you repair it?

4. What ethical issues have you seen surface in relation to scapegoating, coercion, and subgrouping?
5. What might be some initial ethical approaches to dealing with culture and subculture populations different from your own about which you have limited knowledge and experience?
6. How may group leaders with less awareness around power dynamics lead to possible boundary violations?
7. What might be some internal reactions that would hinder a therapist from addressing the competence problems of a colleague.

Vignettes/Role-Plays

1. Monique called the therapist and indicated that unbeknownst to her, she had an unrecognized relationship with Aisha. Monique was a speech and language therapist and she realized she was treating a child who was also being treated by another member who was a physical therapist. Their contact had been via the telephone. She expressed to the therapist that she was well aware that members were not permitted to socialize outside of the sessions. Yet, she knew that this extra-group contact was non-intentional. She was convinced that Aisha did not realize that it was she with whom that member was interacting. The member wondered how she should proceed. What considerations should guide how the therapist addresses this issue with the member?
2. Kenny is a new group member who identifies as a gay African American male. He informs the leaders during the pre-group meeting that he wants to come out to the group fairly quickly so that he can feel authentic. The two group leaders are experienced in addressing issues of identity, but two group members react with distance and discomfort. One of those members, Aaron, asks how the group members can help each other if they are so different. How might the group leaders respond?
3. A therapist hears one of his group members recommend a particular stock to another group member before a session begins. The therapist knows that the member making the recommendation is extremely financially successful. Would the therapist violate any ethical principle by acting on the member's recommendation? What are the considerations in allowing versus disallowing one member to give another stock advice, given that it is occurring outside of the bounds of the session? Would it make a difference if the advice was given within a session?

References

Agazarian, Y., & Peters, R. (1981). *The visible and invisible group: Two perspectives on group psychotherapy and group process*. London: Routledge & Kegan Paul Ltd.

American Counseling Association. (2014). *2014 ACA code of ethics*. https://www.counseling.org/Resources/aca-code-of-ethics.pdf

American Group Psychotherapy Association. (2002). *AGPA and IBCGP guidelines for ethics*. http://ethics.iit.edu/codes/AGPA%202002.pdf

Barkowski, S., Schwartze, D., Strauss, B., Burlingame, G. M., & Rosendahl, J. (2020). Efficacy of group psychotherapy for anxiety disorders: A systematic review and meta-analysis. *Psychotherapy Research*, *30*(8), 965–982. 10.1080/10503307.2020.1729440

Barlow, S. H. (2012). An application of the competency model to the group-specialty practice. *Professional Psychology: Research and Practice*, *43*(5), 442–451. 10.1037/a0029090

Barnett, J. E. (2015). A practical ethics approach to boundaries and multiple relationships in psychotherapy. *British Psychological Society Psychotherapy Section Review*, *56*(1), 27–37. https://www.researchgate.net/profile/Justin_Karter/publication/304495518_Big_Pharmakos_The_ stigmatised_scapegoat_of_medicalisation_and_the_ethics_of_psychiatric_diagnosis/links/5aad87-fa458515ecebe7d2a6/Big-Pharmakos-The-stigmatised-scapegoat-of-medicalisation-and-the-ethics-of-psychiatric-diagnosis.pdf#page=29

Bemak, F., & Chung, R. C. Y. (2019). Race dialogues in group psychotherapy: Key issues in training and practice. *International Journal of Group Psychotherapy*, *69*(2), 172–191. 10.1080/00207284.2018.1498743

Brabender, V. (2020). Group psychotherapies. In S. B. Messer and N. J. Kaslow (Eds.), *Essential psychotherapies: Theory and practice* (4th ed., pp. 369–406). Guilford. https://www.guilford.com/books/Essential-Psychotherapies/Messer-Kaslow/9781462540846

Brabender, V. M., Smolar, A. I., & Fallon, A. E. (2004). *Essentials of group therapy*. Wiley. https://www.wiley.com/en-us/Essentials+of+Group+Therapy-p-9780471244394

Burlingame, G. M., Alldredge, C. T., & Arnold, R. A. (2021). Alliance rupture detection and repair in group therapy: Using the Group Questionnaire–GQ. *International Journal of Group Psychotherapy*, *71* (2),1–33. 10.1080/00207284.2020.1844010

Burlingame, G., Gleave, R., Beecher, M., Griner, D., Hansen, K., Jensen, J., Worthen, V., & Svien, H. (2017). *Administration and scoring manual for the group questionnaire*. OQ Measures, LLC.

Burlingame, G. M., McClendon, D. T., & Yang, C. (2018). Cohesion in group therapy: A meta-analysis. *Psychotherapy*, *55*(4), 384–398. 10.1037/pst0000173

Burlingame, G. M., Svien, H., Hoppe, L., Hunt, I., & Rosendahl, J. (2020). Group therapy for schizophrenia: A meta-analysis. *Psychotherapy*, *57*(2), 219–236. 10.1037/pst0000293

Carter, E. F., Mitchell, S. L., & Krautheim, M. D. (2001). Understanding and addressing clients' resistance to group counseling. *The Journal for Specialists in Group Work*, *26*(1), 66–80. 10.1080/01933920108413778

Chang-Caffaro, Sp., & Caffaro, J. (2018). Differences that make a difference: Diversity and the process group leader. *International Journal of Group Psychotherapy*, *68*(4), 483–497. 10.1080/00207284.2018.1469958

Chen, E. C. (2013). Multicultural competence and social justice advocacy in group psychology and group psychotherapy. *APA Division 49 Newsletter: The Group Psychologist (April 2013)*. https://www.apadivisions.org/division-49/publications/newsletter/group-psychologist/2012/07/social-justice

Chen, E. C., Boyd, D. M., & Cunningham, C. A. (2020). Demarginalizing stigmatized identities of transgender and gender nonconforming individuals through affirmative group therapy. *International Journal of Group Psychotherapy*, *70*(4), 552–579. 10.1080/00207284.2020.1755291

Chen, E. C., Kakkad, D., & Balzano, J. (2008). Multicultural competence and evidence-based practice in group therapy. *Journal of Clinical Psychology*, *64*(11), 1261–1278. 10.1002/jclp.20533

Chung, R. C. Y., & Bemak, F. (2002). The relationship of culture and empathy in cross-cultural counseling. *Journal of Counseling & Development*, *80*(2), 154–159. 10.1002/j.1556-6678.2002.tb00178.x

Clark, A. J. (2002). Scapegoating: Dynamics and interventions in group counseling. *Journal of Counseling & Development*, *80*(3), 271–276. 10.1002/j.1556-6678.2002.tb00191.x

Comas-Diaz, L. (2012). *Multicultural care: A clinician's guide to cultural competence*. American Psychological Association. https://www.apa.org/pubs/books/4317279

Cone-Uemura, K., & Bentley, E. S. (2018). Multicultural/diversity issues in groups. In M. D. Ribeiro, J. M. Gross, & M. M. Turner (Eds.), *The college counselor's guide to group psychotherapy* (pp. 21–33). Routledge. https://www.taylorfrancis.com/chapters/multicultural-diversity-issues-groups-karen-cone-uemura-eri-suzuki-bentley/e/10.4324/9781315545455-3?context=ubx&refId=3b73ea41-ea9f-4ad8-b71f-1e9dc290de0a

Cross, W. E., Grant, B. O., & Ventuneac, A. (2012). Black identity and well-being: Untangling race and ethnicity. In J. M. Sullivan and A. M. Esmail (Eds.). *African American identity: Racial and cultural dimensions of the black experience* (pp. 125–146). Lexington Books.

D'Andrea, M. (2014). Understanding racial/cultural identity development theories to promote effective multicultural group counseling. In J. L. DeLucia-Waack, C. R. Kalodner, & M. T. Riva (Eds.), *Handbook of group counseling and psychotherapy* (2nd ed., pp. 196–208). Sage Publications. 10.4135/9781544308555

Davies, G., Whelan, S., Foley, A., & Walsh, M. (2010). Gifts and gifting. *International Journal of Management Reviews*, *12*(4), 413–434. 10.1111/j.1468-2370.2009.00271.x

Dies, R. R. (1973). Group therapist self-disclosure: An evaluation by clients. *Journal of Counseling Psychology, 20*(4), 344–348. 10.1037/h0034808

Edwards, C. E., & Murdock, N. L. (1994). Characteristics of therapist self-disclosure in the counseling process. *Journal of Counseling & Development, 72*(4), 384–389. 10.1002/j.1556-6676.1994.tb00954.x

Fallon, A. E., & Brabender, V. (2018). *The impact of parenthood on the therapeutic relationship: Awaiting the therapist's baby* (2nd ed.). Routledge. https://www.routledge.com/The-Impact-of-Parenthood-on-the-Therapeutic-Relationship-Awaiting-the-Therapists/Fallon-Brabender/p/book/9781138119611

Fenster, A. (1996). Group therapy as an effective treatment modality for people of color. *International Journal of Group Psychotherapy, 46*(3), 399–416. 10.1080/00207284.1996.11490787

Fleming, L. M., Glass, J. A., Fujisaki, S., & Toner, S. L. (2010). Group process and learning: A grounded theory model of group supervision. *Training and Education in Professional Psychology, 4*(3), 194–203. 10.1037/a0018970

Fors, M. (2018). Afterword: The unthought known. In M. Fors, *A grammar of power in psychotherapy: Exploring the dynamics of privilege* (pp. 157–159). American Psychological Association. 10.1037/0000086-008

Gantt, S. P. (2021). Systems-centered theory (SCT) into group therapy: Beyond surviving ruptures to repairing and thriving. *International Journal of Group Psychotherapy, 71*, 224–252. 10.1080/00207284.2020.1772073

Gelso, C. (2014). A tripartite model of the therapeutic relationship: Theory, research, and practice. *Psychotherapy Research, 24*(2), 117– 131. 10.1080/10503307.2013.845920

Greene, L. R., & Kaklauskas, F. J. (2020). Anti-therapeutic, defensive, regressive, and challenging group processes and dynamics. In F. J. Kaklauskas & L. R. Greene (Eds.). *Core principles of group psychotherapy: An integrated theory, research, and practice training manual* (pp. 71–85). Taylor and Francis.

Grenon, R., Schwartze, D., Hammond, N., Ivanova, I., Mcquaid, N., Proulx, G., & Tasca, G. A. (2017). Group psychotherapy for eating disorders: A meta-analysis. *International Journal of Eating Disorders, 50*(9), 997–1013. 10.1002/eat.22744

Gross, J. M. (2010). The nine basic steps for a successful group. In S. S. Fehr (Ed.), *101 interventions in group therapy* (Revised ed., pp. 421–423). Routledge. http://docshare01.docshare.tips/files/26655/266559357.pdf

Gutheil, T. G., & Gabbard, G. O. (1998). Misuses and misunderstandings of boundary theory in clinical and regulatory settings. *American Journal of Psychiatry, 155*(3), 409–414. 10.1176/ajp.155.3.409

Guthrie, C. (2006). Disclosing the therapist's sexual orientation: The meaning of disclosure in working with gay, lesbian, and bisexual patients. *Journal of Gay & Lesbian Psychotherapy, 10*(1), 63–77. 10.1300/J236v10n01_07

Haen, C., & Thomas, N. K. (2018). Holding history: Undoing racial unconsciousness in groups. *International Journal of Group Psychotherapy, 68*(4), 498–520. 10.1080/00207284.2018.1475238

Hanson, J. (2005). Should your lips be zipped? How therapist self-disclosure and non-disclosure affects clients. *Counselling and Psychotherapy Research, 5*(2), 96–104. 10.1080/17441690500226658

Hays, P. A. (2008). *Addressing cultural complexities in practice: Assessment, diagnosis, and therapy* (2nd ed.). American Psychological Association. 10.1037/11650-000

Helms, J. E. (2008). *A race is a nice thing to have: A guide to being a White person or understanding the White persons in your life* (2nd ed.). Hanover, MA: Microtraining Associates.

Henretty, J. R., & Levitt, H. M. (2010). The role of therapist self-disclosure in psychotherapy: A qualitative review. *Clinical Psychology Review, 30*(1), 63–77.

Hook, J. N., Davis, D., Owen, J., & DeBlaere, C. (2017). *Cultural humility: Engaging diverse identities in therapy.* American Psychological Association. 10.1037/0000037-000

Horowitz, L. M., Alden, L. E., Wiggins, J. S., & Pincus, A. L. (2000). *Inventory of interpersonal problems (IIP).* Mind Garden, Inc. https://marketplace.unl.edu/buros/inventory-of-interpersonal-problems.html

Horowitz, L. M., Rosenberg, S. E., Baer, B. A., Ureño, G., & Villaseñor, V. S. (1988). Inventory of interpersonal problems: Psychometric properties and clinical applications. *Journal of Consulting and Clinical Psychology*, *56*(6), 885–892. 10.1037/0022-006X.56.6.885

Horowitz, L. M., & Strack, S. (Eds.). (2010). *Handbook of interpersonal psychology: Theory, research, assessment, and therapeutic interventions.* Wiley. https://www.wiley.com/en-us/Handbook+of +Interpersonal+Psychology:+Theory,+Research,+Assessment,+and+Therapeutic+Interventions-p-9780470471609

Horvath, A. O., Del Re, A. C., Flückiger, C., & Symonds, D. (2011). Alliance in individual psychotherapy. *Psychotherapy*, *48*(1), 9–16. 10.1037/a0022186

Kaklauskas, F. J., & Greene, L. R. (2020). Finding the leader in you. In F. J. Kaklauskas & L. R. Greene (Eds.). *Core principles of group psychotherapy: An integrated theory, research, and practice training manual.* Routledge. https://www.routledge.com/Core-Principles-of-Group-Psychotherapy-An-Integrated-Theory-Research/Kaklauskas-Greene/p/book/9780367203092

Kaklauskas, F. J., & Nettles, R. (2019). Towards multicultural and diversity proficiency as a group psychotherapist. In F. J. Kaklauskas, & L. R. Greene (Eds.), *Core principles of group psychotherapy: A training manual for theory, research, and practice* (pp. 25–46). Routledge.

Kaslow, N. J. (2004). Competencies in professional psychology. *American psychologist*, *59*(8), 774–781. 10.1037/0003-066X.59.8.774

Knapp, S., Younggen, J. N., VandeCreek, L., Harris, E., & Martin, J. N. (2013). *Assessing and managing risk in psychological practice: An individualized approach* (2nd ed.). The Trust.

Knox, S. (2008). Gifts in psychotherapy: Practice review and recommendations. *Psychotherapy: Theory, Research, Practice, Training*, *45*(1), 103–110. 10.1037/0033-3204.45.1.103

Knox, S., & Hill, C. E. (2003). Therapist self-disclosure: Research-based suggestions for practitioners. *Journal of Clinical Psychology*, *59*(5), 529–539. 10.1002/jclp.10157

Lane, R. C., & Hull, J.W. (1990). Self-disclosure and classical psychoanalysis. In G. Stricker & M. Fisher (Eds.), *Self-disclosure in the therapeutic relationship*. Springer. 10.1007/978-1-4899-3582-3_3

Lefforge, N. L., Mclaughlin, S., Goates-Jones, M., & Mejia, C. (2020). A training model for addressing microaggressions in group psychotherapy. *International Journal of Group Psychotherapy*, *70*(1), 1–28. 10.1080/00207284.2019.1680989

Lewis, M. E., Hartwell, E. E., & Myhra, L. L. (2018). Decolonizing mental health services for indigenous clients: A training program for mental health professionals. *American Journal of Community Psychology*, *62*(3-4), 330–339. 10.1002/ajcp.12288

MacNair-Semands, R. R. (2007). Attending to the spirit of social justice as an ethical approach in group therapy. *International Journal of Group Psychotherapy*, *57*(1), 61–66. doi:10.1521/ijgp.2007.57.1.61

Mahalik, J.R., Van Ormer, E.A., & Simi, N.L. (2000). Ethical issues in using self-disclosure in feminist therapy. In M. M. Brabeck (Ed.), *Practicing feminist ethics in psychology* (pp. 189–201). American Psychological Association. 10.1037/10343-009

Marcus, H. E., & King, D. A. (2003). A survey of group psychotherapy training during predoctoral psychology internship. *Professional Psychology: Research and Practice*, *34*(2), 203–209. 10.1037/0735-7028.34.2.203

Marmarosh, C. L. (2021). Ruptures and repairs in group psychotherapy: From theory to practice. *International Journal of Group Psychotherapy*, *71*(2), 205–223. 10.1080/00207284.2020.1855893

Mbroh, H., Najjab, A., Knapp, S., & Gottlieb, M. C. (2020). Prejudiced patients: Ethical considerations for addressing patients' prejudicial comments in psychotherapy. *Professional Psychology: Research and Practice*, *51*(3), 284–290. 10.1037/pro0000280

Miller, S. D., Duncan, B. L., Brown, J., Sparks, J. A., & Claud, D. A. (2003). The outcome rating scale: A preliminary study of the reliability, validity, and feasibility of a brief visual analog measure. *Journal of Brief Therapy*, *2*(2), 91–100.

Miller, S. D., Hubble, M. A., Chow, D., & Seidel, J. (2015). Beyond measures and monitoring: Realizing the potential of feedback-informed treatment. *Psychotherapy*, *52*, 449–457. 10.1037/pst0000031

Moreno, J. K. (2007). Scapegoating in group psychotherapy. *International Journal of Group Psychotherapy*, *57*(1), 93–104. 10.1521/ijgp.2007.57.1.93

Ohrt, J. H., Ener, E., Porter, J., & Young, T. L. (2014). Group leader reflections on their training and experience: Implications for group counselor educators and supervisors. *The Journal for Specialists in Group Work, 39*(2), 95–124.

Owen, J., Jordan, T. A., Turner, D., Davis, D. E., Hook, J. N., & Leach, M. M. (2014). Therapists' multicultural orientation: Client perceptions of cultural humility, spiritual/religious commitment, and therapy outcomes. *Journal of Psychology and Theology, 42*(1), 91–98. 10.1177/009164711404200110

Owen, J., Tao, K. W., Drinane, J. M., Hook, J., Davis, D. E., & Kune, N. F. (2016). Client perceptions of therapists' multicultural orientation: Cultural (missed) opportunities and cultural humility. *Professional Psychology: Research and Practice, 47*(1), 30–37. 10.1037/pro0000046

Platt, L. F. (2020). The presenting concerns of transgender and gender noncomforming clients at university counseling centers. *The Counseling Psychologist, 48*(3), 407–431. 10.1177/001100001 9898680

Quirk, K., Miller, S., Duncan, B., & Owen, J. (2013). Group Session Rating Scale: Preliminary psychometrics in substance abuse group interventions. *Counselling and Psychotherapy Research, 13*(3), 194–200. 10.1080/14733145.2012.744425

Rapin, L. S. (2010). Ethics, best practices, and law in group counseling. In R. K. Conyne (Ed.), *The Oxford Handbook of Group Counseling* (pp. 61–82). Oxford.

Ribeiro, M. D. (Ed.). (2020). *Examining social identities and diversity issues in group therapy: Knocking at the boundaries.* Routledge. 10.4324/9780429022364

Rutan, J. S. (2021). Rupture and repair: Using leader errors in psychodynamic group psychotherapy. *International Journal of Group Psychotherapy, 71*, 310–331. 10.1080/00207284.2020.1808471

Rutan, J. S., Stone, W. N., & Shay, J. J. (2014). *Psychodynamic group psychotherapy* (5th ed.). Guilford Press. https://www.guilford.com/books/Psychodynamic-Group-Psychotherapy/Rutan-Stone-Shay/9781462516506

Sensoy, Ö., & DiAngelo, R. (2017). *Is everyone really equal? An introduction to key concepts in social justice education* (2nd ed.). Teachers College Press. https://www.tcpress.com/is-everyone-really-equal-9780807758618

Shapiro, E. L., & Ginzberg, R. (2002). Parting gifts: Termination rituals in group therapy. *International Journal of Group Psychotherapy, 52*(3), 319–336. 10.1521/ijgp.52.3.319.45507

Shechtman, Z. (2002). Child group psychotherapy in the school at the threshold of a new millennium. *Journal of Counseling & Development, 80*(3), 293–299. 10.1002/j.1556-6678.2002.tb00194.x

Shechtman, Z., & Kiezel, A. (2016). Why do people prefer individual therapy over group therapy? *International Journal of Group Psychotherapy, 66*(4), 571–591. 10.1080/00207284.2016.1180042

Smolar, A. I., & Eichen, A. E. (2013). A developmental approach to gifts in long-term group psychotherapy extending from an anniversary ritual. *International Journal of Group Psychotherapy, 63*(1), 77–94. 10.1521/ijgp.2013.63.1.77

Spandler, H., Burman, E., Goldberg, B., Margison, F., & Amos, T. (2000). A double-edged sword: Understanding gifts in psychotherapy. *European Journal of Psychotherapy, Counselling and Health, 3*(1), 77–101. 10.1080/13642530050078574

Sue, D. W. (2010). Microaggressions, marginality, and oppression: An introduction. In D. W. Sue (Ed.), *Microaggressions and marginality: Manifestation, dynamics, and impact* (pp. 1–22). Wiley.

Sue, D. W., Capodilupo, C. M., Torino, G. C., Bucceri, J. M., Holder, A. M. B., Nadal, K. L., & Esquilin, M. (2007). Racial microaggressions in everyday life: Implications for clinical practice. *American Psychologist, 62*(4), 271–286. 10.1037/0003-066X.62.4.271

Taloyo, C. A. & Neal, D. W. (2020). Teaching group within a social constructionist framework. In M. D. Ribeiro (Ed.). *Examining social identities and diversity issues in group therapy: Knocking at the boundaries* (pp. 161–172). Routledge. 10.4324/9780429022364

Tervalon, M., & Murray-Garcia, J. (1998). Cultural humility versus cultural competence: A critical distinction in defining physician training outcomes in multicultural education. *Journal of Health Care for the Poor and Underserved, 9*(2), 117–125. 10.1353/hpu.2010.0233

Vásquez, D., Ponte, L., Andrews III, A. R., Garcia, E., Terrazas-Carrillo, E., Ojeda, L., & de Arellano, M. A. (2020). Más allá de las barreras: Competency and practice considerations in language, cultural, and social issues when delivering group CPT to Hispanic immigrants. *International Journal of Group Psychotherapy, 70*(2), 212–243. 10.1080/00207284.2019.1677469

Wampold, B. E. (2015). Routine outcome monitoring: coming of age–With the usual developmental challenges. *Psychotherapy, 52*(4), 458–462. 10.1037/pst0000037

Yalom, I., & Leszcz, M. (2020). *The theory and practice of group psychotherapy* (6th ed.). Basic Books. https://www.basicbooks.com/titles/irvin-d-yalom/the-theory-and-practice-of-group-psychotherapy/9781541617575/

Zur, O. (2004). To cross or not to cross: Do boundaries in therapy protect or harm. *Psychotherapy Bulletin, 39*(3), 27–32. https://www.zurinstitute.com/media/to_cross_or_not_to_cross.pdf

4 Selection, Preparation, and Norm Development among Members

An ethical approach to shaping the group norms from the very first client encounter is central to the success of the group. Because members impact each other significantly, it is important to be thorough about issues such as client selection, pre-group preparation, and responding if a member is not appropriate once placed in a group. The methods and tools that we use to gather information from potential group members should also reflect current knowledge and research so leaders may make informed and ethical decisions.

Pre-group meetings allow leaders to better understand the potential member and learn more about how they might react to the work of the particular group. The labels *Pre-group Meeting* (PGM), *Group Screening*, or *Group Screen* have been widely used, but *Pre-group Meeting* has become more common recently in some agencies. The connotation of being "screened out" may lead group candidates to nervously anticipate an interview-type process, potentially contributing to more anxiety. To avoid this implication, clinicians often explain that the meeting's purpose is for the leader to learn more about the potential member and to help the client learn more about how the leaders and group function, emphasizing that both parties can contribute to decisions about fit and appropriateness of the treatment. The PGM not only promotes the initial formation of the therapeutic alliance between the group leaders and prospective group members but also provides an opportunity for the leader to set the foundation for later bonding with the group and its members. For example, a member could be given ideas about ways that one could approach rather than avoid feelings of intimidation in relation to individual members and the group as a whole. These sessions can also explore the candidate's interpersonal problems and how the group might specifically be helpful.

One way to address the question of who will benefit from group psychotherapy and who should likely be excluded from participation is to consider the concept of *appropriate fit*. To build a well-functioning therapy group, the leader makes both clinical and administrative decisions that need careful and thoughtful attention (Turner, 2018). One of the purposes of the PGM is that it helps determine if an individual is compatible with the developmental goals and tasks for the particular group. The prevailing wisdom is that too much incompatibility between the prospective member and the group can be disruptive, such as adding a grandiose attention-seeking member to a newly forming group, or a withdrawn and dismissive patient to a higher functioning group (Kealy et al., 2016; Rutan et al., 2019). Practical and logistical factors should also be considered during the meeting, particularly variables that may affect attendance such as work schedules, finances, and transportation issues (Gans & Counselman, 2010; Yalom & Leszcz, 2005, 2020).

The ethical principle of Autonomy, and a heightened awareness of avoiding coercion with less assertive or hesitant clients, are important considerations for leaders during the selection process. We also know that when member preferences are not heard and the members cannot fully explore their fears or reservations, they may be less likely to attend the first meeting (Carter et al., 2001). For example, Allison may be worried that she will

DOI: 10.4324/9781003105527-4

stay quiet in a group and thus, she may initially state a preference for individual therapy. Once Allison learns more about how leaders encourage quiet members to jump in—and how practicing such a skill with peers can be life-changing outside of the group in building her social skills—she may be more open to the idea of attending a group treatment. Similarly, when leaders are in the position of needing one more member to fill a group vacancy or be able to start a new group in a timely fashion, they should be aware of the need to define the best treatment for a client and balance that with the need to fill a group. Giving priority to the client's needs rather than clinician's needs is also consistent with the principle of Fidelity.

While most of the PGM literature has focused on clinical dimensions (e.g., whether a narcissistic patient would fit into a mature group), an important recent development is to consider how sociocultural variables could affect selection and composition. The literature on PGMs has been sorely lacking in exploring power differentials and our larger societal systems of oppression that can influence these meetings. An understanding of identities that provide some members with privilege related to race, nationality, language, gender, sexual orientation, socioeconomics, ability, and religion—compared to those identities treated with marginality in society (including intersections across identities)—must be developed and considered in our pre-group processes. Many authors are now expressing the need for more information around how cultural insensitivity in such clinical encounters might be experienced or predicted by members, particularly by those who have experienced racism or discrimination (Kaklauskas & Nettles, 2019; Ribeiro et al., 2018; Yalom & Leszcz, 2020).

The overriding question to be explored is how differences in sociocultural dimensions between a prospective new client and the current group members will be handled—whether the differences (in race, religion, etc.) can be tolerated and explored and contained, or not. The leaders must be conscious of the larger cultural systems at play, particularly when candidates' beliefs, values, and identities may conflict with other members in the group. Conflicts may surface when members with multiple identities come together in one group and the ultimate work for the leader is to judge whether the differences and likely conflicts can be sufficiently contained in the group or not. Some formal pre-group measures such as the Group Therapy Questionnaire-Short Version can be very useful in these PGM sessions to facilitate explorations with potential candidates about aspects of their identities that they would like to share with the group, or those identities that might be challenging to discuss or explore (GTQ-S; MacNair-Semands, 2002; Whittingham, 2015, 2018). Specific examples of diverse identities are provided to prompt the candidate and feelings related to the important aspects of the self are explored. Once a decision is made about inclusion, detailed information on microaggressions (Sue, 2010) and acceptance can be shared by the leaders. Orienting and preparing members for the specific group during the PGM is then approached with attention to these dynamics and other group norms (see later section in this chapter).

Selecting Members Who Can Benefit From Group Participation

This section on selection will focus on the prototypical, unstructured therapy groups with attention to interpersonal learning, insight, and personal change. Similar to other authors (Kealy et al., 2016; Rutan et al., 2014; Yalom & Leszcz, 2020), this section also emphasizes groups that involve relatively heterogeneous membership, an emphasis on exploration rather than education, and an application of addressing characterological and interpersonal difficulties. Selection criteria and procedures for highly structured psychoeducational groups would be quite different from those seeking membership in psychotherapy groups (Brown, 2018).

Process-oriented psychotherapy groups are typically more likely to be composed *heterogeneously* in terms of personality style, psychopathology, and, as we shall discuss, sociocultural variables. Not uncommonly, however, groups that are composed *homogeneously* in terms of gender, culture, ethnicity, sexual identity, or presenting problems may also address similarly broad therapeutic objectives (Bernard et al., 2008). Findings suggest that group interventions that aspire to influence identity development processes, including cognitive- and emotion-focused interventions, have been found to improve self-constructive and self-discovery processes (Giannone et al., 2020). Hence, selection criteria and procedures for therapy groups focused on identity development are included in this section as well. We also discuss how selection and composition intersect with attention to differing identities.

Inclusion Criteria

We start this section with an emphasis on clinical variables and move into the important issues tied to ethics around social justice and sociocultural variables. It is much easier to specify exclusion criteria than inclusion criteria because one problematic characteristic may exclude a person, but numerous complex factors must be present to support inclusion (Yalom & Leszcz, 2020). The most general rule of thumb is that the greater the divergence in level of psychopathology between the potential candidate and the current group members, the more likely negative outcomes for the candidate, and possibly others in the group. Thus, when significant pathology is present, predictions of poor outcomes are more likely to be consistent and certain among leaders. However, Yalom and Leszcz add the caveat that human interaction behaviors are so complex and subtle that such predictions should always be considered tentative.

Considerations and hypothesizing about how the candidate will bond with the leader and potential co-members are important determinants of suitability for group therapy (Bernard et al., 2008) and whether the group will likely be helpful or harmful. Highly reactive clients, for example, could be helped to understand that engaging first in individual therapy or a structured psychoeducational group can assist in learning coping skills that will benefit the client for an intensive therapy group experience. Supervision and consultation can be extremely helpful in weighing the internal and external factors that inform the choices we make at this formative stage (Rutan et al., 2019).

Early on, it was believed that members who do well in group psychotherapy include those with positive expectations, motivations, and other insight-oriented factors. Based on astute clinical observation and empirical study, authors now discuss a more specific ideal prototype member as one with a capacity and willingness to examine one's interpersonal behaviors, to self-disclose, to reflect psychologically on self and others, to give and receive feedback, and to be capable of engaging with other group members (Yalom & Leszcz, 2020). Similarly, Ogrodniczuk et al. (2003) found that extraversion, conscientiousness, and openness were all associated with positive outcomes.

Other authors focus on insight and self-understanding, including the client's (1) understanding of connections between past and present experiences, (2) relationship patterns, and (3) the connections between interpersonal challenges, emotions, and symptoms (Crits-Christoph et al., 2013). This may help explain why having previous therapy of any kind has been found to be a protective factor related to group dropout (Bernard et al., 2008; MacNair & Corazzini, 1994; MacNair-Semands, 2002; Yalom & Leszcz, 2020).

A capacity for interpersonal relationships is certainly required to work in the interpersonal milieu, a finding demonstrated in early psychotherapy trials (Joyce et al., 2000) and replicated over the years (see Bernard et al., 2008). Studies using validated selection instruments have expanded the notion that member expectations and a level of interpersonal skills are essential for successful group work (Burlingame et al., 2011; Söchting et al., 2018). Yalom and Leszcz (2020) point out that conflicts in the domain of intimacy could be considered both an inclusion and exclusion criteria; group therapy can be beneficial for the member but if such intimacy conflicts are extreme, the member may drop out or be extruded by other members.

Early research by Kivlighan and Angelone (1992) used the interpersonal circumplex model and original measure, Inventory of Interpersonal Problems (IIP; Horowitz et al., 1988), and found that group members who perceived themselves as overly dominant experienced the group climate as more avoiding and tense. MacNair-Semands and Lese (2000) also found that highly dominant members viewed the group as less altruistic and rated several therapeutic factors lower than other members, discounting some of the beneficial aspects of the group. More recent research has replicated these findings: Fjelstad et al. (2017) found that those who are dominant and cold are more challenging to engage, and Hammond and Marmarosh (2011) found that those who are affiliative tend to engage well compared to those with an anxious or avoidant attachment style. Nevertheless, it has also been determined that with appropriate pre-group preparation and supportive and active leaders, such cold or distant clients can make significant and efficient progress (Fjelstad et al., 2017). It is clear today that understanding the role of early attachment in our group members helps group leaders foster safety in their groups and hence facilitates growth (Marmarosh, 2017). Marmarosh et al. (2013) provide stimulating case examples that demonstrate how attachment theory can be used to benefit clinical practice. More information on using attachment measures for selection and group preparation is provided later in this chapter.

While all of this clinical and research literature seems to suggest that the greater the psychological health of the candidate, the greater the likelihood of positive outcome, many clients who need group therapy and may benefit from it are also particularly challenged in essential interpersonal domains. The ethical principle of Beneficence may apply here—by orienting the candidate to the kinds of interpersonal challenges that are likely to be experienced and how they could be handled—such healing treatment experiences could be useful. The principle of Justice also requires us to make group psychotherapy available to people with varied backgrounds, not only those whose backgrounds prepare them to quickly install themselves in a group. Skilled group leaders often note that many group therapy members who do not meet these prototypical characteristics can still benefit substantially from group therapy; following a comprehensive phase of preparation, a group therapy trial may be more successful (Bernard et al., 2008). Failure to recognize this potential will likely mean many clients who do not meet these selection criteria would be excluded from a meaningful and effective therapeutic opportunity.

There are crucial ethical issues regarding how the therapist thinks about and decides who is in and who is out, based on both psychological and sociocultural variables. How does the therapist decide, for example, whether a Black candidate for an all White all-White group would be constructive or destructive? While research has identified some important variables such as attachment styles, there are no clear-cut answers to the very complex question of appropriateness of fit between the candidate and the particular current group that is being considered. But it behooves the ethical therapist to hypothesize about how the mix of psychological and sociocultural variables will play out—for the betterment or deterioration of the candidate and the group. Related to the principles of Non-maleficence and Justice, Cone-Uemura and Bentley (2018) advise group therapists who are considering including only one member from a minority group of the potential for prejudice, marginalization, or scapegoating that may recapitulate past injustices and harm. However, the authors also acknowledge that in some settings, it might not be possible to compose groups with more than one member from a particular underrepresented identity. Cone-Uemura and Bentley suggest that a single minority participant may do well in a group if their primary presenting problem is not tied to their minority status (e.g., a member with a minority sexual identity whose primary reason for group therapy is not related to concerns about labeling themselves). Along those lines, minority group members whose identity development is advanced (e.g., who feel secure in and strongly value their cultural identity) are more likely to feel included in a therapy group as long as others in the group do not express prejudicial attitudes.

Exclusion Criteria

In general, members who drop out of a group tend to leave before making progress; dropouts may have consequences for the remaining members in terms of trust, cohesion, and group morale. Any potential member deemed at risk for dropping out should also be carefully considered for exclusion to protect the other members (i.e., serving the principle of Non-maleficence). Clients who tend to prematurely terminate from group include those with low motivation, poor insight, or angry hostility (including those who provoke negative reactions from others); clients displaying denial and defensiveness also are at risk for poor attendance or dropping out of group (MacNair-Semands, 2002; Yalom & Leszcz, 2020).

Yalom and Leszcz (2020) emphasize that although dropout rates are not higher for group treatment than for other therapies, group dropout is more significant because of the deleterious effects on the rest of the group. They highlight the importance of assessing for high levels of external stress; examples of clients who have difficulty finding the energy to respond to others in group included those with marital discord or facing an impending divorce, impending career or academic failure, family conflict, bereavement, and severe physical illness. Yalom and Leszcz also propose that poor attendance can be the result of unpredictable work schedules and demands, so clients who must travel for their work should likely be excluded.

Clients should be excluded from group therapy if they cannot engage in the primary work of the group—interpersonal engagement, interpersonal learning, and acquiring insight—due to logistical, intellectual, psychological, or interpersonal reasons (Yalom & Leszcz, 2020). When considering inclusion and exclusion criteria for a specific group, however, some interpersonal factors must be considered relative rather than absolute (Bernard et al., 2008).

Certainly, some leaders also use diagnoses as exclusion criteria to avoid harm to their members, but a complicated variable such as a diagnosis will not be consistently predictive. For example, pathological narcissism is a common exclusion variable for many group leaders. Research involving group members has found that high levels of narcissism were associated with not only dropping out of group therapy prematurely, but also with domineering, vindictive, and intrusive interpersonal behaviors (Ogrodniczuk et al., 2009). Of course, traits such as narcissism exist on a continuum; individuals with less extreme elevations may well benefit from a group experience. So, while ethical group leaders will want to be aware of the research findings on factors that can impact the whole group, they will also need to be mindful of such things like negative countertransference reactions that can affect the decision-making process (Greene et al., 1980).

Personality traits have also been known to affect outcomes in groups. One example, socially-prescribed perfectionism, and the need to *appear perfect* in particular, seem to be associated with negative attitudes toward seeking help, fears of therapy and therapists, increased anxiety in initial clinical interviews, and with reduced benefit in group therapy (Hewitt et al., 2020; Hewitt, 2020). Moreover, clinicians tend to have more negative impressions of perfectionistic patients as measured by clinician-rated hostility, suggesting that the therapeutic alliance might be compromised by the perfectionistic behaviors of clients and potentially negatively impact outcomes. So, group leaders should be aware that the trait of perfectionism is negatively associated with the likelihood of benefit from group treatment. Findings highlight the importance of evaluating and addressing trait and self-presentation components of perfectionism early in the therapeutic process, such as in a PGM.

Furthermore, exclusion criteria studies indicate that a candidate with acute substance use or significant social inhibition may not benefit from interpersonal therapy groups and indeed tend to have fewer positive expectations for these groups (Fenger et al., 2011; MacNair-Semands, 2002). If candidates have negative expectations about what group treatment offers them, the fundamental therapeutic alliance is undermined (Horvath et al., 2011). Other considerations for exclusion are clients who are unable to participate in the tasks of the group due to an acute crisis (Rutan et al., 2014) and those who may be actively suicidal, requiring intensive risk management. Suicidal members may require an intensive approach both in and outside of the group and can be overwhelming to the other members.

Social functioning, alcohol problems, and antisocial behavior were also found to be related to group dropout in a study based in a public outpatient agency in Denmark offering time-limited psychodynamic groups (Jensen et al., 2014). Additionally, Jensen and colleagues further compared early (in the first month of group, or 12 sessions) and late dropouts to examine potential differences. Their findings demonstrated that early terminators had significant agoraphobic symptoms, lower interpersonal sensitivity, and compulsive-type personality traits, whereas late dropouts had more cognitive and somatic anxiety symptoms and antisocial personality features.

If group candidates are extremely lacking in interpersonal sensitivity, overly silent or angry, or avoidant of emotional immediacy, we would want to consider their exclusion. Exclusion might be considered if they also fail to appreciate the therapy process, are either disengaged or concrete and directive, and are disconnected from here and now dynamics (Burlingame et al., 2011; Krogel et al., 2013; McCallum et al., 2002; Yalom & Leszcz, 2005). Those who disagree with group norms may be disliked by other members, affecting cohesion (Yalom & Leszcz, 2020). One possibility is for the person to be placed in a social skills training group where these features are very systematically targeted prior to admission to a therapy group.

An individual with an extreme lack of interpersonal sensitivity can harm the group's sense of safety. For example,

> Dave often looked withdrawn and sullen much of the time in the first group session. When he interrupted another member and spoke, he expressed strong anger toward the men in his life. When other males in the group tried to relate to his history with his father in the second session, he minimized their experiences by stating that, "at least *your* fathers stuck around." He then stated his experience was both different and worse, insulting their "lame attempts" to connect. He left the group after the two sessions and some of the males in the group struggled with trust and cohesion before fully exploring the sting of their encounters with Dave.

Thus, the ethical therapist needs to be aware of the *helpful research findings around selection* to better serve the whole group. Other considerations, however, can also affect the decision-making process, including the therapist's affective responses to the candidate. When therapists are aware of emotional reactions to group candidates, the potential to respond with personal curiosity rather than quick judgment can benefit the decision-making process.

Choosing Selection Criteria While Considering Composition

In addition to the issue of selecting members who can benefit from and contribute to a group, the issue of group composition is core to forming a cohesive blend of clients that will be effective in reaching individual and group goals. Composition in group psychotherapy refers to the blend of personal and sociocultural characteristics among individual group members (Ribeiro, 2020; Rutan et al., 2014). Bringing a new member into an ongoing group therapy can significantly impact the quality of the experience for both the new member and the existing members. The selection and composition decision-making processes have the potential for clinical errors that have somewhat unique implications compared with other mistakes in psychotherapy, including deleterious effects not just for a member but also for the therapeutic progress of other members (Kealy et al., 2016). Poor judgment in selection and composition, or simply not being capable of making accurate predictions given the complexity of the phenomena and the many unknown and unanticipated factors involved, has been found in some cases to impair the overall climate and work of a group (Gans & Counselman, 2010; Marmarosh et al., 2013).

The ethical principle of Non-maleficence is relevant when making selection decisions, in that members with mental health issues seek a healing group experience rather than one that is damaging or overly distressing. Thus, having relevant selection criteria for decision making, based on research findings and clinical wisdom, as well as some predictions of how members may connect or have conflicts with each other can be useful. Kealy et al. (2016) argue that even the addition of one or two volatile members later deemed selection errors can alter the composition of the group from a combination that works to one that does not, taking the group off its intended course.

A primary question regarding composition is whether the group is an *adequate container* for the inevitable conflicts and clashes that will occur. An essential task of the leader is to consider the composition of members with sufficiently-developed awareness and communication skills to engage in the work of the specific group, and who can tolerate and benefit from the process of interpersonal feedback and other interventions. Candidates often display different presenting symptoms during the pre-group meeting, but if they are similar to other group members around motivation to self-disclose, insightfulness, and communication skills, they are more likely to build co-member connections (Bernard et al., 2008). The leader's goals around composing groups are to gather a diversity of individuals who will take risks to both emotionally support one another and provide challenging feedback with honesty and authenticity, building group cohesion.

To that end, many leaders value the idea of choosing a few initial members with group experience when forming a new group. For example, Beth was in a group the previous semester at a university counseling center. She might be placed in a newly-forming group with another fellow veteran group member, Trey. As Beth and Trey previously learned to be more open, they more comfortably take self-disclosure risks early in the new group. They quickly become popular in the group and encourage disclosure and feelings of safety in the other members (Yalom & Leszcz, 2020). This reflects the principle of Beneficence for the members.

We strive for Justice, Beneficence, Non-maleficence, and Autonomy in our composition decisions by considering both clinical and sociocultural factors. Kealy et al. (2016) put forth that composition is usually discussed in terms of the relative homogeneity or heterogeneity of group members' characteristics; these range from concrete variables—such as gender, race, and presenting problem—to abstract features like interpersonal patterns or capacity for reflective functioning. They argue that group composition can be adjusted over time to serve the objectives of a group, with more specific aims typically calling for greater homogeneity among members. For example, a group with many dominant and talkative members may demonstrate better functioning after the addition of members who are willing to jump in to express themselves when appropriate but not compete for dominance. These *moderately* dominant members might curiously invite the quieter members to join the conversation, which could present quite differently from the dynamics that might surface by adding a few more highly dominant members.

The observation that some volatile or difficult members can improve if added to a well-functioning group with stable membership complicates selection decisions. Early research demonstrated that factors such as the mixture of members' levels of quality of object relations (QOR) can make a difference in treatment response. Piper et al. (2007) found that complicated grief groups composed of a greater proportion of high-QOR members produced greater improvement for their members, regardless of the members' level of QOR. Thus, the presence of members with high QOR influenced the group sufficiently to benefit even those with lower levels of relational functioning. Such results highlight the need for careful attention to the composition of groups so that higher functioning members can influence other members when highly defensive or splitting behaviors surface (Kealy et al., 2016). In accommodating these more challenging patients in the group—provided they have potential for benefitting from the group—we are serving the principle of Justice by making the therapy more broadly available.

Similarly, Kivlighan et al. (2015) found results suggesting that a composition of members with an optimistic bias about group engagement and climate may allow some other group members to be more fully involved with the group, even in a less favorable group climate. They argue that if members were categorized by perception into "optimistic bias" and "pessimistic bias" (where a particular member's perception of engaged group climate is lower than the group's average ratings), it seems that an optimistic bias would likely lead to the member feeling more involved and valued in the group. See Yalom and Leszcz (2020) for more detailed inclusion and exclusion information. See Box 4.1 for a vignette that helps leaders weigh the various factors in making composition decisions.

Measures for Selection and Screening of Group Members

Prior to the turn of the century, making treatment decisions about group versus individual modalities based on empirical evidence had been almost impossible in our field (Burlingame et al., 2011; MacNair-Semands, 2002). When selecting members for a group, the therapist is constrained by the existing group composition and has much less flexibility than the individual therapist. Attention to both fit and interpersonal impact is also challenging for most leaders, as members tend to reveal problematic interpersonal patterns only slowly over time in a group. Predicting fit with other members is undeniably difficult within the brief assessment portion of a PGM. Additionally, even when members are asked specifically about their typical interpersonal patterns during the PGM, candidates may not have the capacity to identify them. And, of course, conflict and difficulties can arise during the group as when a new member—assessed in a PGM as being emotionally stable or well regulated—becomes emotionally abusive in the group and is unwilling to be redirected or respond in line with the contracted group agreements.

The use of screening and selection instruments can serve the principle of Justice in that measures can expand the therapist's perspective on the prospective member and potentially compensate for therapist bias. Such measures can allow the leaders to understand the client's cultural context and history more fully, leading to a deeper knowledge of the intimate concerns that have developed for the potential member. Whereas we are certainly not advanced enough in our field to be able to fully predict the success of a potential

Box 4.1   Vignette on Selection and Preparation

As we contemplate the complexity of our selection and composition decisions, leaders weigh multiple factors that may each have benefits and/or costs for the group. Consider the following example:

> There is one spot left for a new member in a therapy group at a university counseling center. Dante, a client with many personal and therapeutic rejections in his history, is seeking a group to learn why he is often excluded or socially avoided. As he tends to tell long stories without noticing social cues, he has also frustrated two pre-doctoral intern therapists-in-training over the last 2 years, losing one therapist who felt he'd make better progress in another format and losing another structured group that ended due to Covid-19 closures. Dante had previously used up his yearly allotment of individual sessions. He would also add cultural diversity to the group.

> Nancy is also referred to the group; she is a client 'willing to try' group but prefers individual therapy. She can join a group later in the year if fitting, but the leaders think she would add insight and safety to the currently struggling group dynamics, as she appears as an appropriately self-disclosive person. The group could also use more LGBTQ+ members for balancing member sexual identities, and she identifies as bisexual. With some support from other members, the leaders predicted she would make progress quickly in the group.

Because we know that members tend to progress at their own pace and vary in their outcomes, the protection of more vulnerable persons should demand a crucial focus. Focusing on the welfare of the most vulnerable clients means addressing requests for group services with an awareness that potential members have different positions of *control and vulnerability* (Koocher, 2007). We must remain mindful of appreciating the relative strengths and weaknesses of the parties involved. Nonetheless, we must recognize that some clients may experience feelings of harm resulting from participation in multiple-client treatment interventions like group therapy.

In the examples above, many would respond that Dante is likely to need the group membership to improve his overall well-being, more so than Nancy. The leaders must consider that he has fewer options for treatment and is more likely to be hurt by being referred out for off-campus resources. However, the overall group dynamics might improve more by including Nancy, which in turn may lead to a more cohesive and interactional process for all members. If the group is not currently functioning well, the therapists must also consider that members may choose to leave the group if they feel a lack of progress or lack of attraction to the group. The leaders must weigh the potential for all group members to remain committed to the group and to function in a more effective manner, as discussed in the section on selection of members. Rutan et al. (2014) remind us that if a client does not join willingly, that client is a poor candidate despite a therapist's perspective that group is the best treatment.

In thinking about this material, reflect on the following questions: (a) Which factors might influence your decision to accept Dante? Nancy? (b) In order to minimize harm, what options might the leaders consider for the overall group membership? and (c) How do you weigh the need for more diversity in identity against the need to minimize harm to the group?

member (Rutan et al., 2014), we are making progress in that arena. However, some argue that our research and science will never be so deterministic, given the complexity of the phenomena, as to allow us to rely solely on empirical findings for decisions about selection and composition.

It has also become more evident in the last two decades that using a valid screening measure or other assessment tools can help build groups with solid membership, consistent attendance, and positive outcomes. While having specific selection criteria and guidelines can be of help in the choosing of members for group therapy, the leader also may consider several researched selection instruments that are available to help in appropriately composing groups (Burlingame et al., 2006; Rutan et al., 2019). Group leaders need to rely on two diverse but related approaches—clinical assessment and judgment, and empirical tools—to better choose an appropriate member for a specific group. As we have established that our clinical capacities to accurately judge and predict positive group membership are limited, it has become more common to administer group selection measures to supplement our clinical judgment; neither one alone is as good as using both approaches together (Bernard et al., 2008; Burlingame et al., 2011).

Measures Related to Dropout and Expectations

Other selection measures can serve the principles of Justice, Autonomy, Beneficence, and Non-maleficence by increasing the information leaders have about each member. We provide examples of how these principles apply throughout this section. One approach to selection has been to focus on factors associated with premature termination, as well as those interpersonal characteristics related to attendance and outcome. Strauss et al. (2008) described how the selection measures included in the CORE-R Battery produced by the American Group Psychotherapy Association (Burlingame et al., 2006) could be used by a group leader. They reviewed how two selection instruments can help clinicians assess client characteristics to determine fit for group therapy and clarify client needs for pre-group preparation. These two measures are the Group Readiness Questionnaire (GRQ; Burlingame et al., 2011; Cox, 2008; Cox et al., 2004; Krogel et al., 2009) and the Group Therapy Questionnaire (GTQ; MacNair & Corazzini, 1994; MacNair-Semands, 2002). As numerous studies have determined that people need a degree of interpersonal competence to make use of group therapy (Bernard et al., 2008; Rutan et al., 2019; Piper, 2008; Yalom & Leszcz, 2020), it has become clear that interpersonal intimacy factors must be considered more closely.

GROUP READINESS QUESTIONNAIRE

The GRQ (Burlingame et al., 2011; Cox et al., 2004; Krogel et al., 2009) was originally rationally derived to identify people who are likely to do poorly in group psychotherapy because of problems related to inappropriate expectations of group therapy (Expectancy subscale), inability to participate in the group (Participation), and negative interpersonal traits (Demeanor). The GRQ is a self-report instrument of 19 items rated on a five-point Likert-type scale. Beginning with groups of children with trauma in Bosnia, it was then cross-validated using other adult populations (Burlingame et al., 2011; Cox, 2008; Cox et al., 2004). In Europe, the measure was then tested in German inpatient groups (Loeffler et al., 2007).

The general factor structure has been confirmed in multiple studies, and scores adequately predicted group member attrition, process, and outcome. It has also been found to be predictive of group process and outcome over a variety of periods in groups. The convergent validity of the GRQ was also tested in a United States college counseling center population (Baker, 2010). In this study, clients were administered the GRQ at intake, along with the original version of the GTQ (MacNair & Corazzini, 1994; MacNair-Semands, 2002). Convergent validity of the GRQ was generally supported. The original GRQ scales labeled Demeanor, Expectancy, and Total scale scores correlated significantly with the GTQ Expectations about Group scale. Also, GRQ Participation, Expectancy, and Total scale scores correlated with the GTQ Interpersonal Problems scale.

It can be helpful to target specific social skills and behaviors for group selection, and the GRQ wisely included this emphasis. Krogel et al. (2009) found that those rated as the most prepared for group treatment (GRQ low scorers) viewed themselves as being engaged and actively participating in groups, not likely to interrupt other group members, and open and willing to share their thoughts and feelings in a group. In addition to scale and Total scores, three items may now be used as critical indicators. Items 7 (If I disagree with what someone is saying, I will interrupt them before they can finish what they are saying.), 13 (I am abrupt with others if I feel strongly about what I'm saying.), and 17 (I argue for argument's sake) can be used for clinical follow-up.

Thus, the critical items on the GRQ can reflect a low level of social skills and can be further assessed and explored during a PGM. It is currently recommended that GRQ score profiles be utilized at both a scale level and an item level (Burlingame et al., 2012). At a scale level, a client who receives scores in the extremely high range should be considered with more caution in group referral and preparation. Overall, the GRQ is an efficient and easily scored selection measure that has been studied across many populations, making it easy to incorporate for many agencies. Settings can particularly benefit from using the critical items and scale scores in screening out problematic members.

THE GROUP THERAPY QUESTIONNAIRE

The GTQ and GTQ-S, original and short versions (MacNair & Corazzini, 1994; MacNair-Semands, 2002; MacNair-Semands & Lennon, 2017), were initially developed as a clinical tool to identify client characteristics that might impact successful treatment for Yalom-based interpersonal psychotherapy groups. The GTQ has been through several revisions since 2002 to (1) add prompts for discussions of how identity and culture might impact revealing oneself in group, (2) for additional brevity, and (3) to simplify scoring and develop an electronic version (GTQ-E; on the Titanium platform of measures commonly used in college counseling centers). The GTQ-S is currently used more often than the original GTQ, particularly in university counseling center settings but also with focused brief group therapy models (FBGT) globally and in outpatient and hospital settings (Söchting et al., 2018; Whittingham, 2018). The GTQ-S takes approximately 25 minutes to complete and is generally administered at the end of an initial intake session. The information can be brought to a PGM to be reviewed and expanded on together with the leaders for selection decisions.

As a clinical tool, the GTQ has a focus on narrative questions that address capacity to examine interpersonal behavior patterns, ability to self-disclose, and ability to reflect on oneself and others. Yalom and Leszcz (2020) argue that these are some of the significant traits that clients must possess to fully engage in interpersonal therapy groups. Thus, the GTQ allows the clinician an interpersonal window into the relational world of the group candidate. The prompts about whether a client is in crisis or currently having suicidal thoughts can be also used to explore these variables and screen out clients who may need more comprehensive care (MacNair-Semands & Lennon, 2019).

The GTQ-S includes 25 major items across five subscales, with both quantitative (ratings of items on a scale of 1-not at all to 7-very much) and narrative responding. Subscales consist of: (1) Counseling (Experiences and Expectations: e.g., *I look forward to beginning group therapy*), (2) Family (*e.g., What role do you play in your current family or intimate relationships that contributes to difficulties?*), (3) Health/Mental Health (e.g., *Are you feeling suicidal? □ No □ Yes, with thoughts only □ Yes, with intent/plan; Somatic Symptom Checklist*), (4) Interpersonal Problems (*a 34-item interpersonal problem checklist*), and (5) Therapy Considerations (e.g., *What are your goals for the group? What are you most afraid of about group therapy?*).

The first study of the GTQ demonstrated that it successfully predicted group member dropout (MacNair & Corazzini, 1994). Variables related to premature termination from the group included factors labeled Angry Hostility, Alcohol and/or Drug problems, Somatic Complaints, and Social Inhibition. The GTQ successfully classified about 76% of clients as dropouts or continuers. In a subsequent study, group therapy participants (N = 310) from two university counseling centers over a 7-year period completed the GTQ for a study examining interpersonal style, expectations, and attendance in group therapy (MacNair-Semands, 2002). Angry Hostility and Social Inhibition (from the interpersonal checklist factors) were predictive of low group attendance. Additionally, clients with previous therapy reported more positive expectations about group therapy, whereas those reporting greater substance use and more somatic symptoms had fewer positive expectations about groups.

The GTQ has been found to have good psychometric properties, with test-retest reliability ranging from 0.60 to 0.93 for the Likert-rated items (MacNair-Semands, 2002). Although the GTQ was designed for use with interpersonal therapy groups, Söchting et al. (2018) used the GTQ with five types of CBT groups. Findings revealed that patients' expectations of group were associated with attendance and participation as expected. However, in CBT groups, levels of Interpersonal Problems, Health Issues, and Drug and Alcohol Use were not associated with attendance. Therefore, the GTQ may be most useful for interpersonal therapy groups and in settings in which clients can complete the comprehensive measure in a private space. The GTQ and manual can be obtained at no cost by downloading from: https://www.routledge.com/Core-Principles-of-Group-Psychotherapy-An-Integrated-Theory-Research/Kaklauskas-Greene/p/book/9780367203092 (using the button entitled *Support Materials* and choosing the folder entitled *Pre-group 1–10*).

Measures of Attachment Styles and Personality Traits

As newer group approaches move toward the integration of attachment and interpersonal theories, a second empirical approach to selection has been emerging that specifically serves the principle of Autonomy. A variety of diagnostic tools may now assist leaders' assessments by determining the type of interpersonal difficulties that their clients experience and help create better combinations of members with different interpersonal styles. Providing them the information about their styles means members can use *autonomy* to choose to set specific interpersonal goals based on new information from the measures. Inventories categorizing individuals' interactional styles can also create important opportunities for interpersonal learning at the very start of treatment (Whittingham, 2018). Hewitt et al. (2018, 2020), for example, use psychometric data in conjunction with clinical impressions to help group candidates focus on their specific interpersonal goals.

Attachment and interpersonal theories and therapies have significant overlap with regard to theoretical underpinnings and overlapping factor structure of the instruments used. Consequently, the concepts can be more easily conveyed to and accepted by members (Tasca et al., 2021; Whittingham, 2017). For example, FBGT (Whittingham, 2015, 2018) emphasizes both the underlying motivation (attachment style) and inter-personal behaviors (interpersonal theory) in the pre-group assessment process. Other re-searchers use psychodynamic and object relations concepts (i.e., triangles of attachment) to develop a formulation that includes the maladaptive interpersonal patterns of the member (see next section on preparation for more details; Tasca et al., 2021).

INVENTORY OF INTERPERSONAL PROBLEMS (IIP-64 AND IIP-32)

The use of such inventories as the IIP-64 and IIP-32 (Barkham et al., 1996; Horowitz et al., 1988, 2000) provide the leader and member with a visual way of understanding how their interpersonal distress is manifested. It uses a circumplex organization that displays the individual's tendencies to relate on two interpersonal domains: Dominance/Agency (from non-assertive/submissive to highly assertive/domineering) and Affiliation (from overly warm/nurturant to cold/distant). The interpersonal circumplex is a solid and validated measure of interpersonal functioning (Horowitz & Strack, 2010). Leaders generally use the IIP-32 to facilitate a straightforward, collaborative focus on the mechanisms of change thus generating efficient movement in members' insight.

Whittingham (2018) provides an excellent example of a member scoring high on the Focused on the Needs of Others scale of the IIP-32, who is also identified as in a high level of distress. Leaders first investigate the personal history of the client's focus on the needs of others and gain an understanding of the typical contexts of the problems arising in this arena. They then suggest setting goals of adding new *assertive* behaviors, such as sometimes talking first in the group. The leaders also use information from the GTQ-S that asks about salient multicultural identity issues to discuss and explore *how culture might be impacting interpersonal distress*. Once the links between interpersonal distress and culture and context have been established, the therapist inquires as to whether this issue is affecting the client's symptoms on an outcome measure. By identifying attachment styles and transparently making clinical predictions about how the member might react in group, therapists are better able to help members to anticipate potential problems in the group and respond well; the leaders can also develop strategies to smooth the resulting sting of feelings (Yalom & Leszcz, 2020). The IIP-32 is available for a cost at www.mindgarden.com.

OTHER SELF-ASSESSMENTS OF RELATIONAL STYLE

Using formal measures to help members progress more quickly has recently gotten more efficient and client-friendly and thus serves the principle of Beneficence. Adding a measure of attachment has been streamlined with quick and effective measures available online, providing automatic scoring procedures that are easily understood by clinicians and members. Yalom and Leszcz (2020) note that simple self-reports can be accessed online at "The Self-Assessment Kiosk" in the Sinai Health System and at the University of Toronto (see Survey Gizmo; www.surveygizmo.com/s3/2998552/The-Self-Assessment-Kiosk).

As mentioned earlier, personality inventories such as the NEO-FFI (Costa & McCrae 1992) have also provided good information on which personality tendencies contribute to positive group behaviors and negative outcomes. Those with poor group outcomes scored high on the neuroticism scale, reflecting a tendency toward negative emotional reactivity (Ogrodniczuk et al., 2003). Research on the personal capacities or styles of members, such as perfectionism, has also been found to be important for selection (see Hewitt et al., 2020; Piper et al., 2011; Whittingham, 2018). Again, the length of time available for adminis-tration of these instruments is often worth the effort in many settings, especially when balanced with the depth of knowledge captured about the potential member. *An ethical approach is often the more thorough assessment*, leading to more positive outcomes as a result of taking the time needed to fully gather client information.

Ethical Obligations When a Client is Deemed Inappropriate for the Group

When a potential member is not found to be a good fit for a particular group using assessment, ethical issues are raised. If the member is not accepted in the PGM, the leader has the obligation to reduce the potential harm of rejection (i.e., serving the principle of Non-maleficence). We also discuss here the ethical issues around how to reduce harm if it is determined that a member needs to leave an ongoing group during treatment.

When it becomes clear that a selection error has been made, such as when a member exhibits a pattern of causing toxicity, distress, or destructive dynamics in a group, the leaders should carefully consider the decision to refer the client to a more fitting treatment (Kealy et al., 2016). This decision should not be made lightly and should happen relatively rarely, especially because of the potential of provoking anxiety in the other members as well as the shame or distress of the kicked-out member. Leaders need to first examine their own possible countertransference reactions toward the challenging member and may consider consulting with other professionals to ensure the dynamics could not be effectively shifted within the group treatment (Rutan et al., 2014). If a therapist encounters multiple problems of this nature, a re-evaluation of the selection process should be undertaken.

Obligations to the Member

If either the member or the leader has a strong reservation about the fit for group, recommendations for other types of treatments to better prepare the client for future groups may be made, avoiding the perception of a potentially harmful clinical rejection. An ethical approach entails communicating authentically in a caring manner and avoiding harsh judgments that could cause harm. Also, the principle of Autonomy certainly comes into play when the leaders make a decision for a member, even when it may be deemed to be in the best interest of the individual. If interpersonal skills are lacking, for example, the leader may need to reframe the decision about a general therapy group to instead discuss what *kind* of preparatory group would be suitable for the particular individual (Bernard et al., 2008). Consultation with supervisors or professional peers, however, may first promote trying new interventions or approaches that have the potential to shift patterns and provide new insight for all involved. The leader should strive to be honest but reparative in an ethical approach.

The literature has only modest guidance about how to approach the member and whether or how to involve the other group members. Once the leader decides to refer a member out, however, proactively acknowledging the selection error and tactfully communicating with transparency about the need for a more effective and suitable treatment is recommended (Kealy et al., 2016; Motherwell & Shay, 2005; Yalom & Leszcz, 2005, 2020). Protecting the departing member from any further scapegoating that may be occurring is another benefit to removing a member who cannot contribute in a positive fashion (Brown, 2008). The therapist should also attend to the risk of colluding in a scapegoating process by kicking out the scapegoat.

Although processing the decision *within* a group might seem more transparent, a respectful and ethical approach might involve an initial individual meeting with the member so they are able to absorb the decision privately and adequately prepare to process the change. Yalom and Leszcz (2005, 2020) advise that this is best managed during an individual meeting in part to reduce the client's sense of shame and also to avoid other group members' potential counterproductive protestations about the decision. They suggest that taking a hopeful stance around optimizing the individual's treatment can actually lead to relief for the client. Rutan et al. (2014) make the point that removing a disruptive client, if framed within the context of that member's psychodynamic history, can be a therapeutic intervention for the member and also for other group members.

Obligations to the Group

The decision to have a troublesome client leave the group requires serious ethical analysis, not only in relation to the particular individual involved but to the remaining group members. For example, some members might fear that they, too, will be asked to leave the group. The clinical and ethical issues here critically entail thinking through, possibly with consultation, how the group likely will respond, for better or worse in the short term and long term.

Avoiding all harm is impossible (Koocher, 2007) and we should strive instead to minimize harm resulting from our work. Our ethical obligation, Koocher observed, involves foreseeing potential difficulties and maintaining our professional integrity as we strive to advance common interests and outcomes in group. Rejecting a member from group treatment could clearly cause harm, particularly for those who have experienced numerous exclusions in their history. But at the same time, it can also increase the possibility of growth in the remaining members when dynamics have been derailed by a problematic member. The difficult decision to remove such a member *and benefit the work of the remaining members* thus potentially adheres to the principles of Beneficence, Non-maleficence, and Justice.

Exploring inevitable reactions to feeling responsible for pushing another away or of "being left" may also be helpful to the working through process. If the leaders decide that a final goodbye session would likely be healing or provide important closure, the members can be encouraged to respond with honesty and kindness, while actively considering what level of feedback the departing member may be able to hear. Remaining group members may express relief once the member is gone and group functioning improves; each member can then be encouraged to learn something about their own reactions of silence, anger, hurt, conflict, or guilt.

Preparing Members

Because the working alliance and therapy processes (i.e., interpersonal openness, increased self-disclosure) are improved by preparation, an ethical approach to treatment means allocating attention to this step as leaders. Much convincing evidence now exists that pre-group preparation is vital to the health of the group (Yalom & Leszcz, 2020). Preparation generally occurs during a PGM, but can also involve watching videos or participating in *practice* groups in some settings. Pre-group preparation is related to:

- a more rapid development of group cohesion
- less deviation from the tasks and goals of group
- increased attendance
- less attrition
- reduced anxiety
- a better understanding of objectives, roles, and behavior
- a stronger bond with the leader
- increased faith in group as an effective mode of treatment (see Bernard et al., 2008; Piper et al., 2011; Yalom & Leszcz, 2020)

Further, pre-group preparation appears to be dose-related in that more preparation sessions with experiential and emotional intensity are more likely to produce a positive impact (Yalom & Leszcz, 2020). In carefully preparing members, the therapist observes the principle of Non-maleficence, recognizing the harm that can occur when members depart precipitously merely because they do not understand how the group works. Conversely, by helping the member get down to work quickly, the therapist acts in accord with the principle of Beneficence.

Appropriate pre-group preparation has been put forth as a cornerstone of evidence-based group therapy in comprehensive literature reviews (Burlingame et al., 2013; Burlingame & Strauss, 2021). Pre-group preparation is usually provided across a spectrum from passive to more active or interactive formats with behavioral, cognitive, and experiential components (Burlingame et al., 2006). Currently, there is enormous variation in the clinical practices of both selection and pre-group preparation. Variations with regard to the assessment (e.g., the duration of preparation needed, methods of preparation) have been found to be related to premature terminations and to affect the specific ways in which the group and members benefit (Bernard et al., 2008; Gross, 2010; Piper & Ogrodniczuk, 2004; Turner, 2018). It is important to acknowledge, however, that our settings often limit what can be done vis-à-vis selection and preparation, e.g., many groups take place in inpatient units where members often stay for only three to five sessions before being discharged. Even so, therapists should do what they can to prepare members even if it entails only conducting an orientation at the beginning of the session.

Preparing for Diversity and Difference: A Cultural Assessment

Topics related to Justice and Non-maleficence are now more regularly integrated into discussions of ethics in the PGM and group therapy in general, reflecting the mounting belief that social justice is a dynamic issue that inevitably surfaces whenever people of diverse backgrounds meet in groups. Consider this example:

> Fatima states in her pre-group meeting that she generally wears her hijab on campus but had noticed that her ability to meet others increased when she was not wearing it. Fatima felt torn because she wanted to expand her social connections, particularly with men. The leaders explored whether she might discuss this dilemma in the group and ask her to anticipate responses she might get from other members. Fatima then expressed her need for validation around being in the position of choosing between her values and her social goals. This exploration led her to identify other losses and frustrations around being a minority with her peers that she might address in group as well. The leaders anticipate with Fatima that they will encourage other members who have been silenced or rejected in various ways due to culture and religion to share these experiences and thus be able to validate such costs (MacNair-Semands, 2014). Furthermore, if Fatima was a new member joining an existing group, the veteran members should be adequately prepared with the opportunity to process feelings around assimilating a new member; the leaders can then have a positive impact by providing the structure to aid the transition for the whole group (Gross, 2010).

Group leaders should highlight in the PGM that they strive to create a respectful, accepting climate, with a norm of having explorations of differences in culture and identity within a safe group context. Clients should be informed that members come to group with multiple identities and this specific group is a place where all identities are welcome. Kivlighan et al. (2019) suggest starting this process in the PGM to prepare members for the multicultural orientation of the group, noting that group leaders can facilitate this climate by modeling cultural humility (Hook et al., 2017) with openness and comfort.

Adapting preparation to be culturally attuned to the member is an important consideration (Whittingham, 2018). From the first encounter, the leader must monitor the dual processes of assimilation and accommodation to assess for the possible adjustment between the new member and the group and to predict and manage processes such as discrimination, scapegoating, or dropout (Kaklauskas & Nettles, 2019). Chen et al. (2008) note that leaders should attend to the incoming members' beliefs on psychological care that are rooted in that person's culture, whilst being aware of the leader's own culturally determined styles that may impact the member. The therapist and the new member need to be attuned to the culture of the group (the way it works, the way it thinks about psychological problems) and how those fit with the culture of the incoming client.

When leaders focus on selecting and orienting, it is helpful to include members who can share specific social identities, especially if these are minoritized identities related to race, nationality, and sexual orientation (Ribeiro, 2020). Ribeiro proposes that utilizing the PGM to assess for racial identity development is particularly beneficial when populating groups with varied racial groups and could be a good time to assess for sensitivity to issues around dominance and marginalization. D'Andrea (2014) stresses that trust across racial groups and developing safe group attachments can often be accomplished by having several minority group members share a cultural identity. He describes that those connections to one's ethnic group can often facilitate a sense of belonging in the group.

Chen et al. (2008) suggest that during the PGM the therapists can engage in a systematic cultural assessment of potential group members by asking about the client's cultural identity (e.g., cultural or ethnic reference groups, degree of involvement with the culture of origin), the role of the cultural context in the presenting problems (e.g., the perceived source of distress), and the impact of cultural differences on the therapist–client relationship. Other questions can be posed to help determine how flexible the potential group member could be regarding certain topics involving race and difference. Some example questions (Cone-Uemura & Bentley, 2018, p.29) for the potential member include:

1.   How do you feel about being in a group with people different from you?
2.   We're all impacted by what is happening in our society, and sometimes people want to talk about cultural issues like their experience of racism and discrimination. How would that be for you?

Group leaders must also be sensitive to the potential for clashing values of existing and prospective group members (e.g., religious values and sexual identity). Cone-Uemura and Bentley (2018) suggest that leaders consider exploring specific topics as part of the pre-group preparation for some group candidates. These topics might include providing information about the diverse backgrounds and values of other group members, asking whether any offensive stereotypes concern the individual, exploring whether some values held by others might offend them, and asking how they feel about being the only minority member in the group.

It may also be prudent during pre-group preparation to explore with any prospective member, including those from the dominant cultural group, regarding the need to be respectful of individual differences even if the values and beliefs expressed by others clash with those of the member (Kaklauskas & Nettles, 2019; MacNair-Semands, 2014; Ribeiro, 2020; Tasca et al., 2021). The group leader works to create a climate where members understand that all thoughts, feelings, and reactions can be discussed safely if members avoid attacking each other and are invested in understanding the other members' experiences; leaders can also promote a climate in which the spirit of being an *ally* is valued (Kaklauskas & Nettles, 2019). Allies can then advocate for another person in group who is being misunderstood, mistreated, or marginalized.

Yalom and Leszcz (2020) argue that contemporary group leaders must build groups that mirror our society and model openness and acceptance so that group members from minority or oppressed backgrounds can be accepted as individuals and not as stereotypes. Goals for therapy may also drive the decision to include certain identities in group; while some transgendered people may seek group treatment specifically to process issues of identity, others may have wide-ranging needs that are responsive to inclusion in mixed-gender groups (Israel et al., 2008). Additionally, teaching group participants about microaggressions, dynamics of power, and vulnerability are central to establishing a tone of warm acceptance regarding differences.

> A member named Andy, who identified as a trans*man, expressed some desire to increase his confidence now that he was more secure in his identity. During the pre-group meeting, he was informed that he might be the only transgender person in group, but he thought being accepted might be possible. Andy stated that unlike other places in his life, he wanted to share his identity early in the group so he could be authentic. The members learned about Andy's history, including how hard he worked each day to change his appearance before leaving his apartment. Other members disclosed their sexual identities as minorities and provided early empathy in the group. Andy also educated other members about the need for gender neutral bathrooms on campus. Although the members noted that they hadn't known a transgender person before Andy, they embraced his social actions with affirmations and offers of support. He found these responses heartwarming after being rejected by his family. By the end of the group, not only was Andy popular due to his quick and high level of self-disclosure and his support for others, but he gained the confidence to seek a leadership position at his workplace. It was clear that the collaborative decision to include Andy and prepare him for self-disclosure risks was the correct one in this case!

As LeFay (2020) proposes, such gender challenges should be specifically explored with the client to assess their experiences with bias/discrimination and transphobia, and a decision made as to whether the group would represent an affirming space for the trans* individual.

Brabender (2006) expounded on a useful lens for the examination of ethical dilemmas, referencing the principle of Justice because of its relevance to the group therapist's consideration of the many sources of diversity. She observed that leader awareness of Justice includes both being responsive to the particular needs of those subjected to oppression and attending to one's own culturally-based identity issues.

In a society marked by racism, heterosexism, and other "isms," we have opportunities to transform the group's experience rather than perpetuating these dynamics. As these dynamics arise in our PGMs and later group sessions, therapists are given the chance to assist in the creation of healing experiences rather than allowing potentially hurtful interactions to occur or repeat (Turner, 2018). When appropriate, therapists can challenge new group members to expand their perspectives to include consideration of culture and identity; an overarching social justice paradigm applied to group therapy can also increase leader sensitivity to nuances in the interactions of diverse members (MacNair-Semands, 2007). Additionally, addressing social privilege together with knowledge of systemic change can be important for group leaders to explore within their organizations (Chen, 2013).

For example, Dick is a CEO of a local company while earning his Master's degree and is joining a new group. In the second session, he declares to the group that he would need to miss some sessions because of his pressing work commitments. The leaders had failed to pick this up earlier and were immediately concerned that other members were having nonverbal reactions that Dick was seeing himself as in an entitled position vis-à-vis them. Another member, Jean, then complains that her parents are sending her "to the islands again during spring break with my cousin." Although other members had mentioned financial hardships and difficulties paying rent, both Dick and Jean seem unaware of their class privilege. If other members are unable or unwilling to bring up the reactions or differences, leaders might raise the topic and ask how it might feel to those in the group with less wealth. Jean might even become aware that she actually just wanted her parents, who are busy CEOs, to want to be *with her* rather than shipping her off during her break. The leaders help Jean identify both her privileged financial status alongside her poverty of emotional support, which helps other members relate to her with more empathy. If Dick stayed silent, the leaders might again ask if he has a perspective on his position and guide him toward insight by connecting him with Jean and the other members.

Members such as Dick and Jean frequently are oblivious to their privilege given its constancy in their lives. Having privilege identified in the group potentially increases members' social sensitivity. It allows members to consider in a more active way how they will or will not respond to their possession of privilege.

Goals and Norms

The PGM involves both sharing important information (content about the group) and creating the underlying processes (e.g., building an alliance with the leaders, orienting the client to the interpersonal approach of the group, and exploring how the member may reveal themselves and respond to others). The goals of preparation include: describing therapeutic group norms, including regular attendance and punctuality; preparing the client for exploring diverse identities and differences; forecasting that discomfort might surface in early sessions to inoculate the members; and nurturing positive expectations of the group (Whittingham, 2018; Yalom & Leszcz, 2020). With a collaborative approach and confidence about how effective group therapy can be, the client should feel understood and respected from the very start of this first meeting.

Group therapy is a difficult modality for many individuals to accept as their first treatment, so it is important to include the *specific interpersonal goals* the client wants to address. A more intensive individualized preparation, with some skill-building before entering into the group, may increase the scope of clients treated effectively in group therapy. Individuals who have had a prior successful course of therapy will likely do better in group psychotherapy than clients for whom the group is their first psychotherapy experience (MacNair-Semands, 2002; Rutan et al., 2014). Though good composition can increase the likelihood of important here-and-now interactions and interpersonal engagement, leaders also create these dynamics through direct teaching and modeling of group norms. As early as the PGM, leaders can highlight and reinforce members who are (1) eager for engagement, (2) willing to take social risks, and (3) express emotions with curiosity, which will later increase the likelihood of the group becoming cohesive and effective (Yalom & Leszcz, 2020).

Leaders can emphasize ways that members should begin to reveal themselves gradually and appropriately. On the one hand, they work to ensure that each member is active in sharing personal information with the group (Tschuschke et al., 1996). On the other hand, they discourage members from making excessive self-disclosure before trust has developed in the group. Leaders can mention that they initially often serve as "coaches or advocates" to help invite the member into group interactions that are related to personal goals. This coaching role can be viewed as an initial supportive alliance that assists the member to connect with others with similar issues, leading the client to feel as though they belong and are accepted by others as they reveal themselves.

> Vonda states in her PGM that she is not assertive and is afraid of conflict. Explaining how the group norms can support Vonda's personal goals of approaching conflict (rather than avoiding it) provides a framework for the upcoming group process. Vonda can be informed about how leaders tend to intervene when destructive conflict arises in the group. Telling Vonda that gathering the member's personal history behind the angry reactions and helping group members to recognize when feedback is based on personal *history* rather than interpersonal *rejection* can help her to better understand the feedback and reflection processes.

Additionally, having an informative and comprehensive PGM can prepare Vonda to learn the group norms and thus ease her anticipatory anxiety. It also saves the member from an adverse experience early in that person's participation in the group. Setting the stage for the group norms during the PGM also includes assessing Vonda's responses and agreement with the expectations, format, and functioning of the group. As mentioned, members generally do well in group therapy when their personal goals also align with the communicated goals of the specific group around interpersonal functioning. For example, if Vonda's stated goals are initially too vague or difficult to put in behavioral terms, the meeting can help her hone and specify these goals prior to the first session. Instead of saying she wants to "learn to be assertive," she might be encouraged—through a collaborative pre-group discussion—to tell her fellow members that she wants to initiate conversations with others when in disagreement and to speak up to authority figures more often. The leaders might even invite her to consider openly and authentically disagreeing with a leader's perspective when fitting.

An ethical approach means clearly describing and offering a rationale for the group norms during the PGM so that the prospective client can make an informed decision. In general, such norms include (Turner, 2018):

- Using respectful tone and language
- Using "I" language
- Avoiding shaming and blaming of others
- Adhering to confidentiality, including limitations and differences from individual context
- Revealing risk factors and safety issues both within group and outside of group
- Informing the leader of absences and remaining in group for a certain period of time
- Expectations regarding extra-group contacts
- Responding to microaggressions
- Handling premature terminations, to attempt a respectful ending process
- Refraining from using electronic devices during group

Other norms can include restrictions on eating or drinking during group, disallowing the use of social media to discuss group member identities or experiences, electronic recordings of the group and how they may be used for training in clinical case conferences, and details about fee structure including any cancellation or no-show fees. Norms around punctuality and attending group under the influence of substances should also be discussed (Burlingame et al., 2006). Additionally, the PGM is a time for candidates to learn more about leader experience and credentials related to group and clinical work, including any information about students who may be under supervision. Credentials and training details should also be mentioned during the intake or initial consultation to provide the potential member with advanced information that might affect their attraction to the group. Sharing all of this information honors the principle of Respect for Autonomy.

Expectations for precipitous terminations often include that the member will attend a final group session to give the group an opportunity for closure and feedback. This relates to the principles of Non-maleficence, Beneficence, and Autonomy. The final meeting would support Autonomy in providing the departing member space for non-impulsive decision-making and the other members the space to communicate their reactions to the person directly. It serves Beneficence in that benefit can come from this type of processing; it also serves Non-maleficence in that harm can come from closing off communications abruptly. Leaders should also explain what contact will be made after the PGM and before the group start date, particularly for those in ongoing individual counseling who need more support prior to the group.

Other ways to honor a client's Autonomy include providing information about social relationships with other members. Leaders can emphasize that blurring those boundaries could hinder group members from achieving their goals and fully benefiting from group therapy. Specific examples of non-disclosure in a group associated with outside processing of group material with another member can be provided so members can fully understand how these dynamics might play out if the agreement is broken.

Fears and Myths

Typically, members have certain fears about what they will experience (e.g., being rejected, offending others), and until those fears are acknowledged and explored, the ethical principle of Beneficence cannot be honored as little productive work can occur. However, if the group candidate is asked and then can voice any negative assumptions or myths about group treatment (such as with a handout from the CORE-R battery of measures or a selection measure), these stigmatizing views can be challenged and shifted.

Members can experience a greater sense of safety and comfort by learning more about how leaders will intervene to address any tense or conflictual processes and move toward interactional healing, reflection, and understanding. If the leaders are not using a selection measure, the client's interpersonal patterns can be highlighted through careful attention to the interactional processes that happen in the here-and-now of the pre-group preparation meeting, as well as a review of the candidate's interpersonal history. This not only helps to provide clarity about the client's goals but it can also prepare the member experientially for the group's focus on learning through interpersonal interactions (Yalom & Leszcz, 2020).

The PGM process also includes answering any questions potential members have and taking the time to provide specific examples of how the particular client's interpersonal patterns might present and be responded to in the group. Sharing examples about how members learn to hear feedback and reflect on it, for instance, may allay some of the fears and even lead to a member's excitement for practicing real-life change through relating to peers.

Because many PGM processes include exploring both the relational strengths and problems of members, the encounter provides an opportunity for the leaders to build an alliance with the client. For example,

Doug knows he was heavily criticized as a child and struggles with worthlessness; he may assume he is too fragile for group treatment and will be rejected by members. This is exactly his work in the group! Doug may only be able to identify that he is a loyal friend. The leaders can provide reassurance that other members are more likely to see his positive qualities than Doug is himself. Doug may be informed that he will eventually be able to accept and acknowledge the positive qualities and strengths of the self over time. The leaders may choose to highlight for Doug the positive qualities they notice during the PGM. The therapists may also invite Doug to imagine that he could begin to believe he offers kindness, humor, and generosity both in and outside the group.

Hence, the PGM can also help Doug to *envision the types of co-member relationships* he hopes to build and maintain over time.

Similarly, if clients are provided with clear guidelines for effective group behavior and here-and-now interaction, they can feel less threatened by the notion of gradually revealing personal information. One primary goal of pre-group preparation is to help prospective group members manage the anxiety that usually accompanies starting a group (Shechtman & Kiezel, 2016) through clarification and demythologizing of the group experience (Bernard et al, 2008). Because anxiety about entering a group is universal and intrinsic, it is helpful to eliminate anxiety caused by the lack of clarity about goals, tasks, roles, or the direction of the group (Yalom & Leszcz, 2020). Anticipating frustrations or setbacks by normalizing and addressing them during preparation sessions can ultimately prevent premature terminations. Research has also documented that addressing such negative expectations (e.g., my needs will not be met, I will be attacked) about a group significantly contributes to improved outcomes (Söchting et al., 2018).

Describing the Work of Group

Therapists can educate the members that group is an opportunity to increase awareness about how they relate to others so they can learn more beneficial ways to make social connections, while engaged in forming a therapeutic community. The interpersonal process of the group should also be discussed (Ribeiro, 2020). Therapists should provide a clear conceptual framework regarding interpersonal patterns and how they are formed and maintained, with honesty about the amount of time it may take to revise or replace such long-standing patterns. Individual concerns should be addressed with attunement to the client's level of sophistication regarding the treatment process, especially for members new to therapy or from non-Western cultures (Yalom & Leszcz, 2020).

A concise, simple set of instructions about how a group works provides a conceptual framework for understanding the roles that the group leader and group members are expected to fulfill. Information is geared toward correcting misconceptions and promoting group development by identifying common stumbling blocks and mitigating unrealistic expectations about group treatment (Brabender & Fallon, 2009). Key aspects of appropriate group participation, including self-disclosure, interpersonal feedback, confidentiality, extra-group contact, and the parameters of termination should all be defined (Yalom & Leszcz, 2020).

For the full potential of group participation to develop, members also require an understanding of the various methods and processes of the group. Yalom and Leszcz (2020) propose that leaders spell out that each member will often face the common difficulty of establishing and maintaining intimate and rewarding relationships with others. The group is then described as a social laboratory involving working directly with honest exploration between members, which in turn can lead to generalizing the learning into the social world outside of the group. These authors prompt members to share their immediate feelings toward other members and leaders in the group, a process that involves taking interpersonal risks. Members are informed that this process is crucial to making life-changing pattern shifts that allow for more authenticity and acceptance of the self.

In this classic model, Yalom and Leszcz (2020) also remind members that the main task is to learn as much as possible about the way each individual relates to each other person in the group. In addition to normalizing that self-disclosure can feel quite vulnerable and frightening, the member should be cautioned about what opportunities they could miss if they instead withdraw in comfortable silence. These authors also remind leaders, however, that it is the member who must choose to bring in the information disclosed in the PGM rather than the leaders doing so, which could be an ethical violation and also damage trust and the alliance. For instance, leaders may be tempted to urge Kathleen to reveal her fluid sexual orientation if another member identifying as queer later discloses and seeks to use peer support. Instead, the leaders brainstorm with Kathleen in the PGM about ways that she might know when she is ready to reveal (i.e., serving the principle of Autonomy as well as Kathleen's confidentiality), considering the various responses she might receive and how she may give help to others.

A Model for Preparation Using Assessments for Interpersonal Attachments and Culture

Tasca et al. (2021) describe an excellent method of pre-group preparation for group psychodynamic-interpersonal psychotherapy (GPIP) based on a case formulation of the individual. Leaders directly share the client's case formulation based on the model's central concepts of object relations and cyclical maladaptive interpersonal patterns. Therapists then provide the member with information on how the group works and what to expect, as well as a sense of how change may occur in group therapy. They troubleshoot in advance any potential issues that are consistent with the interpersonal and intrapersonal dynamics identified in the case formulation that may surface in the group (i.e., inoculation). This is consistent with the goals of providing clients with a new understanding of themselves and then giving them new experiences and practice in relationships in group (Levenson, 2017; Whittingham, 2018).

In line with what Yalom and Leszcz's (2020) classic text on group therapy proposes, the pre-group preparation for GPIP typically takes place in one or two meetings that may be combined with a pre-group assessment. Tasca et al.'s (2021) emphasis on pre-group preparation is also consistent with recommendations from experts in the clinical group practice. For example, the American Group Psychotherapy Association Clinical Practice Guidelines (Bernard et al., 2008) devote a significant amount of attention to the assessment and preparation of clients for group therapy. Similar to the Kaklauskas and Greene support materials (which can be found and downloaded from the Kaklauskas & Greene 2019 book's website by clicking the button "Support Materials" at https://www.routledge.com/Core-Principles-of-Group-Psychotherapy-An-Integrated-Theory-Research/Kaklauskas-Greene/p/book/9780367203092) and the CORE-R Battery (Burlingame et al., 2006), Tasca et al. (2021) also provide sample written descriptions and handouts related to client goals, the group therapy agreement (contract), and the group model.

Another inspiring emphasis from the GPIP model, similar to the Whittingham (2018) FBGT model, is exploring aspects of member identities and addressing them thoroughly in the pre-group session. Most individuals from ethnic and racial minorities have experienced blatant prejudice and rejection or more subtle forms of discriminatory messages such as microaggressions. GPIP therapists are encouraged to honestly examine their implicit

---

Box 4.2   Summary of Pre-group Preparation and its Benefits

1. Both empirical research and expert consensus consistently endorse the value of pre-group preparation.
2. Successful preparation will help modulate client anxiety and communicate information that enables the client to provide appropriate, ethically-based informed consent.
3. Successful preparation includes teaching the members about respectful behaviors for differing identities and eliciting responses about how members might react to differences.
4. Effective preparation enhances the therapeutic alliance with the leaders.
5. Effective preparation promotes agreement between the leader and prospective group members on the goals and tasks of group therapy.
6. Clients who are well prepared for group are significantly more likely to participate meaningfully, comply with treatment, and are much less likely to stop therapy prematurely (Bernard et al., 2008; Yalom & Leszcz, 2020).

---

biases and values related to the minority group with which the member identifies. A classic study found that successful discussion and resolution of a microaggression can result in a heightened therapeutic alliance (Owen et al., 2014). One of the core issues in the assessment and pre-group preparation phase, therefore, is to explore how minority status might impact an individual's work and demeanor in a therapy group and on the functioning of the group as a whole (Ribeiro et al., 2018; Tasca et al., 2021). See Box 4.2 for a summary of pre-group preparation and its benefits.

Preparing for Extra-Group Contact

Leaders should set clear norms around extra-group or outside contact. While many leaders believe that agreements are crucial to creating a safe and healthy group climate, therapists also find such agreements challenging to describe and enforce. Gumpert and Black (2006) describe an important study of 90 social workers (20 years of experience on average) which involved presenting them with a list of 17 ethical issues thought to be relevant to work with groups. Therapists were then asked to rate the frequency with which they had faced each of these issues in their group practice. Surprisingly, at the top of the list was the issue concerning communication among group members outside of group meetings. The authors found this difficult to explain at the time, and yet recent group training programs continue to emphasize such norms to help prevent the destructive dynamics that can surface with such extra-group contact. So how do leaders best inform members of the risks of extra-group communication?

Such agreements and contracts represent an ethical approach and respect member autonomy by informing potential members of the norms before they join a group. Even more recent updates are provided by the Oregon State University's Group Therapy Participation Agreement in 2020 (see Kaklauskas & Greene, 2019 book's website referenced earlier), and include the following language:

> Group is not a place to make social friends, and if you use it this way, you may not have the desired benefits you want out of your experience. Group is a chance to have

therapeutic relationships in which you learn more about yourself and the ways in which you relate to others. You may have strong feelings toward some members of the group, as you do with people in your life; however, group can be a safe environment to explore those feelings and how you act on them. If you do have contact with someone outside of group (e.g., see someone on campus), we ask that you share that contact with the group at the next meeting. As a guideline, however, please no social media, texting or out of group socializing with any members while you are a member of group.

When discussing this agreement, leaders can provide examples such as the following:

Imagine that you want to invite two members of your group to go get coffee after the session. Several things might result: 1) One member agrees, but the other member has to go to work. Even though the second member was invited, they might feel left out or even envious because they couldn't be a part of a potential new social connection. Other members could also view the pair leaving together and feel excluded as a result; 2) Once at the coffee shop, the conversation naturally turns to group dynamics and other members because those are shared experiences. One member may talk about another member rather than address their concerns in the group, missing out on practicing their goal of providing direct feedback; and 3) One member decides to reveal deeper emotions and personal history to the other member. The member feels supported and thus does not feel the need to use the group to work through these issues, withdrawing from the group. This contributes to the group members staying on a more superficial level.

There are numerous clinical examples to draw on relating to extra-group contact, including members who begin dating and consequently leave the group prematurely. Each leader can tailor examples that might relate to the prospective member's clinical issues to help them better understand the potential consequences.

Providing examples to help potential members understand how extra-group contact can affect other members may also be complex in some settings. Rutan et al. (2019) note how socializing and extra-group contacts will be handled generally depends on the nature of the group. They argue that while most ongoing psychodynamic groups strictly discourage contact and socializing—since they can lead to secrets, collusive relationships, or verbal withdrawal—certain groups related to sobriety or abstinence may instead encourage ongoing connection and support. Extra-group contact may also be inevitable in certain environments, such as inpatient hospital units, prisons, or small-town communities. Many group agreements also suggest that group members who have contact with another member, especially if an interaction elicits emotions, commit to talking about this in the next group session. Rutan et al. (2019) further purport that such an agreement can build an overt, dependable, and clinically-guided approach to handling these situations.

Final Note

One example of leader competence is in the selection and preparation of clients for a group. An understanding of privileged identities and those identities treated with marginality in society must be explored and considered in our pre-group processes. Selection instruments can help clinicians assess client characteristics to determine fit and clarify client needs for the pre-group preparation. How potential members respond to differing identities should also influence selection decisions. The sample questions provided earlier in this chapter can be used for the leader to elicit the client's approach to differing identities. Assessing the client's history of discrimination and bias is also helpful.

Another essential leader competency is carefully considering the *composition* of members who can tolerate and benefit from interpersonal feedback. Leaders should tailor the inclusion and exclusion criteria when forming a specific group; however, some interpersonal factors must be considered relative rather than absolute. If group candidates are overly silent, overly angry, or avoidant of emotional immediacy, exclusion should be considered. Also, exclusion can be considered if the client also fails to appreciate the therapy process, is overly dominant, lacks interpersonal sensitivity, or is either disengaged or concrete. Exclusion can be difficult because shame, hurt, and threat may arise for the excluded member. An ethical approach attempts to minimize harm with a caring but authentic approach while finding alternative treatments.

Appropriate pre-group preparation is described as a cornerstone of evidence-based group therapy. Adapting preparation to be culturally attuned to the member is an important consideration; leaders can also create a climate in which being an *ally* is appreciated and reinforced. Typically, members have fears about what they will experience, and until those fears are explored, the ethical principle of Beneficence cannot be honored as little fruitful work will occur. However, if the group candidate is invited to voice their negative assumptions about a group, the views can be disputed and changed. Intensive individualized preparation, with some skill-building before entering into the group, may increase the scope of clients treated effectively in group therapy.

CEU Questions

1. It is unethical for either leaders or members to use undue pressure to keep members in the group who may be considering leaving, even if they are at risk for deteriorating. (T/F)
2. Contracts and disclosure forms should include (a) degrees and licenses of the leader, (b) fees, billing, and scheduling practices, (c) confidentiality and its limits, (d) information about the nature of group and of the risks, benefits, rights, and agreements as a member of a therapy group, or (e) all of the above.
3. When a group leader informs new members about the norms of the group, it is a good idea to present information about norms for extra-group contact and when it is necessary for members to report the contact to the group. (T/F)
4. It would be unfair to consider how potential members respond to differing identities when making selection decisions since some clients have little exposure to diversity. (T/F)
5. Intensive pre-group preparation may increase the range of clients treated effectively in group therapy. (T/F)
6. Leader awareness of Justice includes being responsive to the particular needs of those subjected to oppression but does not apply to attending to one's own culturally-based identity issues. (T/F)
7. Expectations that a terminating member will attend a final group session to give the group an opportunity for closure relates to the principles of (a) Autonomy and Fidelity, (b) Fidelity and Non-maleficence, (c) Autonomy, Non-maleficence, and Beneficence, or (d) none of the above.
8. Extra-group contact may be inevitable in certain environments, such as inpatient hospital units and prisons. (T/F)

Answer Key: 1. T; 2. e; 3. T; 4. F; 5. T; 6. F; 7. c; 8. T

Discussion Questions

1. What are the most common client fears about group therapy and how do you explore them?
2. In exploring sociocultural identities, how do you approach each potential member's responses to differences?
3. In the PGM, what benefits may come from exploring cultural and social issues that impact our group members?
4. How might you discuss the power differential between you and your group members?
5. What ethical issues have you seen surface in relation to selection or composition decisions?
6. How can leaders prepare clients around issues of coercion or scapegoating without creating undo anxiety?
7. What are the ethical and legal issues involved in premature termination by members?

Vignettes/Role-Plays

1. A therapist is about to disband her group due to her retirement. Some members will be placed in other groups and some members will terminate altogether. In the final sessions, some members discuss the possibility of developing friendships outside of the group. What might be some important considerations for the therapist to foster as members pursue this issue?
2. Erica and Aayla have been in a long-term open group together for over five months and begin dating. Others notice that they both reveal less to the group and attend less regularly. Soon, Rachel mentioned that she had seen them out dancing and wondered if their relationship had shifted to be more than friends, though this violates the norms of their group. How might the leaders approach them both if they confess to dating? Please address and consider the following: a) Leaders may ask one or both to leave the group; if so, the leaders could consider giving Erica and Aayla autonomy to decide who leaves; b) the leaders could keep the member who has been in the group the longest, or c) the leaders could keep the member with less outside support.
3. A new therapist learns in a PGM that the potential member has not had much exposure to people with physical disabilities and might feel anxious related to another member previously accepted in the group. What factors might the therapist consider in response and what ethical principles might apply?

References

Baker, E. L. (2010). *Selecting members for group therapy: A continued validation study of the group selection questionnaire* [Unpublished doctoral dissertation]. Brigham Young University. https://scholarsarchive.byu.edu/cgi/viewcontent.cgi?article=3127&context=etd

Barkham, M., Hardy, G. E., & Startup, M. (1996). The IIP-32: A short version of the Inventory of Interpersonal Problems. *British Journal of Clinical Psychology*, *35*, 21–35. 10.1111/j.2044-8260.1996.tb01159.x

Bernard, H., Burlingame, G., Flores, P., Greene, L., Joyce, A., Kobos, J. C., Leszcz, M., MacNair-Semands, R. R., Piper, W. E., Slocum McEneaney, A. M., & Feirman, D. (2008). Clinical practice guidelines for group psychotherapy. *International Journal of Group Psychotherapy*, *58*(4), 455–542. 10.1521/ijgp.2008.58.4.455

Brabender, V. (2006). The ethical group psychotherapist. *International Journal of Group Psychotherapy*, *56*(4), 395–414. 10.1521/ijgp.2006.56.4.395

Brabender, V. M., & Fallon, A. (2009). Ethical hot spots of combined individual and group therapy: Applying four ethical systems. *International Journal of Group Psychotherapy*, *59*(1), 127–147. 10.1521/ijgp.2009.59.1.127

Brown, N. W. (2008). Troubling silences in therapy groups. *Journal of Contemporary Psychotherapy*, *38*(2), 81–85. 10.1007/s10879-007-9071-z

Brown, N. W. (2018). *Psychoeducational groups: Process and practice* (4th ed.). Routledge. 10.4324/9781315169590

Burlingame, G. M., Cox, J. C., Davies, D. R., Layne, C. M., & Gleave, R. (2011). The Group Selection Questionnaire: Further refinements in group member selection. *Group Dynamics: Theory, Research, and Practice*, *15*(1), 60–74. 10.1037/a0020220

Burlingame, G. M., Davies, D. R., Cox, J. C., Baker, E. L., Pearson, M., Beecher, M., & Gleave, R. (2012). *The Group Readiness Questionnaire manual* [Unpublished manuscript]. Provided by author.

Burlingame, G. M. & Strauss, B. (2021). Efficacy of small group treatments: Foundation for evidence-based practice. In M. Barkham, W. Lutz & L. G. Castonguay (Eds.), *Bergin & Garfield's handbook of psychotherapy and behavior change* (7th ed.). Wiley. https://www.wiley.com/en-us/Bergin+and+Garfield%27s+Handbook+of+Psychotherapy+and+Behavior+Change%2C+7th+Edition-p-9781119536581

Burlingame, G. M., Strauss, B., & Joyce, A. S. (2013). Change mechanisms and effectiveness of small group treatments. In M. J. Lambert (Ed.), *Bergin and GarfielFd's handbook of psychotherapy and behavior change* (6th ed., pp 640–689). Wiley. https://www.researchgate.net/publication/303105298_Change_mechanisms_and_effectiveness_of_small_group_treatments

Burlingame, G. M., Strauss, B., Joyce, A., MacNair-Semands, R., MacKenzie, K. R., Ogrodniczuk, J., & Taylor, S. (2006). *CORE Battery—Revised: An assessment tool kit for promoting optimal group selection, process and outcome.* American Group Psychotherapy Association.

Carter, E. F., Mitchell, S. L., & Krautheim, M. D. (2001). Understanding and addressing clients' resistance to group counseling. *The Journal for Specialists in Group Work*, *26*(1), 66–80. 10.1080/01933920108413778

Chen, E. C. (2013). Multicultural competence and social justice advocacy in group psychology and group psychotherapy. *APA Division 49 Newsletter: The Group Psychologist (April 2013)*. https://www.apadivisions.org/division-49/publications/newsletter/group-psychologist/2012/07/social-justice

Chen, E. C., Kakkad, D., & Balzano, J. (2008). Multicultural competence and evidence-based practice in group therapy. *Journal of Clinical Psychology*, *64*(11), 1261–1278. 10.1002/jclp.20533

Cone-Uemura, K., & Bentley, E. S. (2018). Multicultural/diversity issues in groups. In M. D. Ribeiro, J. M. Gross, & M. M. Turner (Eds.), *The college counselor's guide to group psychotherapy* (pp. 21–33). Routledge. https://www.taylorfrancis.com/chapters/multicultural-diversity-issues-groups-karen-cone-uemura-eri-suzuki-bentley/e/10.4324/9781315545455-3?context=ubx&refId=3b73ea41-ea9f-4ad8-b71f-1e9dc290de0a

Costa, P. T., & McCrae, R. R. (1992). The five-factor model of personality and its relevance to personality disorders. *Journal of Personality Disorders*, *6*(4), 343–359. 10.1521/pedi.1992.6.4.343

Cox, J. C. (2008). Selecting members for group therapy: A validation study of the Group Selection Questionnaire. *Dissertation Abstracts International: Selection B: The Sciences and Engineering*, *69*(3-B), 1947. https://psycnet.apa.org/record/2008-99180-219

Cox, J. C., Burlingame, G. M., Davies, D. R., Gleave, R., Barlow, S., & Johnson, J. (2004, February 23-28). The group selection questionnaire: Further refinements in group member selection. [Symposium]. American Group Psychotherapy Annual Meeting, New York, NY, United States.

Crits-Christoph, P., Gibbons, M. B. C., & Mukherjee, D. (2013). Psychotherapy process-outcome research. In M. J. Lambert (Ed.). *Bergin and Garfield's handbook of psychotherapy and behavior change* (6th ed., pp. 298–340). Wiley. https://pennstate.pure.elsevier.com/en/publications/psychotherapy-process-outcome-research

D'Andrea, M. (2014). Understanding racial/cultural identity development theories to promote effective multicultural group counseling. In J. L. DeLucia-Waack, C. R. Kalodner, & M. T. Riva (Eds.), *Handbook of group counseling and psychotherapy* (2nd ed., pp. 196–208). Sage Publications. 10.4135/9781544308555

Fenger, M., Mortensen, E. L., Poulsen, S., & Lau, M. (2011). No-shows, drop-outs and completers in psychotherapeutic treatment: Demographic and clinical predictors in a large sample of non-psychotic patients. *Nordic Journal of Psychiatry, 65*(3), 183–191. 10.3109/08039488.2010.515687

Fjelstad, A., Høgelend, P., & Lorentzen, S. (2017). Patterns of change in interpersonal problems during and after short-term and long-term psychodynamic group therapy: A randomized clinical trial, *Psychotherapy Research, 27*(3), 350–361. 10.1080/10503307.2015.1102357

Gans, J. S., & Counselman, E. F. (2010). Patient selection for psychodynamic group psychotherapy: Practical and dynamic considerations. *International Journal of Group Psychotherapy, 60*(2), 197–220. 10.1521/ijgp.2010.60.2.197

Giannone, Z. A., Cox, D. W., Kealy, D., & Ogrodniczuk, J. S. (2020). Identity-focused group interventions among emerging adults: A review. *North American Journal of Psychology, 22*(1), 41–62. 10.1080/09515070.2020.1870438

Greene, L. R., Abramowitz, S. I., Davidson, C. V., & Edwards, D. W. (1980). Gender, race, and referral to group psychotherapy: Further empirical evidence of countertransference. *International Journal of Group Psychotherapy, 30*(3), 357–364. 10.1080/00207284.1980.11491698

Gross, J. M. (2010). The nine basic steps for a successful group. In S. S. Fehr (Ed.), *101 interventions in group therapy* (Revised ed., pp. 421–423). Routledge. http://docshare01.docshare.tips/files/26655/266559357.pdf

Gumpert, J. & Black, P. N. (2006). Ethical issues in group work: What are they? How are they managed? *Social Work with Groups, 29*(4), 61–74. 10.1300/J009v29n04_05

Hammond, E. S., & Marmarosh, C. L. (2011). The influence of individual attachment styles on group members' experience of therapist transitions. *International Journal of Group Psychotherapy, 61*(4), 596–620. 10.1521/ijgp.2011.61.4.596

Hewitt, P. L. (2020). Perfecting, belonging, and repairing: A dynamic-relational approach to perfectionism. *Canadian Psychology/Psychologie Canadienne, 61*(2), 101–110. 10.1037/cap0000209

Hewitt, P. L., Chen, C., Smith, M. M., Zhang, L., Habke, M., Flett, G. L., & Mikail, S. (2020). Patient perfectionism and clinician impression formation during an initial interview. *Psychology and Psychotherapy: Theory, Research and Practice, 94*(1), 45–62. 10.1111/papt.12266

Hewitt, P. L., Mikail, S. F., Flett, G. L., & Dang, S. S. (2018). Specific formulation feedback in dynamic-relational group psychotherapy of perfectionism. *Psychotherapy, 55*(2), 179–185. 10.1037/pst0000137

Hook, J. N., Davis, D., Owen, J., & DeBlaere, C. (2017). *Cultural humility: Engaging diverse identities in therapy.* American Psychological Association. 10.1037/0000037-000

Horowitz, L. M., Alden, L. E., Wiggins, J. S., & Pincus, A. L. (2000). *Inventory of interpersonal problems (IIP)*. Mind Garden, Inc. https://marketplace.unl.edu/buros/inventory-of-interpersonal-problems.html

Horowitz, L. M., Rosenberg, S. E., Baer, B. A., Ureño, G., & Villaseñor, V. S. (1988). Inventory of interpersonal problems: Psychometric properties and clinical applications. *Journal of Consulting and Clinical Psychology, 56*(6), 885–892. 10.1037/0022-006X.56.6.885

Horowitz, L. M., & Strack, S. (Eds.). (2010). *Handbook of interpersonal psychology: Theory, research, assessment, and therapeutic interventions.* Wiley. https://www.wiley.com/en-us/Handbook+of+Interpersonal+Psychology:+Theory,+Research,+Assessment,+and+Therapeutic+Interventions-p-9780470471609

Horvath, A. O., Del Re, A. C., Flückiger, C., & Symonds, D. (2011). Alliance in individual psychotherapy. *Psychotherapy, 48*(1), 9–16. 10.1037/a0022186

Israel, T., Gorcheva, R., Burnes, T. R., & Walther, W. A. (2008). Helpful and unhelpful therapy experiences of LGBT clients. *Psychotherapy Research, 18*(3), 294–305. 10.1080/10503300701506920

Jensen, H. H., Mortensen, E. L., & Lotz, M. (2014). Drop-out from a psychodynamic group psychotherapy outpatient unit. *Nordic Journal of Psychiatry, 68*(8), 594–604. 10.3109/08039488.2014.902499

Joyce, A. S., McCallum, M., Piper, W. E., & Ogrodniczuk, J. S. (2000). Role behavior expectancies and alliance change in short-term individual psychotherapy. *Journal of Psychotherapy Practice & Research, 9*(4), 213–225. https://psycnet.apa.org/record/2000-16107-005

Kaklauskas, F. J., & Greene, L. R. (Eds.). (2019). *Core principles of group psychotherapy: An integrated theory, research, and practice training manual.* Routledge. https://www.routledge.com/Core-Principles-of-Group-Psychotherapy-An-Integrated-Theory-Research/Kaklauskas-Greene/p/book/9780367203092

Kaklauskas, F. J., & Nettles, R. (2019). Towards multicultural and diversity proficiency as a group psychotherapist. In F. J. Kaklauskas, & L. R. Greene (Eds.), *Core principles of group psychotherapy: A training manual for theory, research, and practice* (pp. 25–46). Routledge. https://www.taylorfrancis.com/chapters/towards-multicultural-diversity-proficiency-group-psychotherapist-francis-kaklauskas-reginald-nettles/e/10.4324/9780429260803-2

Kealy, D., Ogrodniczuk, J. S., Piper, W. E., & Sierra-Hernandez, C. A. (2016). When it is not a good fit: Clinical errors in patient selection and group composition in group psychotherapy. *Psychotherapy, 53*(3), 308–313. 10.1037/pst0000069

Kivlighan, D. M., Jr., & Angelone, E. O. (1992). Interpersonal problems: Variables influencing participants' perception of group climate. *Journal of Counseling Psychology, 39*(4), 468–472. 10.1037/0022-0167.39.4.468

Kivlighan, D. M., III, Adams, M. C., Drinane, J. M., Tao, K. W., & Owen, J. (2019). Construction and validation of the Multicultural Orientation Inventory—Group Version. *Journal of Counseling Psychology, 66*(1), 45–55. 10.1037/cou0000294

Kivlighan, D. M., Jr., Li, X., & Gillis, L. (2015). Do I fit with my group? Within-member and within-group fit with the group in engaged group climate and group members feeling involved and valued. *Group Dynamics: Theory, Research, and Practice, 19*(2), 106–121. 10.1037/gdn0000025

Koocher, G. P. (2007). Twenty-first century ethical challenges for psychologists. *American Psychologist, 62*(5), 375–384. 10.1037/0003-066X.62.5.375

Krogel, J., Beecher, M. E., Presnell, J., Burlingame, G., & Simonsen, C. (2009). The Group Selection Questionnaire: A qualitative analysis of potential group members. *International Journal of Group Psychotherapy, 59*(4), 529–542. 10.1521/ijgp.2009.59.4.529

Krogel, J., Burlingame, G., Chapman, C., Renshaw, T., Gleave, R., Beecher, M., & MacNair-Semands, R. (2013). The Group Questionnaire: A clinical and empirically derived measure of group relationship. *Psychotherapy Research, 23*(3), 344–354. 10.1080/10503307.2012.729868

LeFay, S. (2020). Gender identity in group. In M. D. Ribeiro (Ed.), *Examining social identities and diversity issues in group therapy: Knocking at the boundaries* (pp. 41–52). Routledge. 10.4324/9780429022364-3

Levenson, H. (2017). Time-limited dynamic psychotherapy. In M. J. Dewan, B. N. Steenbarger, & R. P. Greenberg (Eds.). *The Art and Science of Brief Psychotherapies: A Practitioner's Guide-3rd ed.* (pp. 259–300). American Psychiatric Association.

Loeffler, J., Bormann, B., Burlingame, G., & Strauß, B. (2007). Auswahl von Patienten für eine Gruppenpsychotherapie: Eine Studie zur Überprüfung des GSQ an klinishchen Stichproben aus dem deutschen Sprachraum. *Zeitschrift für Psychiatrie, Psychologie und Psychotherapie, 55*, 77–86. 10.1024/1661-4747.55.2.75

MacNair-Semands, R. R. (2002). Predicting attendance and expectations for group therapy. *Group Dynamics: Theory, Research and Practice, 6*(3), 219–228. 10.1037/1089-2699.6.3.219

MacNair-Semands, R. R. (2007). Attending to the spirit of social justice as an ethical approach in group therapy. *International Journal of Group Psychotherapy, 57*(1), 61–66. 10.1521/ijgp.2007.57.1.61

MacNair-Semands, R. R. (2014, August 7–10). Using an ethical framework to promote transformation in group. In MacNair-Semands, R. R. (Chair), Marmarosh, C. & Riva, M., *Ethical issues in working with individual and cultural differences in groups* [Symposium]. American Psychological Association 122nd Annual Convention, Washington, DC, United States.

MacNair, R. R., & Corazzini, J. G. (1994). Client factors influencing group therapy dropout. *Psychotherapy: Theory, Research, Practice, Training, 31*(2), 352–362. 10.1037/h0090226

MacNair-Semands, R. R. & Lennon, E. (2017, March 6–11). *Confidentiality agreements and breaches: Ethical, legal, and clinical considerations in group therapy* [Conference session]. American Group Psychotherapy Annual Meeting, New York, NY, United States.

MacNair-Semands, R. R. & Lennon, E. (2019, February 25–March 2). *Assessing and managing suicide risk in group therapy: Ethical and clinical considerations* [Conference session]. American Group Psychotherapy Annual Meeting, Los Angeles, CA, United States.

MacNair-Semands, R. R., & Lese, K. P. (2000). Interpersonal problems and the perception of therapeutic factors in group therapy. *Small Group Research, 31*(2), 158–174. 10.1177/10464964 0003100202

Marmarosh, C. L. (2017). Attachment in group psychotherapy: Bridging theories, research, and clinical techniques. *International Journal of Group Psychotherapy, 67*(2), 157–160. 10.1080/002072 84.2016.1267573

Marmarosh, C. L., Markin, R. D., & Spiegel, E. B. (2013). *Attachment theory and group psychotherapy*. American Psychological Association. 10.1037/14186-000

McCallum, M., Piper, W. E., Ogrodniczuk, J. S., & Joyce, A. S. (2002). Early process and dropping out from short-term group therapy for complicated grief. *Group Dynamics: Theory, Research, and Practice, 6*(3), 243–254. 10.1037/1089-2699.6.3.243

Motherwell, L., & Shay, J. J. (2005). *Complex dilemmas in group psychotherapy: Pathways to resolution* (1st Ed.). Routledge. 10.4324/9780203021071

Ogrodniczuk, J. S., Piper, W. E., Joyce, A. S., McCallum, M., & Rosie, J. S. (2003). NEO-five factor personality traits as predictors of response to two forms of group psychotherapy. *International Journal of Group Psychotherapy, 53*(4), 417–442. 10.1521/ijgp.53.4.417.42832

Ogrodniczuk, J. S., Piper, W. E., Joyce, A. S., Steinberg, P. I., & Duggal, S. (2009). Interpersonal problems associated with narcissism among psychiatric outpatients. *Journal of Psychiatric Research, 43*(9), 837– 842. 10.1016/j.jpsychires.2008.12.005

Owen, J., Jordan, T. A., Turner, D., Davis, D. E., Hook, J. N., & Leach, M. M. (2014). Therapists' multicultural orientation: Client perceptions of cultural humility, spiritual/religious commitment, and therapy outcomes. *Journal of Psychology and Theology, 42*(1), 91–98. 10.1177/009164711404200110

Piper, W. E. (2008). Underutilization of short-term group therapy: Enigmatic or understandable? *Psychotherapy Research, 18*(2), 127–138. 10.1080/10503300701867512

Piper, W. E., & Ogrodniczuk, J. S. (2004). Brief group therapy. In J. L. DeLucia-Waack, D. A. Gerrity, C. R. Kalodner, & M. T. Riva (Eds.), *Handbook of group counseling and psychotherapy* (pp. 641–650). Sage Publications. 10.4135/9781452229683.n46

Piper, W. E., Ogrodniczuk, J. S., Joyce, A. S., & Weideman, R. (2011). *Short-term group therapies for complicated grief: Two research-based models*. American Psychological Association. 10.103 7/12344-000

Piper, W. E., Ogrodniczuk, J. S., Joyce, A. S., Weideman, R., & Rosie, J. S. (2007). Group composition and group therapy for complicated grief. *Journal of Consulting and Clinical Psychology, 75*(1), 116–125. 10.1037/0022-006X.75.1.116

Ribeiro, M. D. (Ed.). (2020). *Examining social identities and diversity issues in group therapy: Knocking at the boundaries*. Routledge. 10.4324/9780429022364

Ribeiro, M. D., Gross, J. M., & Turner, M. M. (2018). *The college counselor's guide to group psychotherapy*. Routledge. 10.4324/9781315545455

Rutan, J. S., Greene, L. S., & Kaklauskas, F. J. (2019). Preparing to begin a new group. In F. J. Kaklauskas & L. S. Greene (Eds.), *Core principles of group psychotherapy: An integrated theory, research, and practice training manual*. Routledge. 10.4324/9780429260803

Rutan, J. S., Stone, W. N., & Shay, J. J. (2014). *Psychodynamic group psychotherapy* (5th ed.). Guilford Press. https://www.guilford.com/books/Psychodynamic-Group-Psychotherapy/Rutan-Stone-Shay/9781462516506

Shechtman, Z., & Kiezel, A. (2016). Why do people prefer individual therapy over group therapy? *International Journal of Group Psychotherapy, 66*(4), 571–591. 10.1080/00207284.2016.1180042

Söchting, I., Lau, M., & Ogrodniczuk, J. (2018). Predicting compliance in group CBT using the group therapy questionnaire. *International Journal of Group Psychotherapy, 68*(2), 184–194. 10.1 080/00207284.2017.1371569

Strauss, B., Burlingame, G. M., & Bormann, B. (2008). Using the CORE-R battery in group psychotherapy. *Journal of Clinical Psychology, 64*(11), 1225–1237. 10.1002/jclp.20535

Sue, D. W. (2010). Microaggressions, marginality, and oppression: An introduction. In D. W. Sue (Ed.). In *Microaggressions and marginality: Manifestation, dynamics, and impact.* (pp. 1–22). Wiley.

Tasca, G. A., Mikail, S. F., & Hewitt, P. L. (2021). *Group psychodynamic-interpersonal psychotherapy*. American Psychological Association. https://www.apa.org/pubs/books/group-psychodynamic-interpersonal-psychotherapy-sample-chapter.pdf

Turner, M. M. (2018). Nuts and bolts: The group screen. In M. D. Ribeiro, J. M. Gross, & M. M. Turner (Eds.), *The college counselor's guide to group psychotherapy* (pp. 145–155). Routledge. https://www.taylorfrancis.com/chapters/nuts-bolts-group-screen-marc%C3%A9e-turner/e/10.4324/9781315545455-14?context=ubx&refId=fb178c73-436c-4bb4-a1f0-330147b150ec

Tschuschke, V., Mackenzie, K. R., Haaser, B., & Janke, G. (1996). Self-disclosure, feedback, and outcome in long-term inpatient psychotherapy groups. *The Journal of Psychotherapy Practice and Research*, 5(1), 35–44. https://pubmed.ncbi.nlm.nih.gov/22700263/

Whittingham, M. (2015). Focused brief group therapy. In E. S. Neukrug (Ed.), *The SAGE encyclopedia of theory in counseling and psychotherapy* (pp. 420–423). Sage Publications. 10.4135/9781483346502.n144

Whittingham, M. (2017). Attachment and interpersonal theory and group therapy: Two sides of the same coin. *International Journal of Group Psychotherapy*, 67(2), 276–279. https://psycnet.apa.org/record/2017-11037-008

Whittingham, M. (2018). Innovations in group assessment: How focused brief group therapy integrates formal measures to enhance treatment preparation, process, and outcomes. *Psychotherapy*, 55(2), 186–190. 10.1037/pst0000153

Yalom, I. D., & Leszcz, M. (2005). *The theory and practice of group psychotherapy* (5th ed.). Basic Books. https://www.academia.edu/13587158/The_Theory_and_Practice_of_Group_Psychotherapy

Yalom, I. D., & Leszcz, M. (2020). *The theory and practice of group psychotherapy* (6th ed.). Basic Books. https://www.basicbooks.com/titles/irvin-d-yalom/the-theory-and-practice-of-group-psychotherapy/9781541617575/

5   Informed Consent

Informed consent is a legal and ethical term referring to a process wherein a client achieves an understanding of a proposed treatment and states an agreement to pursue that treatment. From the standpoint of Principlism (Beauchamp & Childress, 2013), providing the opportunity for informed consent is consonant with several ethical principles. Respect for Autonomy is served in that the practitioner is offering the information needed by clients to make prudent, reasoned decisions about their treatment. Beneficence is honored in that a well-informed client is likely to be in an optimal position to derive benefit from treatment. For example, through the informed consent, the client has been instructed on those behaviors that contribute to progress and has agreed to engage in them. General Beneficence (Beauchamp & Childress, 2013) is also served: When a member has a positive group experience—in part due to good preparation for group involvement—that member's positive attitude toward group treatment is likely to be carried into the community. Informed consents also support Non-maleficence in that they spare the client the distress likely to be generated by (a) not knowing what to expect from the treatment, or (b) having false expectations for the treatment.

An informed consent process is also required by other ethical frameworks. Feminism (Proctor, 2018) demands that the power differential between client and therapist be as minimal as possible. Providing the client with all the information needed for good decision-making about joining a group serves this end. It is particularly important for women, people of color, individuals representing sexual minorities, and other disempowered groups to be empowered and make authoritative decisions on their own (Bender & Ewashen, 2000).

> Offering information and obtaining agreement for a treatment through the use of an interactional interchange defines the psychotherapeutic venture as a mutual one, altering the who, what, and how of treatment from a more paternalistic endeavor to one in which the power of choice and the burden of responsibility are distributed, noted Fallon (2006, p. 434).

The informed consent invites the client to be a collaborator, and when clients perceive themselves to be partners with the therapist, outcomes tend to be more favorable (Behnke, 2004). Finally, the therapist's openness in presenting not just the benefits but also the risks and alternative treatments is consistent with Virtue ethics.

A Process, Not an Event

Although practitioners often think about informed consent as an event occurring at the beginning of the treatment, it is a process that extends over the duration of treatment (Blease et al., 2016; Knapp et al., 2013; Pomerantz, 2005). Certainly, before joining a

DOI: 10.4324/9781003105527-5

group, the client must consent to it and that consent must be based on information about the treatment in the recruitment and prescreening phases. However, the client's understanding of aspects of the informed consent deepens as treatment progresses:

> Shelley was in both individual therapy and group psychotherapy with the same therapist (combined therapy). She had participated in group psychotherapy for five weekly sessions when in session six, Barry stated that he was disturbed by Alex's comment to him after the last session. Alex responded, "I don't even remember speaking with you after last session." Barry said, "Don't you remember when we were walking down the hall? You said that Aisha's coming out in the group really surprised you. I didn't think it was appropriate to be talking about it outside this space." Looking at the therapist, Aisha said, "Isn't that a violation of confidentiality? I feel that Alex violated my confidentiality." Alex rejoined, "I'm sorry. It's just that I was really moved. You and I were walking down a long hall, and no one was in sight." The group continued to talk about what constituted a violation and converged on the notion that Alex's action had not been prudent and that comments about members' disclosures should be confined to the group sessions. Shelley revealed in her individual therapy session that although initially she was surprised by Barry's confrontation of Alex and thought perhaps it was an overreaction to a minor event, as the discussion progressed, she began to see that such extra-mural conversations could bring harm to a member.

The point is that any important concept such as confidentiality will require continuing clarification over the course of the group. It is one thing for the incoming member to be told about a risk or responsibility and another thing to experience these elements within group sessions. Newer members such as Shelley can see that the therapist's talk about confidentiality involves a vital, ongoing concern to all members of the group. Moreover, sometimes clarifications are needed regarding group rules and other structural features. For example, this group might not have ever discussed the acceptability of speaking about group events while entering or leaving the group.

An informed consent is a process rather than a single event also because, at times, structural aspects of the group can change—members need to be informed of the change and provide consent for continued participation:

> Valeria was referred to a particular psychotherapy group, but as a recent immigrant her English Language Proficiency was limited. No other group was available in the geographic area in her native language. Given the fact that Valeria was otherwise a good fit for the group, the therapist explored bringing in an interpreter who could also serve as an interpreter and cultural broker if particular facets of Valeria's culture were important for the therapist and ultimately the group to understand. The therapist provided informed consent with members on the introduction of the interpreter. The informed consent specified how the interpreter would work in the group, the risks of having the interpreter, and the potential benefits.

Judgment on the part of the group leader is required in determining what changes would necessitate a new or additional informed consent. However, whenever the risks to the members change, a supplemental informed consent is prudent. Another example of a circumstance involving a structural change occurred when, during the Covid-19 pandemic, therapists shifted from conducting groups in-person to online. This transition involved a host of new risks (such as the potential of hacking) and responsibilities for the member (such as the importance of the member participating in the session in a private place). A modification of this magnitude would activate the need for a new informed consent.

Format of the Informed Consent

Generally, the informed consent is presented to the incoming member in two forms—verbal and written. A conversation about the elements of the informed consent is necessary to gear the way information is offered to the client. For example, some vocabulary differences might occur in a verbal informed consent with an adolescent versus a middle-aged person. The characterization of group psychotherapy might vary depending upon an individual's experience with therapy including whether the individual had prior group psychotherapy experiences. However, the major advantage of conducting the informed consent process in the context of a conversation is that this format creates space for the client's reactions, both verbal and non-verbal (Brabender, 2002; Fallon, 2006). For example, in responding to the therapist's characterization of the treatment, the incoming member might reveal some misconceptions that can then be corrected and anxieties that can be addressed. The verbal component should be regarded as complete not when the therapist has covered a certain set of topics but rather when the incoming member has demonstrated an understanding of essential points (Banach & Pillay, 2019).

The written format is needed as a formal recognition that the client has offered consent and willingness to take on the risks and assume the responsibilities of the treatment; that is, it is evidence that the informed consent has occurred. A written informed consent ensures that all group members will be presented with certain basic pieces of information. This format conveys to the incoming member the seriousness with which the therapist takes the contractual understanding between member and therapist. In order to be a useful document, the written informed consent must be readable by the member (cf. Walfish & Ducey, 2007). In attending to reading level, the group psychotherapist is honoring the ethical principle of Justice by making the materials accessible to a wider swath of the population.

While a written informed consent typically is presented at the beginning of the treatment, modifications made to the informed consent may or may not need to be codified in a formal written document. At times, when the therapist is introducing a change in some aspect of the treatment once the group is underway or once a given member has been in the group, it may be sufficient for the therapist to document the presentation of the relevant information and the expression of consent on the part of the members. However, changes that are more complex and involve the introduction of a set of new risks might well warrant a new informed consent to support ethical practice and good risk management. An example of the latter would be the switch from in-person to online group therapy.

Therapists should take care to make appropriate adjustments to the way the informed consent is presented when individuals have special needs (Knapp et al., 2013). For example, some individuals who have difficulty processing extensive verbal information might benefit from seeing a video clip of the group so as to be able to envision its workings.

Elements of the Informed Consent

This section outlines the topics that are typically included in an informed consent with recognition that contexts, circumstances, and populations make a difference in what is included. The major categories to be considered are (a) therapist credentials; (b) treatment goals; (c) the risks of treatment; (d) the responsibilities of members including financial obligations; and (e) alternate treatments the prospective member might consider.

Credentials of the Group Psychotherapist

Incoming group members have a right to know that the therapist is appropriately credentialed to run the group. Some members will be more interested than others in learning about the specifics of the therapist's credentials. However, all members should be apprised of certain basic aspects such as the practitioner's licensure status. Given that some states require that the therapist provide new clients with particular information in writing about therapist credentials (Pomerantz & Handelsman, 2004), group psychotherapists should become informed about regulations within their jurisdictions of practice.

If the group psychotherapist is a student working under supervision, the incoming member should be apprised of this fact (Fisher & Oransky, 2008). Generally, the name of the supervisor and contact information should be made available to the member. If the group members at any point communicate a misimpression about the trainee's credentials, that misimpression should be corrected (Fisher & Oransky, 2008).

Goals and Potential Benefits of Treatment

The selection and preparation processes entail a discussion of how the group might benefit the individual and how changes that the individual is seeking could be pursued in the psychotherapy group. A beneficial outcome of this pre-group exploration is a joint understanding on the part of the therapist and new group member about the member's specific goals. At times, the incoming member might have in mind goals that cannot be served by a particular group. For example, an individual might expect to make friendships with members of a group that disallows socialization outside of the sessions. Another individual might imagine that medication monitoring will occur in the sessions. Skillful inquiry on the part of the therapist leading to the recognition of potentially unrealistic goals is invaluable in providing the prospective member with an accurate picture of what outcomes are likely from group participation. Once the therapist clarifies what can and cannot be done in the group, the candidate might agree to join the group or decline but in either case, the therapist has done justice to that individual's right to self-determination.

Delineating the member goals for group participation is implicitly or explicitly an acknowledgment that eventually the member will terminate from the group. Mangione et al. (2007) note, "Informed consent entails talking to clients from the beginning of the treatment process about the end and how to end the treatment productively" (p. 29). The therapist during the informed consent process should anticipate not only how the member's achievement of the goals will be recognized but also who will participate in the process. For example, will this process engage the member, the therapist, and other members or some other configuration? The therapist should also discuss how the member should leave the group (e.g., should the member offer the group a certain number of sessions notice prior to leaving?).

Risks of Group Treatment

Potential group members may have fears about joining a group but may not be fully aware of the variety of risks of group treatment. The risks to any complex human engagement are many and the therapist will need to be selective in choosing which to present. Attempting to be exhaustive carries two perils. The first is that likely risks might be obscured by improbable risks. The second is that the presentation of risks carries the possibility that an individual who might benefit from group psychotherapy will decide to decline membership in the group. The task of crafting an informed consent creates a tension between Respect for

Autonomy and Beneficence. Apprising members of risks is consistent with the former. Doing so in a way that safeguards a member's interest in being in the group honors the latter.

In deciding which risks in the pool of all possible risks to share, the therapist should consider several factors. The first is whether any laws exist within the therapist's jurisdiction that provide direction on this matter. The second is any empirical evidence about the likelihood that a particular risk will emerge. All else being equal, observable risks are more important to identify to the prospective group member than hypothetical risks. The third factor is the application of one of the traditional standards used to evaluate risks. The *professional standard* entails presenting those risks that are generally disclosed by other practitioners possessing the same skill level and practicing in the same community (Paterick et al., 2008). The *materiality standard* requires disclosure of material risks—risks that involve significant harm—that a prudent patient would wish to know in deciding whether to consent to treatment (Paterick et al., 2008).

Although some risks are common across all types of groups, every group must be analyzed for the particular risks it presents to members. For this reason, group psychotherapists should take care to take guidance from other professionals' informed consent forms but make certain that such forms are appropriately adapted for their individual groups.

The Risk of Discomfort

What is inevitable is that at various times in the group, the member will experience an unpleasant affect. It is not unusual for the members to feel anxiety in their early period of group participation: Is it safe? Will I be attacked? Will the leader be helpful? A range of other negative affects is likely to occur over the course of each member's tenure in the group. Also to be expected are reactions to feedback that the member might regard as negative or dissonant with that member's self-perception. Challenging the members to shift behaviors and engage in new behaviors are part of the group process. By forecasting these occurrences, the therapist inoculates the incoming member against a misimpression that having a negative feeling in the group necessarily means that the group is not working for that member. Helping the patient anticipate these realities can help prevent negative outcomes down the road (Marmarosh, 2016).

Were the therapist to merely anticipate for the member such uncomfortable moments, it might well discourage the candidate's enthusiasm for group participation. However, balance can be achieved by the therapist's addition of several important points. First, all relationships are characterized by positive and negative events and reactions. Second, uncomfortable moments in the group often contribute greatly to members' learning and progress. For example, the therapist can give the instance of a member who learns about a behavior that is distressing to others. The therapist can note that having an off-putting behavior identified is naturally likely to create discomfort, but it also provides information necessary for the member to make positive changes. Third, the therapist should emphasize that positive feedback and positive emotional reactions are also very much a common and powerful part of the group experience.

Risk of Confidentiality Breaches

The incoming group member should be informed of all of the legally mandated reasons the therapist would be obligated to breach confidentiality. Variation exists from state to state with respect to the mandate that the therapist violates confidentiality. Therefore, it is essential that the therapist be aware of state law on this matter (Barnett & Coffman, 2015).

Uncertainty about legal requirements not only impedes the group psychotherapist when a rapid response is needed but also hinders that clinician from offering a sufficiently comprehensive informed consent with respect to confidentiality.

As part of the informed consent, the therapist must disclose to the incoming member that the therapist cannot guarantee that the other members will observe confidentiality. This is a risk that is inherent in group psychotherapy with breaches being caused by a variety of factors such as confusion about boundaries, an effort to diminish the intensity of the group experience, and pleasure in gossiping (Pepper, 2004). New therapists might imagine that once the therapist has emphasized to the incoming member the importance of confidentiality, the member will observe it, but violations of confidentiality are not uncommon (Roback et al., 1992). Therapists should also acknowledge that confidentiality breaches could have real-life negative consequences (such as a gay member who is outed to that member's co-worker and subsequently loses a job in a homophobic organization).

Therapists might fear that apprising the incoming member of the risk of loss of confidentiality could dampen the person's motivation to join the group. However, clients are likely to be reassured by the therapist's communication of the notion that (a) any violation of confidentiality would be taken very seriously with a possible imposition of sanctions considered; and (b) the therapist exercises care to keep the need for maintaining confidentiality in each member's awareness.

Lack of Progress or Deterioration

Most individuals who enter any form of psychotherapy will progress (Prochaska et al., 2020). However, some individuals will fail to show positive change and others will show deterioration in their condition. Group psychotherapy is no different in this regard (Bernard et al., 2008). Consequently, the therapist should let the incoming member know that progress is not guaranteed.

This message—a member's potential lack of progress—could have a particularly chilling effect on a member's desire to enter the group. Accordingly, it is important that this message be coupled with other information about group psychotherapy outcomes. First, the therapist should mention that, as noted above, it is highly likely that the member will benefit from participation in group psychotherapy. Second, the therapist should point out that both the therapist and the member will be monitoring therapeutic progress. Therapists who build in proximal measures, such as the tools in the Clinically-Oriented Research Evaluation (CORE) Battery-R (Burlingame et al., 2006), might point to these indicators. In the case that treatment does not appear to be benefitting the member, the therapist and member can identify changes that might catalyze treatment such as increased participation on the part of the member. Third, emphasis should be given to the ways in which the incoming member can increase the likelihood of a positive group experience, such as by regular and prompt attendance, engagement in judicious self-disclosure, and consideration of group feedback (Brabender, 2002). Fourth, periods can occur in which progress is made even when it is not evident to the member. The member should be encouraged to be open with the group if a concern emerges about a lack of progress in the group.

Risks to Clients' External Relationships

The simple fact that groups can be powerful catalysts for personal change means that they carry risk. Members need to be educated about the costs of change and personal growth (Bernard et al., 2008). For instance, a member may choose to leave a conflictual romantic relationship after sharing some patterns in the group and getting feedback about how the client appears to be treated by the partner. A group leader does members a disservice when not informing members that pain and struggle are often associated with making personal changes.

> Dipti, a member working on expressing anger and assertiveness, is warned by the leader that practicing assertiveness can get messy. The therapist says, "Trying to learn appropriate communication sometimes means that clients swing too far in one direction as they practice change." Providing an example for Dipti of her being overly assertive with her boss at work, especially after withholding her anger for over a year, could help Dipti understand the potential risks of practicing new skills as she makes personal growth.

Other Risks

In the informed consent process, the leader is fulfilling a responsibility to protect the members from adverse outcomes. However, for example, leaders cannot fully assure members that they will not be targets of threatening behavior or verbally abusive comments. Other risks include members being subjected to coercion, scapegoating, harsh and destructive confrontation from peers, breaches of confidence, inappropriate reassurance, attacks, and even physical injury (Bernard et al., 2008; Marmarosh, 2016). While we do not want to scare off potential members by over-focusing on these possibilities, we need to honor that clients may need to consider how they might respond should a harmful action in the group occur. Leaders can collaboratively explore where members might ask for support if necessary (e.g., asking another strongly aligned group member for a perspective, or asking the leaders to weigh in or intervene if feeling hurt or stuck).

Member Responsibilities

An important part of the informed consent process is apprising the incoming member of their responsibilities, ensuring that the responsibilities are fully understood, and obtaining the individual's commitment to fulfill those responsibilities. Members should be apprised of the variety of responsibilities they have to themselves, the other members, and the leader. These responsibilities include attending group sessions consistently and on time, remaining for the entire session, responding to other members' contributions, sharing information about themselves, and expressing feelings and impulses in words rather than actions. Depending upon the group format, other responsibilities might be indicated.

Financial Responsibilities

One of the most important agreements to discuss with potential group members is the expectation to be responsible and prompt with fees and payments to clinicians. Whereas there are a variety of examples and norms about payments in different practice settings that can work well, it is important to communicate directly to each member about how they should be responsible for their bills. Rutan et al. (2014) argue that informing members about how the therapist will manage payments is crucial, observing that therapists also need to be direct and forthright about how missed sessions will be handled and billed. Further, attendance issues and agreements often intersect with payment agreements.

Rutan et al. (2014) point out that clients may need to be reminded that third-party payers do not reimburse for missed sessions. Some therapists also ask for a certain time frame for any cancellations, such as 24–48 hours in advance of the group. At times, leaders may also decide to make exceptions for illness, transportation difficulties, or other valid reasons to miss a session. However, leaders may want to avoid making exceptions at all, as therapists then put themselves in the position to determine whether a reason for an absence is legitimate and unavoidable rather than an acting out or defense. An alternative plan that accommodates client exigencies is one in which clinicians determine in advance a set number of sessions that the member may miss and not be charged (Rutan et al., 2014). Nonetheless, consistency in attendance and payment norms is crucial. Clear agreements in an area that may be ripe for conflict should assist in clinical and ethical decision-making.

The ethical issues around fees may also relate to social justice (MacNair-Semands, 2007). Shapiro and Ginzberg (2006), for example, make a strong case for being direct and honest about money matters and for exploring the unique resistances and defenses that can arise around the charging and collecting of fees. Their comprehensive approach in-corporates individual, familial, societal, and gender influences to understand such re-sistances within both therapist and group member. Classism and culture have the potential to emerge in this context through such dynamics as entitlements, shame about socio-economic status, and lack of awareness about the effects of poverty. Poverty can be a central aspect of identity and a complex experience; it is known to spawn a potent set of mental health challenges (Ziadeh, 2020).

If fees and payment matters are brought into the group process, the intense reactions that some members may have related to the topic of money may be difficult for leaders to handle. Gans (1992) initially pointed out that understanding how our clients view and react to money is an important window into their inner selves. However, this can be particularly delicate when therapists use sliding scale payments, add pro bono members into a group, or make a temporary adjustment based on a member's altered financial situation. The latter options might be used by the therapist to advance social justice ends (Brabender, 2002), but must lead to thoughtful fee and payment processes, and careful documentation of decision-making (Knauss, 2006). Leaders who are respectful and thoughtful around payment concerns can respond with calm, consistency, and pro-fessionalism while valuing the important product that the group offers (Rutan et al., 2019). New group leaders do well to seek consultation from their more senior counterparts about establishing fee policies and managing fee issues that arise in the group.

Similarly, marketing materials must be clear about fees (Kaplan, 2018). Providing group members with information about how fees may change over time is also important. When fees are raised without warnings or knowledge that this may occur, the situation can become precarious if several members protest and collude against the leader. Other risks that may need reporting are discussed in Chapter 6.

Attendance and Punctuality

In the informed consent process, it is useful to specify those normative behaviors that are essential to the group's accomplishing its goals. Of particular importance is that members attend sessions regularly and arrive at sessions on time. Frequent absences and late arrivals compromise the continuity of the group's work. Even when the therapist emphasizes these elements in the informed consent, members can have lapses. At such times, it can be useful to recognize that all had agreed to adhere to these requirements. It is also helpful to have such a policy in place if the therapist needs to make a difficult decision about a member whose circumstances change and can no longer fulfill these requirements. For example, suppose a member wanted to miss once a month due to new work obligations. Having a strict attendance policy enables the therapist to more believably explain to the member that this plan will not be acceptable given how the group is expected to function. Of course, therapists can choose to relax a given policy but should do so only after carefully considering what the rationale is for the exception, the long-term consequences for the group, and the observance of the policy going forward for all members.

Use of Substances

Therapists do well to craft a policy about the use of substances during or prior to group sessions. Group therapy sessions can be stressful, and it is natural for members to consider means by which the stress can be lessened. One route is by using alcohol or other non-prescribed substances prior to the group to achieve a particular state of mind during the session. Members might also partake in oral substances during the session, for example, bringing food or coffee to the meetings, or chewing gum during the session. In some groups, particularly those designed for children (Kahn, 1993) or for very low functioning members, the therapists themselves might provide refreshments during the sessions. It is helpful to the workings of the group for members to know the policy about oral substances prior to each member's joining the group. Beyond simply stating the expectation, the therapist should provide a rationale to the member for why the use of substances prior to or during group sessions is prohibited. The therapist should also specify the consequences to the member of presenting to group sessions under the influence.

Use of Technology and the Informed Consent

Group leaders have been employing technology for decades, if only to contact a potential group member by phone to schedule a meeting for screening. However, in the last decade, the use of technology has increased rapidly (Eonta et al., 2011; Harwood et al., 2011). The ever-burgeoning incorporation of technology holds promise of enhancing members' engagement with treatment, facilitating communications between therapist and group member, reaching underserved populations (Stoll et al., 2020), sparing mental health professionals the risk of being physically present with violent patients (Vogt et al., 2019), enabling members to access psychoeducational information, assisting the tracking of therapeutic outcomes, enabling more economical treatment (Stoll et al., 2020) and protecting the continuity of the group when special circumstances such as a pandemic prevent face-to-face meetings. However, with each technological element comes the introduction of one or more risks to the group member, many of which pertain to privacy and confidentiality. Hence, in the informed consent process the group psychotherapist should describe to the entering member (a) what technology will be employed in the conduct of the group and communications with group members; (b) the major risks attached to those technologies; and (c) any safeguards that the therapist will introduce, or the group member is encouraged to use, to mitigate those risks.

Even the most ordinary uses of technology should be included in the informed consent. For example, the group psychotherapist should obtain permission to leave a message on the member's answering service given that other parties could have access to the member's voicemail. Email and text messaging represent modes of communication with many conveniences but also additional challenges. One challenge is confidentiality: Can the client and therapist retain control over the information that is transmitted via email? As part of the informed consent, the patient and therapist might consider the extent to which the patient's computer is secure: Who has access to the computer? Is it protected by a firewall and a password? Answers to these questions could lead to a tightening of security. The therapist should emphasize in the informed consent the importance of ensuring that email communications are encrypted. Additionally, the therapist should specify what types of information should be exchanged via emails or text messages. Restricting information to business-keeping matters makes sense for the group psychotherapy situation. Matters of substance, i.e., those related to the member's work in treatment, ought to be restricted to sharing in the group so that all can participate.

Social networking (for example, Facebook and Instagram) represents another area of concern. In the absence of rules about making connections on social networks, members are likely to "friend" one another or obtain information about one another through these networks, so embedded are they in the broader culture. The therapist must be forthright about expectations concerning social networking. Although undoubtedly some benefits might be identified with members' engagement in social networking with one another, the perils are far greater. For example, if Delphine has a relationship with Malaika on a social network, Delphine loses the capacity to control what information all the other members have about her—it is now under Malaika's control. The therapist can support the establishment of a "no social networking" rule by refraining from engaging in this activity with members. As for the members, engagement with other clients on social networking sites holds many dangers for the therapist. Gabbard et al. (2011) write:

> Most users see Facebook as a forum for self-expression through posts, affiliations, and photos. These items are, of course, more personally revealing than what is generally disclosed in a treatment relationship. Also, Facebook users may post photos and "tag" or label another Facebook user by name without the knowledge or consent of the individual in the picture. Facebook users may discover that they are tagged in a professionally unbecoming photograph long after numerous others have seen it. (p. 169)

Gabbard et al. warn that even if therapists avoid engaging with patients online, they should nonetheless avoid making derogatory statements about patients or practices, given the myriad ways a patient could access a therapist's online material.

One development that has been catalyzed by the Coronavirus pandemic is the practice of conducting psychotherapy groups virtually. These groups can be either synchronous or asynchronous. A synchronous group is one that takes place on such platforms as Zoom or Skype. It involves moving from the circle to the screen in which all members can see one another and the therapist. Asynchronous groups are text-based and involve having members leave commentaries on one other member's entries. Asynchronous groups are far less researched than their synchronous counterparts (Weinberg, 2020a) and represent more of a departure from traditional group psychotherapy.

It is all but guaranteed that what was born of necessity will become regular practice for some practitioners. Without a doubt, virtual groups have advantages. They allow for the group to be available to individuals who live in remote areas (Harwood et al., 2011). They contribute to the stability of the group in that members and the therapist can attend even when their actual geographic locations change. They offer members greater convenience (Stoll et al., 2020). However, the therapist's decision-making regarding whether to embrace a virtual format as a regular feature of a group must weigh the disadvantages of this medium against its strengths. The disadvantages are not trivial and many pertain to the therapist's loss of control regarding the management of information:

- With the synchronous virtual format, the therapist loses control over the setting (Campbell & Norcross, 2018; Weinberg, 2020b). For example, the therapist can see the member in a frame but might not be able to see other individuals in the member's physical environment, people who could be auditing the communications in the group. Breaches in confidentiality could occur in other ways. For example, if the proper safeguards have not been implemented, the virtual group room could be intruded upon by outsiders. Moreover, distractions can occur during the session such as when pets crawl over group members or a member announces a need to leave to answer the door.

- The therapist has more limited access to visual information about the member, information that usually helps the therapist to discern mood and ongoing reactions to the group (Harwood et al., 2011). When groups are conducted virtually, a great deal of body/postural data is lost to the therapist. Moreover, such usual data as members' seating choices and distance from one another are absent. Members are also curtailed in their ability to learn about another through access to sensory data.

- Paradoxically, for some members, the online sessions might involve contact that is too close. Jurist (2021) points out that details of facial expressions can be seen more readily in online formats, an accessibility that might be disturbing to some group members.

- Still another limitation is captured by the concept of the digital divide (Hoffman et al, 2000). Individuals from higher socio-economic levels have more abundant technological resources and more familiarity with technology. This factor could limit the availability of group psychotherapy to economically disadvantaged individuals.

- Research on the effectiveness of this format in relation to the traditional face-to-face medium is only beginning to emerge in the literature (Stoll et al., 2020). Particularly lacking is information on patient characteristics that do or do not support distance technology applications (Stoll et al., 2020). As Harwood et al. (2011) note, in the absence of a robust empirical basis, a careful case-by-case analysis should be made of the suitability of this format for a given client. Harwood et al. note that a substantial empirical base exists for the notion that the most favorable treatment outcomes occur when treatment is matched to the characteristics of the client. Such matching should occur in decisions about online versus face-to-face group participation.

These disadvantages may or may not compel a group psychotherapist away from a virtual format. However, group psychotherapists who proceed with a virtual application should find means to mitigate the disadvantages. For example, the therapist should establish as part of the informed consent the member's responsibility to participate in the sessions from a location that is secure, that is, in a place where member exchanges are neither visible nor audible (Weinberg, 2020b). The lack of visual information can be partially offset by instructing clients on how to position the camera in relation to the self. Weinberg (2020a) suggests that the lack of connection members might feel in the virtual format might be offset by increased therapist self-disclosure and encouraging members to use their imaginations. The therapist must direct the members to use the maximum privacy settings on their electronic devices.

The informed consent for virtual groups should contain all the information traditionally offered in the informed consent for in-person groups, as well as additional information on the issues addressed above. As Campbell and Norcross (2018) note, the informed consent for virtual treatment should also contain information about emergency services the client can access locally, any respect in which billing departs from in-person practices, limitations in regarding confidentiality particular to virtual treatment, and how the therapist stores and disposes of client data collected through online means.

Alternative Treatments

As members are deciding whether to enter a psychotherapy group, they have a right to be informed about alternative ways in which they might address their difficulties. Therapists who present their groups and no alternative treatments contribute to a misimpression that the current option is the only option. Such a move deprives individuals of exercising self-determination, that is, they see the option as treatment versus no treatment rather than treatment A versus treatment B, C, or D. In specifying the alternatives, the therapist should identify advantages and disadvantages of each, including relative time frames in which particular treatment goals are likely to be met. The comparison of different treatments should be based on the therapist's knowledge of the evidence base of different approaches (Blease et al., 2018).

At times, group psychotherapists will refer to themselves. This circumstance would arise if a therapist has seen a client in another capacity—for individual, couples, or family therapy, or a psychological assessment—and sees the client as potentially benefiting from a group experience, specifically in the therapist's group. In making the referral, the therapist is in a potential conflict of interest in that the therapist stands to benefit from the client's accepting the therapist's recommendation. The question could arise as to whether the therapist is privileging self-interest over the client's well-being. Moreover, if the client has an established relationship with the therapist, the client might feel little freedom to reject the recommendation. Still, compelling reasons might exist for why the client should enter the therapist's group. It might the case that this individual would be unlikely to enter a group in the absence of a strong, pre-existing bond with the therapist. It could be that the therapist's group is far more convenient geographically than other groups. In order to provide the client with maximal autonomy in making the decision, the therapist should identify alternative group experiences the client might pursue. Delineating the advantages and disadvantages of each option is also helpful. The therapist might also encourage the client to get a consultation with another practitioner if the client wishes to explore what group might mesh best with their needs.

Group psychotherapists' presentation of themselves to the public should be consistent with the elements of the informed consent. Box 5.1 highlights the need for this consistency when group psychotherapists advertise their services.

Considerations for Special Populations

Informed consent is not an all-or-nothing phenomenon but exists on a continuum (Bennett et al., 2006; Fisher & Oransky, 2008). This element of continuity is useful when considering how to proceed when an individual is not able to give full legal consent by virtue of age, degree of impairment, or some other factor. Although it might be a third-party who has the legal authority to give consent, the prospective group member should participate in the informed consent process as fully as possible. Although the therapist should always customize the informed consent to the individual, in the case of the populations discussed in this section, particular flexibility and ingenuity is called for on the part of the therapist.

Child and Adolescent Populations

For much of the history of psychotherapy, psychotherapists regarded the informed consent process as irrelevant to children and adolescents. Because the law typically gives parents the right to consent on behalf of their children, once the therapist provided the informed consent to the parents, their obligation was fulfilled. What this perspective ignores is that informed consent is not merely a legal requirement but an ethical duty and a pillar of successful treatment. Clinicians have an ethical duty to respect the autonomy of the person by engaging the juvenile in the informed consent process. Doing so also confers clinical benefits in that—as with adults—a child who understands what the group is about is more likely to participate meaningfully in the group (Knauss, 2007).

Box 5.1   Advertising Considerations

Saul Reddy has decided to form a psychotherapy group. He reviews the group psychotherapy literature and finds studies indicating that group psychotherapy can lessen depression and anxiety and can strengthen members' social skills. He uses this information as the basis for creating an advertisement in which he poses this question, "Do you want to feel better and be more successful in connecting with others? If so, consider joining Dr. Reddy's psychotherapy group." The advertisement also includes a testimonial from a former client as well as Saul's name and degree followed by "Expert in Group Psychotherapy." Finally, he lists his contact information. Saul happens to encounter an acquaintance, Fred, who also conducts psychotherapy groups. In the context of a broader conversation, Fred tells Saul that he had seen his advertisement and was concerned that, perhaps inadvertently, Saul was creating the impression that these positive changes are guaranteed. Saul responded that advertisements do not lend themselves to capturing complexities and he would expect to provide more information when candidates appeared for the initial consultation about joining the group.

In approaching Saul about the content of the advertisement, Fred was honoring the ethical principle of Respect for Autonomy—that is, ensuring that individuals receive accurate information about group psychotherapy to make an informed decision about whether to even take the first step in pursuing it. Indeed, Saul is correct in asserting that what can be achieved in a brief marketing communication is limited and a far greater opportunity would be provided by a one-on-one meeting. Still, Saul's phrasing is not optimal for accurate communication in that the tone suggests that if individuals engage in a particular behavior (pursuing group psychotherapy) then certain benefits will be obtained (for example, improved relationships). No psychological treatment can offer this unqualified assurance. A way to circumvent this potential miscommunication is to talk about what the group seeks to do. Any phrasing that suggests that group psychotherapy *can* achieve certain ends is preferable to that indicating that it *will* achieve them.

Two additional problems are present in Saul's advertisement, one of which is that Saul declares himself to be an expert in group psychotherapy. This designation is highly ambiguous. Does Saul mean that he has achieved some external recognition such as specialist status recognized by a group psychotherapy organization? Has he received a certain number of favorable reviews online? Has he published a particular number of articles in group psychotherapy? In presenting himself as an expert, Dr. Reddy is risking that potential clients will make their own associations to this ill-defined term. Moreover, Dr. Reddy might be unjustified in calling himself an expert depending upon what criterion he is using. Number of publications, for example, does not establish one as an expert; nor does the number of positive online reviews establish expertise. If Dr. Reddy had received a credential from a credentialing organization, it would be appropriate to list it rather than the vague term "expert."

Dr. Reddy's use of a testimonial is also of concern. If Dr. Reddy had approached a current client for a testimonial, it could be seen as coercive. Any current client is dependent upon Dr. Reddy for their well-being and could well not feel free to refuse Dr. Reddy's request. It is for this reason that most professional codes of ethics disallow the solicitation of testimonials from current clients. For example, the Ethics Code of the American Psychological Association states, "Psychologists do not solicit

> **testimonials** from current therapy clients/patients or other persons who because of their particular circumstances are vulnerable to undue influence" (Standard 5.05 Testimonials). Although a former client does not present a challenge to the same degree, the professional would need to ensure that the client did not feel pressured to provide the testimonial. Moreover, the group psychotherapist must make clear that any positive results realized by the endorser are not guaranteed for all.

As this chapter has outlined, informed consent entails multiple processes, only one of which is the act of consent itself. Although the non-adult might be unable to offer consent in a legal sense, the child or adolescent can participate in the other processes we have described. They are able to learn about the group by discussing its goals and methods with the therapist in a developmentally appropriate way. The therapist can describe risks and benefits. The therapist should be careful to talk about the limits of confidentiality and specify what information might be shared with third parties such as parents. Children and adolescents can indicate understanding of the preceding information by explaining that information in their own words. All of these steps are fundamentally the same as with adult patients. It is the last step that is different. Rather than offering consent, the juvenile incoming member can give "assent"—a statement of willingness to enter the group and an ongoing opportunity to state disagreement with one or more aspects (Henkelman & Everall, 2001; Knauss, 2007).

In delivering the "informed" component of the informed consent process, the therapist should consider the capabilities of the child to understand material and gear communications to the child's developmental level (Koocher, 2008). Rather than delivering a long lecture to the child/adolescent—a format that would likely tax many children's attention span—the group psychotherapist should engage the entering member in a conversation that will reveal the child's comprehension. Henkelman and Everall (2001) provide questions that can invigorate the discussion with the child:

> What do you expect to have happen here? How do you understand the issue that brought you here? What do you hope to gain from counselling? What do your parents know about this issue? Do your parents know you were here? If not, why not? Is there a way your parents can be helpful or involved in solving this problem? What are the benefits of being here? What are the drawbacks? Was counseling your idea, or did somebody suggest it to you? How did you decide that counselling might be helpful with this issue? (p. 116)

Although the aforementioned questions could apply to individual therapy as well as group psychotherapy, questions can be added that are tailored to the group situation. For example, the therapist could inquire about how the child feels in various group situations such as with friends or classmates.

Impaired Adults

Some individuals who enter psychotherapy groups lack the legal capacity to give consent due to impaired functioning. Common conditions associated with legal guardianship include dementia, psychosis, and various developmental disabilities, particularly when such conditions are marked or severe. In such instances, a guardian might be appointed by the court to perform healthcare decision-making. Despite this circumstance, group psychotherapists have an obligation to the extent possible to engage the person in an informed consent process (Fisher & Oransky, 2008). All individuals who enter group psychotherapy have a right to learn about the treatment in terms of benefits and risks, goals, and methods. Time should be given to the incoming member who might not be able to offer legal consent to have their questions answered. Particular impairments might make it difficult for the individual to grasp certain elements of the informed consent. The therapist performs an important service in identifying these impairments and finding means to compensate for them in how the informed consent is delivered (Knapp et al., 2013). For example, if the individual's tendency to think concretely creates an impediment to understanding the feedback process, the therapist could conduct a role-play with the entering member in which the feedback process is demonstrated. As Fisher and Oransky point out, in order to obtain a clearer idea of the individual's ability to participate in the informed consent process, clinicians can supplement their observations with the use of tools such as the MacArthur Competence Assessment Tool for Treatment (Grisso et al., 1997). If, in the end, the potential group member does not assent to the treatment, this preference should be given weight by the therapist.

Mandated Treatment

One of the greatest challenges to successful treatment is when an individual is mandated to participate in therapy. Treatment is mandated for a variety of societal and psychological problems including child abuse, domestic violence, and substance abuse. According to Snyder and Anderson's (2009) review of the literature, research findings reveal, unsurprisingly, that individuals who are mandated to treatment come to treatment in a resistive posture. Moreover, such individuals tend to show a lesser motivation to change (Begun et al., 2003). Although intrinsic motivation is necessary for therapeutic progress, it can be nurtured within the therapy itself, including during the informed consent process.

One potentially useful strategy is understanding the entering group member's psychological position relative to treatment by applying the transtheoretical model (Prochaska & DiClemente, 1983; Prochaska et al., 2020). Within this model, individuals are recognized as being at any one of five different stages of change from pre-contemplation through maintenance of change. The therapist using this scheme respects the stage of change in which the person currently resides and gears interventions accordingly. For example, new members in the pre-contemplation stage benefit from being aware of the negative consequences of their behavior. For individuals who are mandated to treatment, the external negative consequences are often easy to identify. However, it is also helpful if the therapist can access the internal concomitants of the external problems, that is, the suffering the person experiences. In the contemplation stage when individuals are considering working toward change, education and feedback are helpful, both of which can be provided in the informed consent process. On the other hand, individuals who are in the action stage—ready to commit to working on a recognized problem—can be directed toward more behaviorally-based processes. Although thinking about the stages of change could be beneficial in working with any entering member, this analysis is especially likely to be useful when the individual has been required by a third party to join the group. It is also beneficial in that it recognizes that mandated participants are not a homogeneous group. Even though the involuntary aspect of group participation is likely to evoke negativity in many, within that population are subgroups of individuals at different levels of readiness to change.

Therapists working with mandated group members should keep in mind three important points. First, the boundary between voluntary and involuntary is not binary (Doel, 2019). Many individuals who are apparently voluntary begin treatment in large part to satisfy external parties. Second, clients can benefit from treatment, even if it is mandated (Rooney, 2009; Snyder & Anderson, 2009). Third, clients mandated to participate in treatment can become voluntary participants if they come to experience the group as valuable.

Final Note

No coverage of the informed consent process can be complete because what is needed in the informed consent depends upon many particulars of the therapist's practice—the purpose of the group, the processes employed, the format (in-person, virtual, textual), and many other factors. Hence, all informed consents must be customized to fit the practice of the therapist even if that therapist uses a template created by other therapists. Moreover, the informed consent process continues throughout treatment as the member's under-standing of the group deepens and as any conditions in the group change. The informed consent protects both client and therapist. The client is protected in that the informed consent process enables the client to make a considered decision about whether to enter the group. The process also protects the therapist in that it provides evidence that the client did receive crucial information. This chapter outlined the many other benefits that ac-company a well-informed consent process such as fostering a strong therapeutic alliance, de-mystifying treatment, eradicating confusion, supporting the formation of realistic ex-pectations, and encouraging members to take responsibility for their progress.

CEU Questions

1. What implications would transferring a group from in-person to online mode have for the informed consent process?
2. What are the two advantages of online groups?
3. Individuals who are unable to give legal consent to treatment can nonetheless provide assent. (T/F)
4. Violations of confidentiality in a psychotherapy group are rare. (T/F)
5. An informed consent is a process, not a single event. (T/F)
6. It is unnecessary for supervisees to disclose the fact that they are working under supervision. (T/F)
7. When therapists apprise entering group members that progress is not guaranteed, how might they lessen the likelihood that such information will discourage participation?
8. A common problem with HIPAA and Informed Consent forms is that they are written at a reading level that is too high. (T/F)
9. Individuals who are mandated to receive group treatment do not benefit from participation in treatment. (T/F)
10. When members enter the group, they should be apprised of the therapist's policy and practices about raising fees. (T/F)

Answer Key: 1. The therapist must develop a supplemental informed consent in light of altered risks and member responsibilities; 2. Examples: Can accommodate members in geographically remote areas; Can be more convenient; Can contribute to the stability of the group; 3. T; 4. F; 5. T; 6. F; 7. Share finding that most people benefit; indicate that progress will be monitored; describe behaviors that lead to more favorable outcomes; 8. T; 9. F; 10. T

Discussion Questions

1. Therapists are sometimes required to violate the confidentiality of the group member to protect another party when a group member makes or implies a physical threat. How might the therapist help the group to process therapist confidentiality breaches?
2. What feelings might be evoked in a group leader who learns that multiple members of the group have been obtaining information about the therapist from online sources, even if the information is not highly personal? How might the therapist manage these feelings?
3. What informed consent processes are possible in brief group treatment in which members might remain in the group for only 2–3 sessions?
4. Are there risks particular to college counseling groups that should be discussed in the informed consent process?
5. Some group leaders have a variable fee and others a fixed fee. Debate the pros and cons of each.
6. Some group leaders require the members to pay for their seat in the group whether they attend the session. Do you agree with this policy? Is it fair?
7. Does the leader have an obligation to serve social justice ends in establishing fees?
8. A prospective member wants to know the characteristics of a group member. What do you feel is appropriate to share with the prospective member?
9. What issues have arisen related to the responsibility for payment by group members in your practice setting? What have you learned from these experiences?

Vignettes/Role-Plays

1. This exercise focuses on various common parts of the informed consent process. All components of this activity involve the trainees pairing off and taking turns playing the therapist and the prospective group member. The following are variations, which the trainer can adapt based upon the particulars of a clinical context:

    1. The therapist (a) describes the group rule of confidentiality; (b) makes clear to the prospective group member why confidentiality is important (i.e., the damages that could ensue from violations); and (c) the consequence(s) for the member of an intentional violation.
    2. One topic that would generally be included in the informed consent is the lack of guarantee that communications in the group will be regarded as privileged. The therapist should explain to the prospective member (a) what privilege is; (b) why it might not be guaranteed; (c) how it might be relevant to the client; and (d) possible remedies to a privilege problem (e.g., the member would be careful about communicating with other members about matters that might be litigated).

2. The therapist is conducting the informed consent process when the new group member tells the therapist that she is transgender. The therapist realizes she had not previously inquired about the client's gender identity. The incoming member says she was stigmatized previously in a psychotherapy group of cisgender members. She wonders whether one of the risks of group participation is that she will again be stigmatized. How would you respond?

3.   Vonda changes her job and loses her insurance coverage for group therapy after being in the group for eight months. She offers to pay out of pocket but can only afford a fraction of the normal fee. Vonda raises the issue in the group and most members are supportive, but two members feel this would be unfair to them. How might the group leaders respond while respecting the group dynamics surfacing?

References

Banach, M., & Pillay, R. (2019). Ethical challenges in group work: Potential perils and preventive practices. In S. M. Marson & R. E. McKinney (Eds.). *The Routledge handbook of social work ethics and values* (pp. 191–197). Routledge.

Barnett, J. E., & Coffman, C. (2015, May). Confidentiality and its exceptions: The case of duty to warn. [Web article]. Retrieved from http://www.societyforpsychotherapy.org/confidentiality-and-its-exceptions-the-case-of-duty-to-warn

Beauchamp, T. L., & Childress, J. F. (2013). *Principles of biomedical ethics* (7th ed.). Oxford University Press. 10.1093/occmed/kqu158

Begun, A. L., Murphy, C. M., Bolt, D., Weinstein, B., Strodthoff, T., Short, L., et al. (2003). Characteristics of the Safe at Home instrument for assessing readiness to change intimate partner violence. *Research on Social Work Practice, 13*, 80–107. 10.1177/1049731502238758

Behnke, S. (2004). Informed consent and APA's new ethics code: Enhancing client autonomy, improving client care. *Monitor on Psychology, 35*(6), 80–83. https://www.apa.org/monitor/jun04/ethics

Bender, A., & Ewashen, A. (2000). Group work is political work: A feminist perspective of interpersonal group psychotherapy. *Issues in Mental Health Nursing, 21*(3), 297–308. 10.1080/016128400248103

Bennett, B. E., Bricklin, P. M., Harris, E., Knapp, S., VandeCreek, L., & Younggren, J. N. (2006). *Assessing and managing risk in psychological practice: An individualized approach.* The Trust.

Bernard, H., Burlingame, G., Flores, P., Greene, L., Joyce, A., Kobos, J., Leszcz, M., MacNair-Semands, R.R., Piper, W. E., Slocum McEneaney, A. M., Feirman, D. (2008). Clinical practice guidelines for group psychotherapy. *International Journal of Group Psychotherapy, 58*, 455–542. 10.1521/ijgp.2008.58.4.455

Blease, C., Kelley, J. M., & Trachsel, M. (2018). Informed consent in psychotherapy: implications of evidence-based practice. *Journal of Contemporary Psychotherapy, 48*(2), 69–78. 10.1007/s10879-017-9372-9

Blease, C. R., Lilienfeld, S. O., & Kelley, J. M. (2016). Evidence-based practice and psychological treatments: the imperatives of informed consent. *Frontiers in Psychology, 7*, 1170. 10.3389/fpsyg.2016.01170

Brabender, V. (2002). *Introduction to group therapy.* Wiley. https://www.wiley.com/en-us/Introduction+to+Group+Therapy-p-9780471378891

Burlingame, G. M., Strauss, B., Joyce, A., MacNair-Semands, R., Mac-Kenzie, K., Ogrodniczuk, J., et al. (2006). *Core battery-Revised.* American Group Psychotherapy Association.

Campbell, L. F., & Norcross, J.C. (2018). Do you see what we see? Psychology's response to technology in mental health. *Clinical Psychology: Science and Practice, 25*(2), Article e12237. 10.1111/cpsp.12237

Doel, M. (2019). Ethics and values in social group work. In S. M. Marson & E. E. McKinney (Eds.). *The Routledge handbook of social work ethics and values* (pp. 181–190). Routledge.

Eonta, A. M., Christon, L. M., Hourigan, S. E., Ravindran, N., Vrana, S. R., & Southam-Gerow, M. A. (2011). Using everyday technology to enhance evidence-based treatments. *Professional Psychology: Research and Practice, 42*(6), 513–520. 10.1037/a0025825

Fallon, A. (2006). Informed consent in the practice of group psychotherapy. *International Journal of Group Psychotherapy, 56*(4), 431–453. 10.1521/ijgp.2006.56.4.431

Fisher, C. B., & Oransky, M. (2008). Informed consent to psychotherapy: Protecting the dignity and respecting the autonomy of patients. *Journal of Clinical Psychology: In Session, 64*(5), 576–588. doi: 10.1002/jclp.20472

Gabbard, G. O., Kassaw, K. A., & Perez-Garcia, G. (2011). Professional boundaries in the era of the Internet. *Academic Psychiatry, 35*(3), 168–174.

Gans, J. S. (1992). Money and psychodynamic group therapy. *International Journal of Group Psychotherapy, 41*(1), 133–152. 10.1080/00207284.1992.11732584

Grisso, T., Appelbaum, P. S., & Hill-Fotouhi, C. (1997). The MacCAT-T: A clinical tool to assess patients' capacities to make treatment decisions. *Psychiatric Services, 48*, 1415–1419. 10.1176/ps.48.11.1415

Harwood, T. M., Pratt, D., Beutler, L. E., Bongar, B. M., Lenore, S., & Forrester, B. T. (2011). Technology, telehealth, treatment enhancement, and selection. *Professional Psychology: Research and Practice, 42*(6), 448–468. 10.1037/a0026214

Henkelman, J. J., & Everall, R. D. (2001). Informed consent with children: Ethical and practical implications. *Canadian Journal of Counselling, 35*(2), 109–121. https://cjc-rcc.ucalgary.ca/article/view/58665

Hoffman, D. L., Novak, T. P., & Schlosser, A. (2000). The evolution of the digital divide: How gaps in Internet access may impact electronic commerce. *Journal of Computer Mediated Communication, 5*, 233–245. 10.1111/j.1083-6101.2000.tb00341.x

Jurist, E. (2021). Mentalizing health. Retrieved from https://elliot4cc.substack.com/p/mentalizing-health?r=39v0q&utm_campaign=post&utm_medium=web&utm_source=copy

Kahn, S. R. (1993). Reflections upon the functions of food in a children's psychotherapy group. *Journal of Child and Adolescent Group Therapy, 3*(3), 143–153. 10.1007/BF00999845

Kaplan, S. A. (2018). The art of the sell: Marketing groups. In M. D. Ribeiro, J. Gross, & M. M. Turner (Eds.), *The college counselor's guide to group psychotherapy* (pp. 117–130). Routledge.

Knapp, S., Handelsman, M. M., Gottlieb, M. C., & VandeCreek, L. D. (2013). The dark side of professional ethics. *Professional Psychology: Research and Practice, 44*(6), 371–377. 10.1037/a0035110

Knauss, L. K. (2006). Ethical issues in record-keeping in group psychotherapy. *International Journal of Group Psychotherapy, 56*(4), 415–430. 10.1521/ijgp.2006.56.4.415

Knauss, L. K. (2007). Legal and ethical issues in providing group therapy to minors. In *Handbook of cognitive-behavior group therapy with children and adolescents* (pp. 75–95). Routledge.

Koocher, G. P. (2008). Ethical challenges in mental health services to children and families. *Journal of Clinical Psychology In Session, 64*(5), 601–612. 10.1002/jclp.20476

MacNair-Semands, R. R. (2007). Attending to the spirit of social justice as an ethical approach in group therapy. *International Journal of Group Psychotherapy, 57*(1), 61–66. 10.1521/ijgp.2007.57.1.61

Marmarosh, C. L. (2016). Can we collaborate? Mistakes made when group and individual therapists ignore multiple realities. *Psychotherapy, 53*(3), 320–324. 10.1037/pst0000067

Mangione, L., Forti, R., Iacuzzi, C. M. (2007). Ethics and endings in group psychotherapy: Saying good-bye and saying it well. *International Journal of Group Psychotherapy, 57*(1), 25–40. 10.1521/ijgp.2007.57.1.25

Orlinsky, D. E., & Howard, K. I. (1986). Process and outcome in psychotherapy. In S. L. Garfield & A. E. Bergin (Eds.), *Handbook of psychotherapy and behavior change* (3rd ed., pp. 311–381). Wiley.

Paterick, T. J., Carson, G.V., Allen, M. C., & Paterick, T. E. (2008). Medical informed consent: General considerations for physicians. *Mayo Clinical Proc., 83*(3), 313–319. 10.4065/83.3.313

Pepper, R. (2004). Confidentiality and dual relationships in group psychotherapy. *International Journal of Group Psychotherapy, 54*(1), 103–114. 10.1521/ijgp.54.1.103.40379

Pomerantz, A. M. (2005). Increasingly informed consent: Discussing distinct aspects of psychotherapy at different points in time. *Ethics and Behavior, 15*, 351–360. 10.1207/s15327019eb1504_6

Pomerantz, A. M., & Handelsman, M. M. (2004). Informed consent revisited: An updated written question format. *Professional Psychology: Research and Practice, 35*(2), 201–205. 10.1037/0735-7028.35.2.201

Prochaska, J. O., & DiClemente, C. C. (1983). Stages and processes of self-change of smoking: toward an integrative model of change. *Journal of Consulting and Clinical Psychology, 51*(3), 390–395. 10.1037/0022-006X.51.3.390

Prochaska, J. O., Norcross, J.C., & Saul, S. F. (2020). Generating psychotherapy breakthroughs: Transtheoretical strategies from population health psychology. *American Psychologist, 75*(7), 996–1010. 10.1037/amp0000568

Proctor, C. (2018). Virtue ethics in psychotherapy: A systematic review of the literature. *International Journal of Existential Positive Psychology*, 8(1), 1–22. http://journal.existentialpsychology.org/index.php/ExPsy/article/view/237

Roback, H., Ochoa, E., Bloch, F., & Purdon, S. (1992). Guarding confidentiality in clinical groups: The therapist's dilemma. *International Journal of Group Psychotherapy*, 42, 81–103. 10.1080/00207284.1992.11732581

Rooney, R. (2009). *Strategies for work with involuntary clients* (2nd ed.). Columbia University Press.

Rutan, J. S., Greene, L. S., & Kaklauskas, F. J. (2019). Preparing to begin a new group. In Kaklauskas, F. J., & Greene, L. R. (Eds.), *Core principles of group psychotherapy: A training manual for theory, research, and practice*. Routledge.

Rutan, J. S., Stone, W. N., & Shay, J. J. (2014). *Psychodynamic group psychotherapy*. Guilford Press.

Shapiro, E. L., & Ginzberg, R. (2006). Buried treasure: Money, ethics, and countertransference in group therapy. *International Journal of Group Psychotherapy*, 56(4), 477–494. 10.1521/ijgp.2006.56.4.477

Snyder, C. M., & Anderson, S. A. (2009). An examination of mandated versus voluntary referral as a determinant of clinical outcome. *Journal of Marital and Family Therapy*, 35(3), 278–292. 10.1111/j.1752-0606.2009.00118.x

Stoll, J., Müller, J. A., & Trachsel, M. (2020). Ethical issues in online psychotherapy: A narrative review. *Frontiers in Psychiatry*, 10, Retrieved from https://www.frontiersin.org/articles/10.3389/fpsyt.2019.00993/full.

Vogt, E. L., Mahmoud, H., & Elhaj, O. (2019). Telepsychiatry: Implications for psychiatrist burnout and well-being. *Psychiatric Services*, 70(5), 422–424. 10.1176/appi.ps.201800465

Walfish, S., & Ducey, B. B. (2007). Readability level of Health Insurance Portability and Accountability Act notices of privacy practices used by psychologists in clinical practice. *Professional Psychology: Research and Practice*, 38(2), 203–207. 10.1037/0735-7028.38.2.203

Weinberg, H. (2020a). From the couch to the screen—Online (group) therapy. *Groupcircle*, 1, 3.

Weinberg, H. (2020b). Online group psychotherapy: Challenges and possibilities during COVID-19—A practice review. *Group Dynamics: Theory, Research, and Practice*, 24(3), 201–211. 10.1037/gdn0000140

Ziadeh, S. (2020). Group interpersonal psychotherapy in the context of poverty and gender. In M. Ribeiro (Ed.), *Examining social identities and diversity issues in group therapy* (pp. 203–222). Routledge.

6 Supervision

For a neophyte group psychotherapist to develop into a competent group psychotherapist, supervision is essential. Supervisors are necessary for trainees' development of a knowledge base concerning group psychotherapy including theory and research, skills for conducting groups, and a set of professional attitudes that lead to ethical group practices. Supervisors are also critical to ensuring that the services supervisees provide advance the welfare of the members of their groups while avoiding any harm to those members (Barnett & Molzon, 2014).

Competence of Supervisors

To responsibly provide supervision of fledgling group psychotherapists, trainers need to be competent group psychotherapists themselves and be knowledgeable about clinical supervision and the supervision of group psychotherapists specifically. Achieving competence as a supervisor is challenging insofar as supervision is given short shrift in graduate training (Falender, 2018; Falender & Shafranske, 2007), often confined to a single course. Moreover, supervision of group psychotherapy might be a topic never broached in formal training. Consequently, group psychotherapists are often in the position of creating their own training program for this professional activity. Fortunately, in recent years, the resources have expanded for clinical supervisors, particularly in the form of guidelines, and these are listed in Table 6.1. An overview of these guidelines suggests that group psychotherapist-supervisors should (a) learn about models of supervision and research on supervision; (b) practice the skills in performing supervision; and (c) have their supervision of group psychotherapy work supervised.

Competence in group psychotherapy is not a unitary quality but varies according to the supervisory tasks undertaken (Barnett & Molzon, 2014). For example, a group psychotherapist who has provided supervision for a long-term outpatient group with a high level of competence will undoubtedly find that supervising an inpatient group demands new learning:

> Dr. Yar was contracted by a psychiatric hospital to supervise various group psychotherapy activities at the hospital. Dr. Yar was a well-known supervisor who had assisted many group psychotherapists launch private practice groups. Dr. Yar got off to a rocky start when supervising two psychology interns who found that their group sessions were poorly attended. The interns reported that several of the group members insisted on watching soap operas in the community room. The staff seemed unwilling to help the interns recruit the members for the session. The interns felt stymied and frustrated.

DOI: 10.4324/9781003105527-6

Table 6.1 Organizational Guidelines in Relation to Supervision

Title	Description	Reference
Guidelines for Clinical Supervision in Health Services Psychology	Seven domains with evidence-supported competencies	American Psychological Association. (2015). Guidelines for clinical supervision in health service psychology. *American Psychologist, 70*(1), 33–46. https://doi.org/10.1037/a0038112
ACA Code of Ethics, Section F	Addresses evaluation of supervisees, gatekeeping and remediation, counseling for supervisees, and endorsements.	American Counseling Association. (2014). *2014 ACA code of ethics.* https://www.counseling.org/Resources/aca-code-of-ethics.pdf
NASW Code of Ethics	Section 3.01 is on Supervision and Consultation and addresses competence, boundaries, dual/multiple relationships, and evaluation of supervisees.	National Association of Social Workers. (2017). *Code of ethics of the National Association of Social Workers.* https://www.socialworkers.org/About/Ethics/Code-of-Ethics/Code-of-Ethics-English
Association for Specialists in Group Work: Best Practice Guidelines	Section A8.b addresses supervision and consultation and establishes that supervisors have the responsibility of ensuring that supervisees adhere to ethical guidelines.	Thomas, R. V. & Pender, D.A. (2008). Association for specialists in group work: Best practice guidelines 2007 revisions. *The Journal for Specialists in Group Work, 33*(2), 111–117. https://doi.org/10.1080/01933920801971184

Relative to a private practice outpatient group, the inpatient group psychotherapist must attend assiduously to the relationship between the group and the treatment environment in which it is embedded (Brabender & Fallon, 2019). Dr. Yar, who enjoyed a high level of competence in supervising outpatient private practice groups, was far less competent in supervising an embedded group. From a virtue ethics perspective, in moving to this new venue, Dr. Yar would have been well-served by humility and honesty, which would have enabled him to realize that his supervisory competence needed bolstering in this new assignment.

Duties of Supervisors

Supervision of group psychotherapy is a complex activity that involves myriad responsibilities, each of which is directed toward assisting the trainee in acquiring the core competencies that group psychotherapy requires (see Barlow's group psychotherapy competency scheme, 2012). The supervisor assists supervisees in conceptualizing their group experiences, formulating interventions, recognizing their own reactions, engaging in ethical decision-making, and monitoring the progress of group members. The supervisor helps the supervisee to "stretch emotional boundaries" as well as contain members' intense affects (Alonso, 1985, p. 40). However, the group psychotherapy supervisor also provides emotional support for the supervisee who is likely to have anxieties and apprehensions about leading a group. Many of these will be the same reactions new group members have such as fear of exposure and worry about being attacked. Malat (2019) develops upon this notion further:

> Because of the large volume of interactions and amount of clinical data that occurs in any group session, supervisees can get overwhelmed and can become too focused on

the content of what everyone said in the group versus the nonverbal process in the group (Zaslav, 1988). In addition, there is much more public exposure in group therapy than individual therapy. Supervisees often have fears that are important to explore (e.g., fears that the group will become out of control (p. 196).

The Supervisory Alliance

The effective supervisor forges with the supervisee a robust supervisory alliance in which both parties recognize their common commitment to the growth of the supervisee as a group psychotherapist. The supervisor must create an atmosphere in which the supervisee feels comfortable acknowledging vulnerability. From a feminist ethics perspective (van Zyl, 2018), a supervisory relationship that has a strong collaborative element—one in which the supervisee's perspectives and reactions are recognized as having value—is more likely to encourage the supervisee's openness than a relationship in which the power differential is emphasized. A collaborative relationship is also one in which the feedback is bi-directional (Ammirati & Kaslow, 2017). The supervisor provides feedback to the supervisee but also invites the supervisee's feedback, which might take the form of the supervisee's observations of the supervisor's group work and the supervisee's feedback on the supervision itself. These demonstrations of supervisory humility (Watkins et al., 2019) are likely to strengthen the alliance between supervisor and supervisee. The supervisor strives to develop multicultural competence in the supervisee, and does so, in part, by demonstrating it in the relationship. For example, some supervisees might be challenged to empathize with group members whose background contrasts greatly with that of the supervisee. The supervisor can manifest the empathy the supervisee is currently lacking by showing curiosity about the supervisee's background and worldview and helping the supervisee to appreciate how the supervisee's experiences shape the group. Finally, but not exhaustively, supervisors inevitably make missteps and when they do, benefit the alliance by taking responsibility for acknowledging the mistake and making efforts to repair the relationship (Watkins et al., 2019); conversely, neglecting to repair a ruptured supervisory relationship can have a long-term detrimental effect on the relationship (Gray et al., 2001).

Provision of Feedback

A core competency for supervisors is to provide feedback in a way that provides the trainee with maximal opportunity to move forward as a group psychotherapist. It should be geared to what trainees are able to absorb at their developmental levels (Worthington, 2006). For example, rather than pointing out to a new group psychotherapist a missed interpretation, the supervisor might work with that trainee to pick up on a feeling expressed by several members. The recognition of patterns that many interpretations require would be appropriate for a more advanced trainee. The supervisor should take care to balance critical feedback with strength-based comments. Continuous negative feedback is demoralizing to a trainee and tends to go unheeded (Brabender, 2006). Weatherford et al. (2008) observed that positive feedback diminishes anxiety, especially in the case of the new supervisee, and increases self-efficacy. Feedback should be formative (ongoing) and summative. For example, after six months of working with a supervisor, a group psychotherapy trainee should not learn that the supervisor has observed the supervisee manifesting consistent problems with empathy. This feedback should have been delivered when the trainee began exhibiting the difficulty. Formative feedback provides the trainee the opportunity to make any necessary changes; withholding it departs from fair and just practice.

Ethical misjudgments should be treated with particular care by the supervisor. In such a circumstance, the trainee can readily feel shame and embarrassment. Such reactions, when intense, can deprive the trainee of the ability to explore the internal and external factors that led to misjudgment. Training is well-served when the supervisor can make clear that ethical judgment requires development, like any other ability. Good supervisors, even when embarrassed by the supervisee's conduct, avoid engaging in blaming behaviors that are unlikely to serve the supervisee's training needs.

The feedback the student is offered is only as good as the material on which the supervisor bases an assessment. The supervisor, rather than relying solely on the supervisee's report, should have direct exposure to the supervisee's work. Of course, if the supervisor is engaged in co-therapy with the trainee, direct observation is built into the arrangement. Otherwise, the supervisor should ask the supervisee to provide audiovisual recordings or the supervisor should be a silent observer in the group. Also, the supervisor might encourage the trainee to obtain client feedback to provide fodder for supervisory discussion and trainee evaluation, to enhance trainee self-efficacy (Reese et al., 2009), and to inculcate in the trainee the value of client feedback. Client outcomes also reflect on the quality of the supervision and therefore, provide feedback to supervisors themselves (Callahan et al., 2009). As the supervisor identifies challenges the supervisee is facing, the supervisor should identify potential learning experiences that might help the trainee to progress. For example, a trainee who is having difficulty remaining engaged in the midst of one or more angry group members could participate in role-plays with the supervisor taking on the role of an angry member.

Training the Supervisee to Be an Ethical Practitioner

The group psychotherapy supervisor must assist the supervisee in becoming an ethical practitioner. This developmental process is nurtured by helping the supervisee to see the basic elements of the group through an ethical lens, assisting the supervisee in learning not just the techniques and procedures of good practice, but in gaining an appreciation of the underlying ethical principles. For example, rather than merely teaching the supervisee how an informed consent is conducted, the supervisor should also cultivate the supervisee's understanding of how a strong informed consent safeguards the new member's autonomy. Likewise, as ethical conundrums emerge, the supervisor should not be so focused on solving the problem at hand as engaging the supervisee in a process of understanding how group psychotherapists deal with ethical problems. Focus on the ethical dimensions of practice should be an ongoing rather than occasional effort (Brabender, 2007; Kaklauskas & Olson, 2020).

Diagnosing Difficulties

The supervisor has an ethical obligation to assist the supervisee in remedying difficulties in achieving competence. Particularly when a supervisee has pervasive and seemingly intractable difficulties, the supervisor might be aided in conceptualizing this problem by considering the Ethics Acculturation model (Handelsman et al., 2005; Knapp et al., 2013, drawing on the work of Berry, 2003). This model's point of departure is the recognition that when individuals pursue training in a profession, they enter a new culture much like an immigrant adjusting to life in a new country (Bashe et al., 2007). When students travel abroad, they might be given a set of rules such as "Don't wear this type of attire," or "In this country, if you tip for services provided, it's considered offensive." Often a sufficiently robust set of rules enables students to navigate with at least a modicum level of success.

However, were the student to relocate for a substantial period, say, a year or two, the list of rules might not suffice. Rather, the student would need to take in the mores, ethos, and values of the culture, which would then enable the student to recognize what ways of comporting the self and relating to others would be regarded as acceptable. In doing so, the student must reconcile his or her own cultural sensibilities with those of the new culture. Some elements might chafe, that is, arouse tension, and the student would need to identify ways of grappling with the disparities between the very familiar and the less so.

The new group psychotherapist is in a similar situation. That person must acclimate to the mores, values, and sensibilities of the profession, including those that are pertinent to the practice of group psychotherapy. The Ethics Acculturation Model (Handelsman et al., 2005) recognizes that individuals come to the task of becoming an ethical decision-maker in that profession having developed their own values and beliefs about what constitutes ethical behavior in their personal lives. When disparities exist between personal and professional ethics, an individual might respond to the conflict in any one of a number of ways. Using an *assimilist strategy*, the individual could adopt wholesale the ethical culture of a profession while ignoring any pre-existing moral ideas. Such an approach leads to a rule-based approach to ethically fraught situations with problems arising when a rule does not exist in relation to a given ethical concern (Knapp et al., 2013). A *separatist strategy*, on the other hand, would direct the person to ignore what is regarded as acceptable to the profession while emphasizing personal morality. Supervisors are likely to regard such trainees as resistant to their input. Employing a *marginalizing strategy*, the person distances the self from both professional and personal frameworks, operating in a rudderless and often inconsistent fashion. Finally, an *integrationist strategy* would compel the person to find ways to harmonize personal and professional ethics:

> Carey began graduate school with a firm intent to help others. This value was consonant with and derived from her familial upbringing and her religious affiliation. In her graduate ethics class, she learned about how an adequate informed consent would entail apprising the potential patient of the risks of a given type of therapeutic involvement such as group psychotherapy. In her mind, the level of detail about possible risks should be titrated to ensure that the client was not discouraged from pursuing treatment. She was surprised to hear her instructor say that even if a detailed informed consent induced some possible clients to forego therapy, it is nonetheless sound ethical practice to provide them with a realistic picture of risks. It seemed odd to Carey that the instructor said that the client should determine what risks are tolerable. Eventually, Carey reasoned to herself that downplaying risks must not serve the well-being of the client because if the client were to feel deceived about this matter, it might diminish what that client could obtain from the treatment experience.

Whether or not Carey achieved the best possible integration of the two points of view, she nonetheless demonstrated openness and commitment to making the two frameworks congruent. Presumably, as Carey advances in experience and knowledge, she will exhibit progressively greater confidence in integrating the personal with the professional. This integration is crucial for a practitioner's achievement of maturity as an ethical decision-maker. For those trainees who evidence non-integrative strategies, substantial focus, and effort within training are needed to help them craft solutions to ethical problems that do justice to both the professional and the personal realms. The supervisor should help the supervisee to understand how ethical codes and guidelines can be helpful by referencing these tools and facilitate an exploration of the relationship between personal and professional codes.

Gatekeeping Responsibilities

At times, the provision of feedback, positive and negative, formative and summative, does not lead to necessary changes. Such occasions call upon the supervisor to take on another core supervisory role—that of gatekeeper. The gatekeeper role entails providing a professional judgment on whether an individual is qualified to proceed through a defined professional gate. The gate could be, for example, advancement in a profession or the ability to run a group independently in a professional setting. In many cases, group psychotherapy supervisors offer their professional opinions to others who are in a gatekeeping role. For example, the supervisor might submit an evaluation to the faculty of a doctoral program who will determine whether the student is permitted to interview for an internship, the next step in the student's program. Whether the group psychotherapy supervisor is an intermediate or ultimate gatekeeper, this role is important to ensure that the public is protected from unqualified practitioners.

Supervisees who show significant difficulties mastering or executing the competencies of the group psychotherapist to a degree commensurate with their developmental levels can be described as having professional competence problems (PCP; Elman & Forrest, 2007). This term, commonly used in professional psychology, represents a terminological advancement upon the longstanding and stigmatizing term "impaired." Were the trainee to fail to show the necessary progress, it would be incumbent upon the supervisor to provide the supervisee with concrete, direct feedback on the identified competency for which progress is insufficient, a process entailing engagement in a difficult conversation (Lichtenberg et al., 2007). Partaking in a difficult conversation can be regarded as an additional core competency of the group psychotherapy supervisor (Jacobs et al., 2011). The supervisor should not succumb to the temptation to pass the problem on to the next supervisor, a common practice that ultimately exposes the public to the risk of incompetent practitioners (Barnett & Molzon, 2014). For example, Johnson et al. (2008) summarize evidence from supervisors and faculty members that both sets of gatekeepers often offer intentionally inflated evaluations of trainees' performance. In taking on the sometimes unpleasant task of being a gatekeeper (or providing information unfavorable to the trainee to another overarching gatekeeper), the supervisor is honoring the principle of Non-maleficence, that is, avoiding harm to the people the trainee might eventually serve.

Just as supervisees carry risk of failing to serve their group members well or even causing harm to them, so too can supervision be harmful to the supervisee. Harmful supervision can occur when the supervisor acts with malice toward the supervisee, violates professional standards, or shows such a low level of conscientiousness that trainees are implicitly called upon to fend for themselves in the group (Ellis et al., 2014).

Training and Supervision in Group Settings

As this section discusses, additional complexity is created when a learner is embedded in a group of others learning, either for purposes of supervision or experiential group participation.

Group Supervision

One common training medium for group psychotherapists is group supervision involving a supervisor and multiple supervisees who typically lead different groups. This method first emerged because it was regarded as an efficient pedagogical medium, that is, multiple supervisees could receive training simultaneously from one supervisor (Fleming et al., 2010; Hanetz Gamliel et al., 2020). Group supervision has many of the strengths of group psychotherapy, among which are the multiplicity of perspectives and the presence of different types of relationships, relationships with authority and those with peers. To realize the potential benefits of group supervision, supervisors must create an atmosphere of safety by, for example, by communicating supervisor's expectations at the outset of supervision (Araneda, 2015), establishing confidentiality of the group's discussion, and ensuring that unwholesome dynamics such as a high level of competitiveness among members are dismantled. In some cases, supervisees might participate in group supervision while also having individual supervision with the same supervisor or a different supervisor. However, in the absence of additional supervisory contact, the group supervisor must glean sufficient knowledge about each group to know that all of the members' treatment needs are being met.

Experiential Training Groups

One common vehicle for the training of group psychotherapists is the experiential group through which members can learn about group dynamics and achieve an empathic grasp of many aspects of being a group member (Anderson & Price, 2001; Shumaker et al., 2011). Such experiences also enable members to recognize and modify biases and assumptions (Kaklauskas & Nettles, 2020). These benefits suggest that experiential groups can operate in the service of Beneficence. However, for this potential to be realized, members must be protected from any risks that could be attached to such groups. Group phenomena such as coercion, intimidation, microaggressions, and discrimination of members based on their identity statuses can occur in experiential groups as in psychotherapy groups (Lefforge et al., 2020). The leader has an ethical obligation to intervene to protect members from these processes:

> A training institute offered experiential groups for trainees. The leader of the group was also the director of the institute who played a major role in members' advancement through their training program. D'Andre was a group member who was inclined to be more reserved than the other members. After a few sessions, his reticence became noticeable to the other group members, and they began to urge him to be more forthcoming. At one point, he dissolved into tears and left the group room. The group leader/director called him in and asked D'Andre what had upset him. D'Andre revealed that he tended to be relatively inactive in group settings, that he takes a long time to "warm-up." He was frightened that his non-disclosive stance in the group would jeopardize his standing in the training program but also concerned about how particular hidden aspects of his identity would be received by the group members and the leader/training director.

Members do at times encourage one another to open up in the group, a process that can be quite helpful. The group leader has an obligation to discern the point beyond which this encouragement becomes undue pressure, a development requiring leader intervention. They must also discern the level of self-disclosure that is appropriate to a training group versus a therapy group, although this boundary at times will be challenging to locate. Leaders must recognize within themselves forces such as curiosity about the silent member that might hinder their recognition of this line. Limiting self-disclosure to here-and-now reactions in the group is a means of avoiding harm to members, particularly those seeking to protect sensitive information (Yalom & Leszcz, 2020). Still another means is to engage members, prior to group participation, in a discussion about judicious self-disclosure.

The vignette, however, revealed another problem—the dual roles held by the leader. Although the group members ought to have autonomy over their self-disclosures, that autonomy is lessened if important consequences ride on the member's degree of disclosure. Members of experiential training groups are most likely to have their autonomy and privacy protected if leaders carefully think about dual role issues in planning the group. In our vignette, D'Andre and likely other members would have been better served by having someone other than the director of the institute to lead the group. Likewise, when an experiential group is part of a course in group psychotherapy or group dynamics, instructors might consider having another individual lead the experiential portion. Given that such a solution might be cost-prohibitive in many programs, another option is to refrain from evaluating individuals on their participation in the experiential component. The experiential portion of a course should incorporate an informed consent document that includes a specification of (a) any areas in which they will be evaluated and (b) whether the evaluations will feed into any larger decision-making or gatekeeping activity. D'Andre along with other members should have been informed of whether a lack of self-disclosure would be used in decisions about his status in the program. The leader should consider how the privacy of members will be protected. For example, a confidentiality rule should be established with a description of sanctions for violations, and this material should be included in the informed consent. Regular reminders about the confidentiality rule should be given in the group.

Supervisory Contracts and Documentation of Supervision

Increasingly, mental health professionals are recognizing that the various benefits that accrue from a therapy contract with informed consent also extend to the supervisory relationship. When both supervisor and supervisee have a shared understanding of how they intend to work together, less opportunity exists for negative events to occur within the relationship. A good contract describes the specifics concerning the supervisory meetings, the mediums used in supervision, and the methods and criteria by which the supervisee's performance will be evaluated (Gilfoyle, 2008). Supervisees benefit from knowing the processes that will be employed in the supervision. For example, supervisors sometimes draw upon the exploration of the dynamics of the group as they are reflected in the supervisor-supervisee relationship (that is, parallel process). Supervisees benefit from being alerted that this type of work does occur in the supervisory sessions and helped to appreciate its benefits. Supervisory contracts are also useful in supervision groups. In this case, ethical issues such as the maintenance of confidentiality within the supervision groups should be incorporated into the contract.

Supervision sessions should be documented as carefully as psychotherapy sessions. For each supervisory session, the issues in the group and the guidance given to the supervisee should be indicated. However, like the group psychotherapist, the supervisor must be aware of issues of confidentiality and privilege, creating notes that will protect the privacy of individual group members. Supervisors should be aware of any state regulations that might guide their record-keeping for supervisory sessions. Pre-licensure supervisees might benefit by maintaining records of dates and times of supervision, as well as the focus of the supervision for each session (Carnahan & Adorjan, 2017).

Key Distinctions Related to Supervision

This section seeks to provide clarity on the meaning of supervision by distinguishing it from activities that are similar to it but nonetheless distinct. It also acknowledges two subtypes of supervision, clinical and administrative.

Supervision versus Psychotherapy

Good supervisors are adaptable and flexible, modifying their methods based on the learning needs of the supervisee. At times, the discussion of trainee reactions in the sessions and difficulties in performing particular functions might lead to the identification of issues that relate to the individual's struggles in personal relationships and problems that the supervisee might recognize as rooted in their past. Here, the supervisor must draw a line between supervision and psychotherapy. Although problems can be spotted in the supervisory environment, it lacks the features (exclusivity of focus, informed consent, freedom of expression without evaluation) that the psychotherapy environment possesses. Moreover, when the supervisee's psychological health becomes the focus, the supervisor's work and the well-being of members are inevitably neglected. Therefore, the supervisor should exercise care that the supervision remains supervision but identify alternate resources for the student when it is warranted.

Clinical versus Administrative Supervision

Clinical supervision should be distinguished from administrative supervision. The former is primarily focused on the clinical work of the trainee, ensuring that it meets the standard of care, a level of practice regarded as adequate by other prudent, and discerning professionals in one's area. Administrative supervision focuses on the trainee's interface with the larger organization (Tromski-Klingshirn, 2007), attending to such issues as whether the trainee is meeting a particular number of client contact hours. In some settings, the two roles are combined, giving rise to possibilities for conflict. For example, the time allotted to supervision might be unduly focused on administrative rather than clinical matters, leaving the clients' care and the trainee's development as a therapist neglected. A clinical supervisor might discuss with the supervisee the limitations that are created when a group grows beyond a certain size. However, when this role combines with administrative supervision, the supervisor, attentive to institutional pressures, might downplay or ignore this factor. When these roles are combined, supervisors have an ethical obligation to anticipate role conflicts, identify ways to circumvent them as much as possible, and to disclose to the supervisee which role is being served at any given moment.

Supervision versus Consultation

Consultation is different from supervision in terms of the authority for doing clinical work. In supervision, the supervisor takes responsibility not only for the supervisee but also the members in the group the supervisee conducts (Brabender, 2006). In consultation, the professional gives guidance but does not have responsibility for services delivered. For example, a group psychotherapist who is a licensed social worker might obtain a consultation when faced with one of the difficult situations presented in this chapter. The social worker is responsible for whatever decision is implemented. Because consultation is a voluntary service, the group psychotherapist need not follow the advice of the consultant (Brabender et al., 2015). Occasionally, a supervisee might receive a consultation. For example, the supervisee might present material from a group session in a graduate course and receive input from the course instructor. The course instructor is not the supervisor, and the supervisee is bound to conform to the direction of the latter, not the former, were the two perspectives to diverge.

Final Note

Skilled supervision is crucial in the development of competent group psychotherapists. Although attending to mastery of theory and technique is crucial, equally important is cultivating good supervisee's ethical judgment. Supervisors do well to use everyday experiences in conducting psychotherapy groups to point out to trainees the ethical and legal dimensions of the work. They also aid trainees by modeling sound ethical behavior. Supervisors can also make an important contribution by using supervisee's lapses in ethical judgment as an opportunity for training rather than for shaming.

CEU items

1. Supervisors and faculty members tend to offer inflated evaluations of trainees. (T/F)
2. The goals of administrative and clinical supervision can conflict. (T/F)
3. Group psychotherapists must adhere to the guidance they receive in consultations. (T/F)
4. Supervision can be helpful, neutral, or harmful. (T/F)
5. Experiential groups held in a training context should make clear to participants whether their performance is evaluated and how the evaluations will be used. (T/F)
6. Group leaders who conduct training experiential groups should be skilled in recognizing and addressing microaggressions. (T/F)
7. A clinical supervisor is legally responsible for the supervisee's work. (T/F)
8. The term "professional competence problems" is generally preferred over "impaired" in today's training environments. (T/F)
9. "I know it was against the law, but I had to follow my conscience." This group leader is likely embracing a separatist approach to ethical decision-making. (T/F)

1 T; 2. T; 3. F; 4. T; 5. T; 6. T; 7. T; 8. T; 9. T

Discussion Questions

1. Discuss some important boundary issues in the supervisor/supervisee relationships.
2. What are the advantages of a supervision contract?
3. What are some possible resistances to the creation of a supervision contract?
4. What supervisory reactions are likely to be evoked by supervisees who exhibit assimilist versus separatist ethical stances?
5. All group psychotherapists should participate in an experiential group as part of their training. Do you agree or disagree?

Vignettes/Role-Plays

1. You have supervised a co-therapy pair for several months. The initial few weeks of the supervision were rocky as the co-therapists ironed out the different views they had for the group. One co-therapist contacted you prior to the session and indicated that the pair felt they could no longer work together. The co-therapist related an event in which her partner engaged in a very high level of self-disclosure about personal problems. She said to the supervisor, "I feel my co-therapist is engaging in an unethical act by visiting his problems on the members. I think he could be harming them."

    1. How might you help the co-therapy process their differences and move forward in a constructive way?

    2.   Role-play the three-way meeting in which the discussion focuses on self-disclosure and settling on a plan for the future of the group.

2.   A supervisor has observed the trainee arrive at group sessions late on multiple occasions. The trainee is given feedback but fails to improve. The supervisor completes in a candid way an evaluation form for the trainee's doctoral program. The administrator to whom the supervisor reports directs the supervisor to characterize the trainee's behavior in less negative ways to avert liability. If you were the supervisor, how might you respond?

3.   Role-play a difficult conversation between a supervisor and a supervisee in which the supervisor conveys that the supervisee is more responsive to the group members that share the supervisee's identity status vis-à-vis race and gender. Help the supervisee explore possible bases for this bias.

References

Alonso, A. (1985). *The quiet profession: Supervisors of psychotherapy*. Macmillan.

Ammirati, R. J., & Kaslow, N. J. (2017). All supervisors have the potential to be harmful. *The Clinical Supervisor, 36*(1), 116–123. 10.1080/07325223.2017.1298071

Anderson, R. D., & Price, G. E. (2001). Experiential groups in counselor education: Student attitudes and instructor participation. *Counselor Education and Supervision, 41*(2), 111–119. 10.1002/j.1556-6978.2001.tb01275.x

Araneda, M. E. (2015). *Clinical group supervision in mental health counseling training: Experiences of supervisors and their supervisees* [Unpublished doctoral dissertation]. University of Rochester. https://urresearch.rochester.edu/fileDownloadForInstitutionalItem.action?itemId=30401&itemFileId=166560

Barlow, S. H. (2012). An application of the competency model to the group-specialty practice. *Professional Psychology: Research and Practice, 43*(5), 442–451. 10.1037/a0029090

Barnett, J. E., & Molzon, C. H. (2014). Clinical supervision of psychotherapy: Essential ethics issues for supervisors and supervisees. *Journal of Clinical Psychology, 70*(11), 1051–1061. 10.1002/jclp.22126

Bashe, A., Anderson, S. K., Handelsman, M. M., & Klevansky, R. (2007). An acculturation model for ethics training: The ethics autobiography and beyond. *Professional Psychology: Research and Practice, 38*(1), 60–67. 10.1037/0735-7028.38.1.60

Berry, J. W. (2003). Conceptual approaches to acculturation. In K. M., Chun, P. B., Organista, &G., Marin (Eds.) *Acculturation: Advances in Theory, Measurement, and Applied Research*, (pp. 17–37). American Psychological Association.

Brabender, V. (2006). On the mechanisms and effects of feedback in group psychotherapy. *Journal of Contemporary Psychotherapy, 36*(3), 121–128. 10.1007/BF02729055

Brabender, V. (2007). The ethical group psychotherapist: A coda. *International Journal of Group Psychotherapy, 57*(1), 41–48. 10.1521/ijgp.2007.57.1.41

Brabender, V., & Fallon, A. (2019). *Group psychotherapy in inpatient, partial hospital, and residential care settings*. American Psychological Association.

Brabender, V., Knauss, L., & Foster, E. (2015). Psychotherapy supervision: Ethical considerations and resources. *Psychotherapy Section Review, 56*, 38–56.

Callahan, J. L., Almstrom, C. M., Swift, J. K., Borja, S. E., & Heath, C. J. (2009). Exploring the contribution of supervisors to intervention outcomes. *Training and Education in Professional Psychology, 3*(2), 72–77. 10.1037/a0014294

Carnahan, B. & Adorjan, M.A. (2017). Document like a clinician: The ins and outs of documenting your training supervision [Online exclusives]. *Counseling Today*. https://ct.counseling.org/2017/01/document-like-clinician-ins-outs-documenting-training-supervision/#

De Cremer, D., Pillutla, M. M., & Folmer, C. R. (2011). How important is an apology to you? Forecasting errors in evaluating the value of apologies. *Psychological Science, 22*(1), 45–48. 10.1177/0956797610391101

Ellis, M. V., Berger, L., Hanus, A. E., Ayala, E. E., Swords, B. A., & Siembor, M. (2014). Inadequate and harmful clinical supervision: Testing a revised framework and assessing occurrence. *The Counseling Psychologist*, *42*(4), 434–472. 10.1177/0011000013508656

Elman, N.S., & Forrest, L. (2007). From trainee impairment to professional competence problems: Seeking new terminology that facilitates effective action. *Professional Psychology: Research and Practice*, *38*(5), 501–509. 10.1037/0735-7028.38.5.501 (Retraction published 1999, *The Counseling Psychologist, 27*[5], 627–686).

Falender, C. A. (2018). Clinical supervision—the missing ingredient. *American Psychologist*, *73*(9), 1240–1250. 10.1037/amp0000385

Falender, C. A., & Shafranske, E. P. (2007). Competence in competency-based supervision practice: Construct and application. *Professional Psychology: Research and Practice*, *38*(3), 232–240. 10.103 7/0735-7028.38.3.232

Fleming, L. M., Glass, J. A., Fujisaki, S., & Toner, S. L. (2010). Group process and learning: A grounded theory model of group supervision. *Training and Education in Professional Psychology*, *4*(3), 194–203. 10.1037/a0018970

Gilfoyle, N. (2008). The legal exosystem: Risk management in addressing student competence problems in professional psychology training. *Training and Education in Professional Psychology*, *2*(4) 202–209. 10.1037/1931-3918.2.4.202

Gray, L. A., Ladany, N., Walker, J. A., & Ancis, J. R. (2001). Psychotherapy trainees' experience of counterproductive events in supervision. *Journal of Counseling Psychology*, *48*(4), 371–383. 10.1037/ 0022-0167.48.4.371

Handelsman, M. M., Gottlieb, M. C., & Knapp, S. (2005). Training ethical psychologists: An acculturation model. *Professional Psychology: Research and Practice*, *36*(1), 59–65. 10.1037/0735-7028.36.1.59

Hanetz Gamliel, K., Geller, S., Illuz, B., & Levy, S. (2020). The contribution of group supervision processes to the formation of professional identity among novice psychotherapists. *International Journal of Group Psychotherapy*, *70*(3), 375–398. 10.1080/00207284.2020.1727747

Jacobs, S. C., Huprich, S. K., Grus, C. L., Cage, E. A., Elman, N. S., Forrest, L., Schwartz-Mette, R., Shen-Miller, D. S., Van Sickle, K. S., & Kaslow, N. J. (2011). Trainees with professional competency problems: Preparing trainers for difficult but necessary conversations. *Training and Education in Professional Psychology*, *5*(3), 175–184. 10.1037/a0024656 (Retraction published 2012, *Training and Education in Professional Psychology, 6*[4], 219).

Johnson, W. B., Elman, N. S., Forrest, L., Robiner, W. N., Rodolfa, E., & Schaffer, J. B. (2008). Addressing professional competence problems in trainees: Some ethical considerations. *Professional Psychology: Research and Practice*, *39*(6), 589–599. 10.1037/a0014264

Kaklauskas, F. J., & Nettles, R. (2020). Towards multicultural and diversity proficiency as a group psychotherapist. In F. J. Kaklauskas & L. R. Greene (Eds.). *Core principles of group psychotherapy: An integrated theory, research, and practice training manual* (pp. 25–46). Routledge.

Kaklauskas, F. J., & Olson, E. A. (2020). The ethical group psychotherapist. In F. J. Kaklauskas & L. R. Greene (Eds.). *Core principles of group psychotherapy: An integrated theory, research, and practice manual* (pp. 143–155). Routledge.

Kaslow, N. J., Borden, K. A., Collins F. L., Jr., Forrest, L., Illfelder-Kaye, J., Nelson, P. D., Rallo, J. S., Vasquez, M. J. T., Willmuth, M. E. (2004). Competencies conference: Future directions in education and credentialing in professional psychology. *Journal of Clinical Psychology*, *60*(7), 699–712. 10.1002/jclp.20016

Knapp, S., Handelsman, M. M., Gottlieb, M. C., & VandeCreek, L. D. (2013). The dark side of professional ethics. *Professional Psychology: Research and Practice*, *44*(6), 371–377. 10.1037/a0035110

Lefforge, N. L., Mclaughlin, S., Goates-Jones, M., & Mejia, C. (2020). A training model for addressing microaggressions in group psychotherapy. *International Journal of Group Psychotherapy*, *70*(1), 1–28. 10.1080/00207284.2019.1680989

Lichtenberg, J., Portnoy, S., Bebeau, M., Leigh, I. W., Nelson, P. D., Rubin, N. J., … Kaslow, N. J. (2007). Challenges to the assessment of competence and competencies. *Professional Psychology: Research and Practice*, *38*, 474–478. doi:10.1037/0735-7028.38.5.474

Malat, J. (2019). Group psychotherapy supervision: Working at multiple levels. In S. G. De Golia & K. M. Corcoran (Eds.), *Supervision in psychiatric practice: Practical approaches across venues and providers* (pp. 195–202). American Psychiatric Association. https://www.appi.org/Supervision_in_Psychiatric_Practice

Reese, R. J., Usher E. L., Bowman, D. C., Norsworthy, L. A., Halstead, J. L., Rowlands, S. R., & Chisholm, R. R. (2009). Using client feedback in psychotherapy training: An analysis of its influence on supervision and counselor self-efficacy. *Training and Education in Professional Psychology*, 3(3), 157–168. 10.1037/a0015673

Shumaker, D., Ortiz, C., & Brenninkmeyer, L. (2011). Revisiting experiential group training in counselor education: A survey of master's-level programs. *The Journal for Specialists in Group Work*, 36(2), 111–128. 10.1080/01933922.2011.562742

Tromski-Klingshirn, D. (2007). Should the clinical supervisor be the administrative supervisor? The ethics versus the reality. *The Clinical Supervisor*, 25(1-2), 53–67. 10.1300/J001v25n01_05

van Zyl, L. (2018). *Virtue ethics: A contemporary introduction*. Routledge. 10.4324/9780203361962

Watkins, C. E., Hook, J. N., Mosher, D. K., & Callahan, J. L. (2019). Humility in clinical supervision: Fundamental, foundational, and transformational. *The Clinical Supervisor*, 38(1), 58–78. 10.1080/07325223.2018.1487355

Weatherford, R., O'Shaughnessy, T., Mori, Y., & Kaduvettoor, A. (2008). The new supervisee: Order from chaos. In A. K. Hess, K. D. Hess, & T. H. Hess (Eds.), *Psychotherapy supervision: Theory, research, and practice* (pp. 40–54). John Wiley.

Worthington Jr, E. L. (2006). Changes in supervision as counselors and supervisors gain experience: A review. *Training and Education in Professional Psychology*, S(2), 133–160. 10.1037/1931-3918.S.2.133

Yalom, I. D., & Leszcz, M. (2020). *The theory and practice of group psychotherapy*. Basic Books.

Zaslav, M. R. (1988). A model of group therapist development. *International Journal of Group Psychotherapy*, 38(4), 511–519. 10.1080/00207284.1988.11491136

7 The Group Psychotherapist as Ethical Decision-Maker: Process and Product

In the previous chapters, the group psychotherapist might appear to be a wholly rational being who systematically and dispassionately proceeds through a set of decision-making steps leading to a solution likely to be embraced by other similarly trained and experienced group psychotherapists. However, the reality is at times distinct from this depiction. In this chapter, we aim to identify those factors and forces outside of rational, deliberate thought that shape the decision-making process. We consider how these factors and forces can hinder or help the leader in making a good decision based on how the leader approaches them.

In this chapter, as well, we look at the product of decision-making activity—the solutions to dilemmas and practices that group leaders adopt. How are these products likely to be evaluated by their peers? We examine these issues in terms of "Standard of Care," which is defined as a level of practice regarded as adequate by other prudent and discerning professionals in one's area.

Challenges to Ethical Decision-Making

Roughly, challenges to sound ethical decision-making might be categorized as external, that is, residing within the situation the group psychotherapist is facing, or internal, elements the situation activates within the person of the therapist. Admittedly, this distinction is artificial in that aspects of the external situation evoke a reaction in the therapist. Nonetheless, the distinction is heuristic in that it supports the adoption of an inward and an outward perspective in considering professional ethics, both of which are essential.

External or Contextual Challenges

In this section, we characterize those challenges that are contextual. The first challenge, "Multiple Stakeholders," pertains to the structure of the modality itself and how it invites the emergence of particular types of ethical problems. "Organizational Influences" concern the broader context in which the group is embedded.

Multiple Stakeholders

Ethical dilemmas across all modalities have multiple stakeholders, individuals who are affected by whatever decision the therapist makes. The recipient of the therapist's services is a primary stakeholder whose well-being must be paramount to the therapist in relation to that of other parties. In group psychotherapy, the therapist has multiple stakeholders—all the group members—whose well-being is primary. Therefore, the therapist cannot solve a dilemma in relation to one group member without thinking about the effects of various solutions on other group members.

DOI: 10.4324/9781003105527-7

Brabender (2021) describes a circumstance in which a member engaged in multiple violations of confidentiality that ultimately the therapist recognized were due to confusion and possible neurodegenerative disease. The member's violations were unintentional. Moreover, she was someone who appeared to derive considerable benefit from group participation. The therapist's decision about the member's status in the group cannot address her well-being independently of that of the other group members. To have a member who lacks the capacity needed to safeguard other members' privacy risks bringing them harm and is an untenable situation. Because therapists have an obligation to protect members' privacy as much as possible, the therapist's obligation in this situation would be to ask the member to leave the group and to find an alternate treatment for the member. However, in other situations, no evident ethical mandate may offer itself to the therapist and will therefore require creative problem-solving, consultation, and an effort to harmonize various interests.

When confronted with the problem of the multiple stakeholders, the group psychotherapist can be aided by distinguishing between the client and collateral parties. Consider the following vignette:

> Victor, a fifteen-year-old adolescent, participated in a group for treatment of depression. Over the course of the group, Victor came to learn about his habitual avoidance of conflict with others, most especially authority figures. He began to make progress in this regard by, for example, joining other members in expressing irritation toward the therapist. The therapist received a call from Victor's father who said to the therapist that the group was making Victor worse. Although his father admitted that Victor seemed less depressed, he reported that Victor had been engaging in a good deal of backtalk with both of his parents, a behavior he saw as thoroughly unacceptable. He suggested that perhaps the others in the group were "bad influences" and asked the therapist to recommend a different group for Victor.

In this case, both Victor and his parents are stakeholders in his treatment in that all can be affected by any changes (or lack thereof) associated with it. A phone call like the one made by Victor's father reminds the therapist of this fact. Therapists easily feel beholden to adolescent and child members' parents because they typically provide the funding and legal consent for the treatment and may offer other forms of needed support such as transportation. New therapists, in particular, might feel so accountable to parents registering complaints that they give the parents' preferences undue weight. Recognizing that Victor is the client and that the parents are the collaterals who help the therapist to devise an ethically defensible solution to the problem of the parents' displeasure with Victor's behavior. Such recognition would help the therapist not to succumb, in some fashion, to the pressures applied by the parents but to adopt an approach that could reduce tensions between Victor and his parents. The therapist might adopt a psychoeducational approach, providing the parents with information about adolescent development while doing so in a culturally sensitive manner.

Organizational Influences

Throughout these chapters, we have written as though the therapist has full decision-making latitude. Generally, it is only in private practice that this is the case and even there, various contextual forces impinge on how the therapist conducts the group and can bear upon ethical decision-making. However, when a group psychotherapist is working in a larger system of care, particularly when the group is one of multiple elements in a treatment program, the therapist's capacity to control all the features of the group is typically much more severely limited. At times, an organization might dictate practices that are at odds with the therapist's view of sound group practice. For example, the organization might require that the therapist accept a particular number of members into the group that is far beyond that which can reasonably be accommodated. At times, the disparity between the therapist's views of how a group ought to be conducted versus how it is mandated to be conducted could raise ethical concerns in the mind of the therapist.

Overall, before settling into an organization, group psychotherapists should ensure that their personal and professional values align, at least roughly, with the organization's values. Otherwise, the group psychotherapist will likely be facing difficult ethical dilemmas with some regularity, possibly in a context of powerful system-level resistances to their resolution. Low job satisfaction can result from such a values clash (O'Donnell et al., 2008). Group psychotherapists also benefit from examining the organizations in which they conduct their groups with a view to identifying elements in the environment that could hinder ethical decision-making and developing ways to lessen their influence.

Emerging research on situational factors within a workplace that affect ethical decision-making has yielded several findings. First, a high level of performance pressure on employees is associated with weaker ethical decision-making (Mumford et al., 2006). Second, a high level of exposure to ethical lapses in the workplace leads to a lower level of ethical reasoning (Mumford et al., 2006). Third, Mumford et al. (2007) found that higher interpersonal conflict in work settings is associated with poorer ethical decision-making. Fourth, when an individual in a work situation responds to an ethical problem involving a supervisor as opposed to a peer, that individual's decision is more likely to be compromised (Stenmark & Mumford, 2011). Fifth, individuals in leadership positions (and conducting a psychotherapy group is a leadership position) who are not accorded a reasonable level of autonomy and who have not achieved a modicum of self-efficacy will make a poorer decision than individuals higher in autonomy and self-efficacy. Sixth, some individuals are in a work environment that calls upon them to engage in a great deal of high-stakes ethical decision-making. Such a circumstance can lead to stress and burnout (Freudenberger, 1990; Mullen et al., 2017), which in turn could lessen the therapist's ability to make good decisions.

Internal Factors

These factors are those the decision-maker brings to the ethical dilemma. Some concern regular features of human information processing and others, styles and preferences of the individual decision-maker.

Decision-Making Biases and Heuristics

In Chapter 1, the step-by-step model for ethical decision-making we presented might suggest that rational thought processes dominate the decider's activity. However, our last section highlighted that stress can easily seep into decision-making activities and alter them, affecting such important elements of ethical problem-solving as the range of solutions the individual considers before making a final decision or whether the decision is based on self-interest or the well-being of others. To appreciate the array of factors that enter both everyday and ethical decision-making, it is helpful to consider the distinction between intuition and deliberate reasoning, made by Kahneman (2011), Bargh et al. (2012), and others. Automatic processing entails intuitive, rapid thought processes, which occur with minimal expenditure of effort and under minimal voluntary control. In our daily lives, much of our cognitive activity falls within this category. The mental operations that one needs to make coffee or tea in the morning are likely governed by automatic thinking. They are so habitual that one can perform them while thinking about something else such as one's agenda for the day. Deliberate thinking involves effortful cognition that engages focused attention and concentration. If we say to another person, "Please stop watching TV and listen to what I'm saying right now," we are asking for deliberate thinking to take precedence in the person's cognitive activities while acknowledging that attention is limited—it is unlikely that the person will register what we say without withdrawing attention from the TV. At times, the group leader might decide to observe some aspect of group behavior such as the nonverbal exchanges between two members. In doing so, the leader is engaging in deliberate processing.

Automatic and deliberate types of processing continually work together as we pursue life's tasks. Automatic processing takes a stronger role when tasks are relatively un-challenging, and as they increase in demand, deliberate processing's contribution becomes more prominent. Even when deliberate thinking dominates, automatic processing offers reactions, impressions, and ideas as fodder for deliberative thinking. To take our earlier example, the individual trying to figure out the workings of a new brewing system (de-liberate processing) will be influenced by past experiences or overlearning with other brewing systems (automatic processing). In fact, some early mistakes might occur because of the misapplication of prior knowledge to the current circumstance. *By recognizing de-liberate thinking's dependence on automatic thinking, we can understand that much more occurs in ethical decision-making than an orderly thought process.* If a group leader senses that an ethical problem exists, it is likely that deliberate thinking will then be engaged. That is, many of the activities we described (e.g., clarifying the problem, identifying re-levant standards, and generating alternative solutions), particularly in Chapter 1 and elsewhere, will occur. However, those activities will be shaped by automatic appraisals of the problem, which themselves are a result of automatic heuristics and biases.

A heuristic is a shortcut. Kahneman (2011) defines it as "…a simple procedure that helps find adequate, though often imperfect answers to difficult questions" (p. 98). We give examples of three types of heuristics to provide the reader with a sense of how they might enter a clinician's decision-making. One major type of heuristic that human beings employ is the *availability heuristic*, a strategy wherein an individual bases a prediction of how likely an event will occur on how easily it comes to mind. Consider:

> Dr. Clate is considering beginning a second psychotherapy group. To design the group, he attempts to predict the level of functioning of individuals who will be referred to him for group psychotherapy in the near future. He immediately bases his estimate on recent referrals. He remembers that the last two individuals were high functioning, and he begins to design the group for high functioning people.

Immediately, the reader might recognize the flaw in Dr. Clate's method. The more recent referrals might be unrepresentative of the referrals Dr. Clate typically gets. Still, Dr. Clate saved himself considerable time and effort. In some circumstances, Dr. Clate might have the thought, "I don't have access to my records right now. I will use the last two referrals I've received as a proxy for the group, just to get an idea." This conscious embrace of a strategy will enable Dr. Clate to know that he might well be off base in his prediction, a useful caution. However, ordinarily, heuristics are automatic—that is, non-intentional—and easily deny the decision-maker of any awareness of their limitations. Moreover, to the extent that Dr. Clate's recollection of these last two referrals was vivid, he is likely to be more convinced of their usefulness as a predictive base. The overall point is that Dr. Clate's thinking is likely to be more effective if he recognizes and considers his decision-making bias.

Another heuristic is the *anchoring-and-adjustment strategy* wherein an individual uses a piece of information as an anchor for making a judgment, particularly in situations in which numerical estimates are sought. Suppose in a workshop on group psychotherapy, a participant asks the presenter, Dr. Tim, "How often do you remind group members of the confidentiality rule—every session?" If the presenter lacks a rule for confidentiality reminders (e.g., reminding members on the first session of the month), that leader will consult memory but do so using the suggestion "every session" as an anchor. Perhaps, Dr. Tim reminds members approximately once every six months about the confidentiality rule. Dr. Tim will nonetheless use "once a month" as an anchor and make an adjustment from there. For example, Dr. Tim might think, "No, I know it's not as frequent as once a month. Maybe I remind them every three months." Had the participant asked, "Do you remind members once a year about confidentiality?" Dr. Tim might have proffered "every nine months" as his response. Dr. Tim has used an anchor without knowing it.

Particularly relevant to group leaders is the *affect heuristic*, which is a shortcut by which we evaluate information according to our feelings about the topic at hand.

> Lakshmi had been in Dr. Nguyen's therapy group for a year and Dr. Branch's individual therapy for three years. Dr. Branch contacted Dr. Nguyen and said he had not observed any positive changes in Lakshmi in the past six months; he felt she was languishing, perhaps in both of the treatments. He shared that Lakshmi herself had described herself as "stalled." Dr. Nguyen found Lakshmi to be a great asset to the group and she felt very warmly toward Lakshmi. Quickly, she asserted that Lakshmi had been very productive in the group and was benefiting from her engagement with the members. When Dr. Branch pushed her to provide specifics, Dr. Nguyen found herself to be at a loss.

Regarding our group members and our decisions about them, we are going to be affected by our feelings, especially those feelings whose presence we do not fully acknowledge. Dr. Nguyen might have been led to see Lakshmi's progress in positive terms because of her positive feelings for Lakshmi. Likewise, Dr. Nguyen's view of Dr. Branch's feedback might have been shaped by her feelings toward Dr. Branch. Again, typically, Dr. Nguyen will have little awareness of the influence of these affective factors. The affect heuristic is especially important for our consideration because its presence in our decision-making highlights that decisions are not an entirely rational matter. This conclusion, though not particularly surprising, should be of concern to all group psychotherapists as they strive to solve ethical dilemmas: the emotional backdrop of a decision could determine how the therapist evaluates various alternatives.

Approaches to Risk

Uncertainty accompanies ethical decision-making. The decision-maker is called upon to project into the future to anticipate what consequences are likely from any course of action. According to prospect theory—a theory that explains how people make choices—individuals are motivated to avoid losses more than to achieve gains (Kahneman & Tversky, 1982). For example, if an individual is given $50 and is told they can either keep it or forfeit it to have a 50% chance of winning $100.00, most people will opt to keep the $50.00. They are more motivated to avoid the loss of $50.00 than by the possible gain of an additional $50.00. However, this effect does not merely apply to money. When Novemsky and Kahneman (2005) asked college students how much they would pay for a candy bar, they said on average 90 cents. They then were given a candy bar and asked how much they would sell it for. The response on average amounted to $1.83. The value of the candy bar had increased upon its acquisition, raising in doubt the truth of the maxim "Easy come, easy go." If a possible risk is the incursion of a loss, individuals (including group leaders) will engage in behaviors to avoid that loss even if it means forfeiting a gain. Consider this example:

> Fred, the leader of a long-term psychotherapy group, had been finding it difficult to maintain the ideal number of members in his group due to a lack of referrals. Recently, he had been preparing a new member, Aaliya, to enter the group and was optimistic about Aaliya's fit with the group. He was encouraged by Aaliya's first session. However, at the end of the session, Aaliya asked to speak with the therapist. She told him that one of the other group members was known to her as a new employee in the corporation for which both worked. Although she did not believe the other member recognized her, she thought it was very likely that they would eventually and inevitably interact with one another outside of the group. She expressed an opinion that given her status as a new member, it would be better for both members if she were to find another group.

A reader considering this scenario might well see Aaliya's position as a prudent one. Why not avoid a potentially tricky situation, one that could invite boundary crossings of various kinds? According to prospect theory, even if this therapist is someone who ordinarily exhibits good judgment, he might search for reasons supportive of the group accommodating this situation. Whatever his reasons might be, or his suggestions for how complications could be avoided, it is likely that these efforts are motivated by a desire to avoid loss. *When encountering loss, individuals are inclined to engage in risky behavior to prevent it.* In our example, the therapist might be tempted to downplay Aaliya's legitimate concern and even provide false reassurances that the group can easily handle any extra-group contacts between the two members that might occur. The point here is not whether the therapist should make a particular decision but rather, whether the therapist's judgment is unwittingly biased by the need to avoid loss, in this instance, the loss of Aaliya as a member.

One key aspect of prospect theory is the importance given to how a problem is framed in individual and group decision-making. Suppose a group psychotherapist were to look at a statistic saying (a) "Five percent of individuals considering entering a psychotherapy group will fail to enter the group if the therapist apprises those members of a given risk of group participation;" or (b) "Ninety-five percent of individuals apprised of a given risk will choose to enter the group." Notice that statement (a) describes a loss in relation to a neutral point and (b) describes a gain, even though they are objectively comparable. The framing in option 'a' is likely to be effective in discouraging group leaders from apprising an incoming member of a risk because the option will stimulate a fear of loss (Kahneman & Tversky, 1982; Rogerson et al., 2011). Although some writers (Gal & Rucker, 2018; Yechiam, 2019) have contended that loss aversion may be overestimated, it is nonetheless a well-evidenced phenomenon guiding human decision-making, and the framing does influence whether a particular situation stimulates loss aversion. Sometimes, the problem will be framed by the group leader but at other times the problem may be framed by others on the treatment team or the group member.

Heuristics and prospect theory helps us to see how a group leader's thinking may be affected by the characteristic ways humans process information. Our account here is by no means comprehensive and the interested reader can find many other examples of processing styles that could lead the leader away from addressing ethical problems most rationally. For example, confirmation bias is a well-established phenomenon wherein an individual selects information that is supportive of their hypothesis over information that might disconfirm it (Croskerry, 2003). One of the encouraging findings in research on problem-solving is that as the clinician's experience accrues, the proneness to errors and biases lessens (Norman et al., 2017). Much of this research, however, concerns medical diagnoses rather than ethical decision-making. It is plausible that with experience, practitioners have opportunities, sometimes painful, to learn from mistakes. For example, a group leader who engages in hasty decision-making and suffers some negative consequences learns about the costs of haste.

Approaches, Techniques, and Tips for Addressing Ethical Challenges

In the last section, a variety of challenges to effective ethical decision-making were identified. The group leader striving to achieve a high level of ethicality should make an active effort to acknowledge these challenges and address them both in everyday practice and when ethical quandaries arise. Whereas external challenges call for outward-facing coping strategies, internal challenges entail self-reflection and the gathering of information to support a review process.

Addressing Stress

The need for stress management exists in an ongoing way in the life of a group leader. Fortunately, graduate programs in the mental health professions are increasingly recognizing the need to train emerging practitioners to monitor stress levels and practice self-care to ensure that stress is kept in a manageable range. Various writers have described that self-care is an ethical imperative for psychologists (Barnett et al., 2007; Wise et al., 2012), and this notion holds true for the other professions from which group psychotherapists are drawn.

Among the principles identified for psychotherapists' self-care is the recognition that the nature of the work is inherently stressful. As Norcross (2000, p. 710) wrote:

> A growing body of empirical research attests to the negative toll exacted by a career in psychotherapy. Although each of us experience distress differently, the literature points to moderate depression, mild anxiety, emotional exhaustion, and disrupted relationships as the common residue of immersing ourselves in the inner worlds of distressed and distressing people
>
> (Brady, et al., 1995).

Group psychotherapy, with all its complexities, can create a level of stress for the leader that is at least comparable to if not greater than for therapists in other modalities. Recognizing the inherent psychological burden that comes with leading a group allows the therapist to allocate more resources to understanding the present problem and addressing it rather than becoming mired in less constructive self-recrimination. Furthermore, knowing that carrying an emotional load is part of the work can motivate the group leader to build-in support mechanisms to carry the load without undue cost to the group members or the leader. For example, engagement in mindfulness can reduce stress (Brown & Ryan, 2003). Participation in a supervision group, even if the practitioner is experienced, provides another means to maintain stress at manageable levels. The group will provide a unique experience of universality, that is, the therapist is not unique in facing dilemmas in group leadership. Sharing issues in a supervision group, when documented, also constitutes good risk management.

Second, "be aware of your stress level and liberate yourself from it when stress runs high" (Norcross, 2000, p. 711). Monitoring stress levels on a continual basis can allow for interventions to be made as needed. Norcross notes that attunement to internal experiences reflecting levels of stress should be checked against and confirmed by others' observations. For the group leader, valuable additions to personal observation and reflection are the observations of group members and co-leader:

> Saul had been running a group for a year when one member, Genevieve, said, "You've been looking haggard lately. Maybe you are not getting enough sleep." Saul's thinking immediately centered upon Genevieve's caretaking role in the group. Saul was formulating an intervention that would enable Genevieve to obtain members' feedback on this group role when two other members chimed in, saying that they had made the same observation. After the session, the co-leader shared with Saul that even though she had not articulated that observation to herself, she had resonated with it. Upon reflection, Saul realized that as a new parent had he had not fully admitted to himself how parenthood was sapping his energies. He vowed to make a plan with his partner to work toward his own self-restoration.

Just as group members benefit from the multiplicity of points of view in the group situation, so also does the group leader.

Third, personal therapy could be a component of a group leader's self-care. Personal therapy is often seen by therapists as a useful way of addressing personal distress, one which enables the therapist to understand the position of being a patient (Daw & Joseph, 2007). Group therapists who seek group treatment might face the obstacle of having a professional connection to many of the group psychotherapists in their communities. However, with the emergence of online group psychotherapy, a greater wealth of opportunities exists.

Self-care strategies are associated with more favorable outcomes when they are pursued in an ongoing way rather than solely in reaction to a particular increase in stress (Rupert & Dorociak, 2019). In some organizations, self-care is promoted in recognition that accrued stress adversely affects both the staff member and that staff member's work. Resources such as in-services about self-care and automatic outreach to staff after critical events (Maltzman, 2011) convey that self-care is a joint responsibility of employer and employee. Still, many organizations continue to value extreme self-sacrifice. In such environments, the notion is often promoted that health care providers are heroic when they radically subordinate their needs to those of the individuals they serve. At times, these notions are promoted for subgroups of staff as when the expectations for subordination of self are gendered (Weinberg, 2014). As Jurist (2021) points out, resistance to the value of attending to the self's care has deep roots in many cultures, particularly Western cultures. If individuals have an ethical mandate to engage in self-care, so do the organizations that employ them. Those seeking employment in an organization would be prudent to learn about the culture of the workplace and the organizational commitment to staff self-care.

Addressing Heuristics and Biases

The heuristics and biases can be highly potent in shaping a group leader's decision-making but generally operate outside of the leader's awareness. In some instances, heuristics can improve ethical decision-making and clinical decision-making more broadly when these are drawing upon the therapist's long-term experience. However, at other times, they can lead us to an unsound choice. Therefore, to improve ethical decision-making, group leaders need to take these biases and heuristics into account. A variety of ways of doing so are available.

Knowing When to Slow Down the Process

Probably one of the most important skills a practitioner can acquire is knowing which decision-making situations demand careful, thorough cognitive processing, bolstered by the collection of relevant information and use of external resources such as supervision. Routine problems frequently emerge and can be pursued through automatic, intuitive activity. As the therapist's experience accrues, a greater range of decisions can be made with relatively little involvement of more deliberate thinking. If therapists could not count on relatively automatic processing for solutions to routine issues they would be hopelessly bogged down. Ethical dilemmas, however, require a great deal of deliberate processing. Generally, these involve circumstances that are high-stakes or unfamiliar. They also tend to reflect problems whose solutions would simultaneously honor one ethical principle but violate another. Sometimes these situations reveal themselves through the clinician's experience of anxiety:

> Dr. Dahlia felt a surge of anxiety when she overheard one member borrowing money from another for bus fare. She had never witnessed any extra-group behavior of this type and did not yet know how she regarded it. She knew the borrowing member would be furious if this interaction were laid bare in the next group session.

Often, anxiety serves as a cue that greater scrutiny is warranted. However, anxiety is unpleasant. It is possible that, if Dr. Dahlia were to focus on this unfamiliar circumstance more extensively, her anxiety might increase. Therefore, she might succumb to ridding herself of the problem and the anxiety by embracing whatever defensive solution occurred to her immediately. ("It probably was just an emergency. No need for me to make a big deal about it.") An important part of training is to help practitioners regard anxiety as a cue to enhance ethical reasoning (Rogerson et al., 2011).

Slowing down is not an invitation to procrastinate or ruminate over the problem. Rather, it is the practice of allowing sufficient time for a careful investigation of the problem. Part of that investigation could be a consideration of what heuristics and biases might be pulling the therapist in given directions. Particularly important is the identification of any self-interest that might make one solution to the problem especially appealing. The fact that self-interest is served by a decision does not make that decision the wrong one. Hopefully, the therapist can be scrupulous in examining the alternatives to ensure that pursuit of self-interest does not drive the decision-making.

Revisiting the Framing of the Problem

Remember that how the problem is framed is exceedingly important regarding the solutions the problem-solver is likely to devise. Therefore, it can be useful to revisit the statement of the problem to ascertain whether it contains bias (Rogerson et al., 2011). For example, a problem stated in terms of potential loss is likely to evoke the therapist's loss avoidance motive. Formulating the problem in other terms can lessen the strength of a bias:

> Ms. Kensey had an opening in her long-term outpatient group when she received a call from a representative of a local professional group asking her to accept a pro bono group member. In fact, Ms. Kensey had indicated to this organization she would

accept pro bono clients. However, when the opportunity to do so arose, she said to herself, "Am I willing to lose that income?" She discussed the matter with her practice partner who said, "I think this is an opportunity. We are always saying we want our practice to be inclusive in serving social needs. Isn't this our chance to do so?"

Notice that the partner presented the alternative of accepting the member as a gain. Although other factors might have been brought to bear in the ultimate decision (e.g.: Was the practice having difficulty paying its electrical bill? Was the individual appropriate for this group?), the mere articulation of a possible gain lessens the intensity of the loss avoidance response. This example also highlights the potential utility of framing a given alternative in terms of the extent to which it would serve the group psychotherapist's professional and personal values. Often, looking for this alignment will reveal new facets of solutions to ethical problems. However, such a values analysis requires that the group therapist be able to identify such values. Professional development can take the form of achieving values clarity, using approaches that have developed in part to serve this aim, for example, the techniques of Acceptance and Commitment Therapy (ACT; Hayes et al., 2012).

Gathering Additional Information

For any significant ethical problem, all the relevant information is rarely immediately available to define the problem fully or recognize and evaluate alternative solutions. Where the information is obtained can vary from situation to situation. In the earlier mentioned example about the member seeking to borrow money from another member, the perspective of the requesting member might be important to appreciate the problem fully. However, information-gathering regarding laws and professional standards might also need to occur. A therapist who believes that a particular circumstance activates a Duty to Warn does well to read the state law in relation to this obligation as well as any professional standards developed by the group psychotherapist's disciplinary affiliation. For example, the American Psychological Association's Code of Ethics (American Psychological Association, 2010) contains material relevant to Duty to Warn (Ethical Standard 4.05, Disclosures). Some information the therapist might need to gather could pertain to the practicalities of different potential solutions. For example, if hospitalization is a potential alternative, the therapist might wish to obtain information about the availability of hospital beds in suitable settings.

Multiple factors might deter the therapist from obtaining relevant information. Therapists at times overestimate their knowledge about the current problem and its remedies. For example, the therapist in our prior example involving Duty to Warn might recall various presentations on this topic. Duty to Warn situations are relatively rare (Knapp et al., 2013) and while a group psychotherapist might have a grasp of the concept, without any recent experience applying it, that professional might not recall all the critical aspects. Therapists might also be hindered by an undue investment in a particular solution. Any information gathered might compel the therapist in a direction that the therapist regards as undesirable. Gathering information takes time, a requirement that might be at odds with the therapist's wish to readily dispense with the anxiety-producing problem. It is essential that the therapist possess a capacity to contain or hold the anxiety without defensive avoidance for the necessary information-gathering.

Obtaining Supervision and Consultation

Supervision is essential in the training of any group psychotherapist. However, throughout the group therapist's career, supervision and consultation can play helpful roles in aiding the group psychotherapist to successfully negotiate ethical problems. Supervision might be sought in instances in which the group therapist sees in the emergence of a particular ethical problem or set of ethical problems the need for more active oversight by a clinician with more training or experience in a given area. For example, a clinician with experience in treating adults agrees to conduct a group of adolescents. Some ethical dilemmas quickly arise. The clinician seeks supervision both to help in the resolution of the dilemmas and to obtain needed training. Once a clinician can work as an independent practitioner, supervision might be necessary on occasion, but consultation should be a presence in the clinician's professional life.

Given all the factors that have been identified as influencing the clinician's decision-making—many of which operate outside of awareness—it is useful to have another trained perspective when facing ethical dilemmas. The consultant's training and experience and, importantly, the independent perspective often help to clarify what the decision-maker cannot. Knapp et al. (2013) recommend that clinicians employ consultants when providing treatment to difficult clients or other circumstances that clinicians experience as challenging their capabilities.

Despite the potential benefits of supervision and consultation, some group leaders might recoil at the idea of using such resources because it opens one's work to the scrutiny of another professional. At times, mistakes that the leader made that set the stage for the current ethical problem become evident to both parties. Although the wish to avoid exposure of one's imperfections is a natural human impulse, acting upon it might occasion a compounding of errors.

Expanding, Specifying, and Testing Solutions

The stress of an ethical dilemma (or any problem) can limit a group leader's capacity to recognize a full range of potential solutions. Potentially helpful are any techniques that would aid the leader in thinking more flexibly. Graber et al. (2012) describe the crystal ball technique, used in military training, wherein a problem-solving team is told that a crystal ball providing a view into the future has revealed that a particular solution will not work, and the team will need to start "from scratch" in solving the problem. Graber et al. hold that this technique facilitates the team to think more expansively, providing sufficient distance from the original solution such that they can critique it. Presumably, if ethics trainers would adopt such an approach, applying such techniques to real-life problems that emerge in the training situation (Yalof & Brabender, 2001), trainees would become independent practitioners with a diminished allegiance to any given approach and an openness to contemplate others.

Specifying the solution involves developing it further so that it is brought into progressively greater alignment with ethical principles. Throughout these chapters, the point has been made that any given solution to an ethical problem could entail observing one ethical principle while violating another. However, group leaders can identify means for lessening the extent to which a given principle is violated by adding features to the solution that take the ethical principle into account. Consider the following:

> Germaine had been in practice for several decades during which time she led three psychotherapy groups. She was increasingly finding that her energy was diminishing, and she was longing to have greater free time. She worried, too, that her current work activity might not be sustainable on a long-term basis. She decided that she would bring one of her groups to a close.

Certainly, group leaders have a right to adjust their workloads and, at times, they have no choice but to modify them (e.g., illness). However, were the therapist in our example to merely announce to members that the group was ending, even if the therapist incorporated an interval for members to make alternate arrangements, the therapist would not be giving due attention to the principle of non-maleficence. However, if the therapist carefully considers what opportunities might be created for members, such as having another therapist run the group or placing individual members in other therapeutic situations, the therapist would be operating in greater consistency with Non-maleficence and Beneficence. If the therapist seeks the input of members in considering possible means to achieve continuity, the therapist is acting in conformity with the principle of Autonomy. In refining solutions to ethical problems, especially those that are at odds with one or more ethical principles, clinicians should ask themselves the question, *"Is the offended principle infringed to the least possible degree?"* (Knapp & VandeCreek, 2007, p. 403).

Testing solutions to ethical problems occur on multiple levels. Sometimes, decision-makers alight on a solution that is appealing in the short run (perhaps because of ease of implementation) but poses significant difficulties in the long run. One way to test a given solution is by identifying the worst-case scenario, how events might play out were they to do so in the worst possible way for one or more parties (Knapp et al., 2013). Even if this step does not lead the group leader to abandon a proposed solution, the leader might be able to introduce precautions to make the worst possible outcome less likely. For example, suppose a group leader decides upon a solution to an ethical problem that entails giving unwelcome information to a group member. However, upon engaging in worst-case scenario thinking, the therapist realizes that the member might respond impulsively, behaving in a way that would be highly detrimental to the member. If so, the therapist could build in extra supports for that member to diminish the probability of that outcome. Part of testing solutions is to note whether the chosen solution produces the desired consequences. An aspect of the therapist's ongoing development as a leader is learning from one's successes and failures. A chosen solution might produce unexpected negative effects. If so, the leader should take any steps possible to lessen their impact and allow knowledge of a negative outcome to improve the therapist's future decision-making efforts.

Achieving Professional Self-Awareness

Group psychotherapists benefit greatly from achieving awareness about their own decision-making style that is likely to extend to ethical decision-making. Individuals are likely to have a proneness to particular challenges in the different stages of addressing a problem. Among the possible challenges are the following:

* Being vulnerable to a high anxiety response to any manifestation of a problem, which then interferes with the process of gauging the problem's extent.
* Succumbing easily to one of the biases identified earlier.
* Struggling to generate a multiplicity of solutions.
* Allowing shame-proneness to lead to an unwillingness to secure the services of a consultant who would examine their work closely.
* Spending a great deal of time contemplating a solution but having difficulty following through, remaining in a state of indecision.

The awareness of one's personal style, including ways of coping with anxiety and problem-solving strengths and weaknesses, is invaluable in finding mechanisms for capitalizing on strengths and compensating for weaknesses. For example, clinicians who recognize a proneness to the confirmation bias (Baron, 2000) might resolve to engage in an active pursuit of disconfirming evidence for their formulation.

The Ethics Acculturation model (Knapp et al., 2013), which describes the ways that the differences between personal and professional ethics are managed, is useful in thinking about how ethical dilemmas arise. An undue emphasis upon personal ethics can lead to violations in professional codes of conduct. Undue emphasis upon professional ethics can result in a rigid application of rules and laws to the neglect of contextual factors. During training, individuals' tendencies to veer in one direction or another should be identified and explored. Learning about one's tendency to see ethical situations through the lens of personal values or rules and standards allows for compensation. That is, the therapist will know to pose the question, "Is there something in this situation that I might be missing?"

Now that we have considered the array of processes associated with decision-making in regard to an ethical problem, we consider how that decision is evaluated. We also take up the topic of how one's ongoing work as a group leader would be regarded when viewed through ethical and legal lenses.

Standard of Care

The *Standard of Care* is one of the most significant concepts in mental health and is used to determine whether group leaders have acted responsibly. But what exactly is the standard of care and how is it used to determine whether elements of treatment are considered acceptable or reasonable? Outside of the broad expectation to respect clients without harming or exploiting them, there is little agreement in the field about what constitutes proper care.

Definitions and Parameters

There is no single set of rules that delineate the standard of care. Because the standard of care is judged by comparing what a *typical* provider with the same or similar education and training would have done under the same or similar conditions, Reamer (2014) highlights the importance of the three concepts of *typical, reasonable, and prudent*, reflecting the practice of courts to determine what a typical, reasonable, caring and careful practitioner would have done under similar conditions. The standard of care is based on community and professional standards; professionals are thus held to the same standard as others of the same profession or discipline, with qualifications consistent across similar localities (Barnett, 2017a). When considering interventions, therapists with an ethical approach ask themselves what a respected colleague, using a similar theoretical orientation and working with a similar type of client in a comparable type of community, would say about their interventions (Zur, n.d.).

Additionally, the standard of care is not a standard of perfection. Functioning within the standard of care allows for typical or simple mistakes to take place during treatment, so it is not a *perfect* standard. In fact, we must be aware that the standard of care is a minimum standard. Making a miscalculation in judgment does not necessarily put a therapist below the standard of care (Zur, n.d.).

Applying the standard of care to a variety of settings is a challenging task. For example, decisions around what constitutes an irresponsible dual relationship may involve different factors for consideration in a prison, a rural hospital unit, or a college campus setting. Appropriate client advocacy and the boundaries of sharing information may be limited or expanded in certain sites; the standard of care is quite different in military settings (Johnson & Johnson, 2017) and police settings (McCutchen, 2017). Zur (2017) even provided a comprehensive book with chapters specifically identifying how the standard of care applies within a variety of settings.

Because there are diverse training approaches and theoretical orientations, and many different types of communities, settings, and cultures, the concept of the standard of care are also elusive and controversial (Zur, n.d.). Employing the same set of values or attitudes in a variety of settings is also not always easy. For instance, numerous loyalties are intrinsic to therapy practices in the military and do not always allow therapists to adhere to ideals concerning clients' welfare (Johnson & Johnson, 2017).

Caveats

The standard of care is not guided by risk management principles, although they are sometimes confused as synonymous (Barnett, 2017a; Younggren & Gottlieb, 2017). While risk management is instead often geared to decrease the impact of therapist negligence and the sanctioning of licensing boards to lessen the liability for insurance companies, the standard of care is based on legal-professional-communal principles. There is even an increased chance that a new standard of care may develop in certain instances; for example, therapists in training can become anxious when attending programs given by inflexible risk management experts and could choose to avoid all physical touch or refuse all client gifts (Zur, 2017). One of the most harmful errors by expert witnesses, attorneys, and licensing boards has been blurring the standard of care with risk management principles (Zur, n.d.).

The standard is also not static. For example, the proliferation of tele-mental health has advanced the standard of care to be relevant to current times. The standard of care continues to evolve as more practitioners practice in new or modified ways. New statutes and case laws often change the standard. Professional ethical codes are often modified and structure an evolving standard. New research findings, practice guidelines, and theoretical innovations frequently lead to shifts in the standard of care (Zur, n.d.).

Examples of Factors Considered

The basic elements are known in our field: The mental health services offered to individuals, conducted in group or individual settings, should be based on a treatment plan and provided by a mental health professional licensed or authorized within the state to provide such services. Whether provided by psychiatrists, psychologists, social workers, or counselors, interventions must be based on sound or proven clinical methods and adhere to legal and ethical standards. Group psychotherapy, crisis intervention, and assessment—in the pre-group, during, and at the termination of treatment—are all considered conditions that must follow the professional standard of care.

To meet these standards, agencies employing mental health providers should have a detailed and established staff orientation process and must also implement a written policy for regular supervision of all unlicensed and licensed staff. Each employee should also be knowledgeable about the range of their clients' diagnoses/problems. Once a policy manual is complete, aspects that fall under standard of care may include specific details, as in these examples:

- obtaining an emergency contact number
- gathering pertinent releases of information
- providing client rights, including the grievance process
- obtaining past records from clients with chronic risk
- stipulating how and when assessments are given

- specifying when treatment plans are reviewed and how they are modified
- providing documentation guidelines
- obtaining consultation with medical providers related to medication management
- describing referral and discharge planning procedures

Legal Considerations

The legal definition of the standard of care is "the degree of care or competence that one is expected to exercise in a particular circumstance or role" (Merriam-Webster, n.d.). For a group leader to be sued by a complainant, a negative outcome such as suicide or harm to a client is not sufficient evidence of sub-standard care unless there was a violation of other laws or evidence of unsound clinical interventions. Further, unless there is an ethical or legal duty, such as the duty to report child abuse, the standard of care emphasizes the *process* of decision-making rather than the *outcome*.

In courts, plaintiffs must determine that the therapist acted below the standard of care. Administrative law judges or licensing boards may sanction a therapist if they find that the therapist operated below the standard. Often, there is no need to prove damage to a client for the licensing boards to sanction the therapist. For instance, therapists who barter with clients in poverty, make visits to those who are unable to leave the home or employ therapeutic interventions with an agoraphobic client outside the office for de-sensitization have been unjustly accused of operating below the standard of care in some states (Zur, n.d., 2017). Hampton (1984) asserts that the level of care required of therapists differs based on whether a particular jurisdiction follows local, national, or specialist standards of conduct. Moreover, Hampton argues that the standard of care should offer assurance to providers of new or unconventional therapies that the law will not reject their methods outright. Hence, he observes the standard may depend on the weight that it assigns to "respectable minorities" (i.e., multiple schools of thought within a discipline) or whether an unconventional therapy falls within the limits of acceptable practice. The most flexible definition of standard of care might thus provide benefit to the greatest range of practice.

Elements from which the Standard of Care is Derived

The following are the eight elements from which the standard of care is derived (Younggren and Gottlieb, 2017; Zur, n.d.):

- **Statutes:** Each state has statutes, such as Child Abuse or Elder Abuse, and other laws.
- **Licensing Boards' Regulations:** In most states, extensive regulations are governing many aspects of mental health practices. These often include the rules about mandated continuing education and supervision. In recent years, licensing boards have also established rules regarding tele-mental health.
- **HIPAA:** HIPAA regulations and standards include items like record-keeping, client access to records, and security of communications with clients.
- **Case Law:** Case law is one of the foundations of the standard of care. The Tarasoff decision of the California Supreme Court in Tarasoff vs. Regents of the University of California is the most known example of case law (Zur, n.d.), articulating the duty to warn of a client's threat to harm a third party.
- **Ethical Codes of Professional Associations:** The codes of ethics of professional associations are an essential, but also controversial, part of the standard of care.

Unlike most statutes, case law, and regulations, the codes of ethics are often vague about what types of behavior are mandated or prohibited. The lack of clarity in the codes has allowed many attorneys and licensing boards to interpret the codes in a way that has led to the sanctioning of therapists who supposedly practiced below the interpreted standard of care. Moreover, though several codes of ethics assert that they are not intended to be a basis of civil liability, some licensing boards incorporate ethics codes of professional associations into their licensing law making the codes legally binding. Group therapists who present themselves as specialists may be likely to be held to the ethical standards articulated by a more specialized professional association (Zur, n.d.).

*   **The Respected Minority Principle:** As a consequence of the legitimate, established and distinct multiple therapeutic orientations in the field of psychotherapy, most experts agree that when it comes to the standard of care, majority approaches should not rule and diversity should be upheld. An additional complexity accord among professionals' part of the standard is what has been called "respected minority." This principle may apply if the research support of the technique is not well established yet (Reid, 1998). An example is Eye Movement Desensitization and Reprocessing, also known as EMDR (Shapiro, 2002). When Dr. Shapiro introduced her methodology there was very little research on the method. By the beginning of the 21st century, EMDR has become one of the most effective and well-researched methodologies for treating PTSD.
*   **Consensus Among Professionals:** In a field that contains numerous therapeutic orientations, a consensus is difficult. Professional associations publish guidelines on different topics, such as the American Group Psychotherapy Association's group therapy practice guidelines (e.g., Bernard et al., 2008; Leszcz & Kobos, 2008). These documents only provide general practice guidelines that are neither always applicable nor always in agreement with state laws or licensing board regulations.
*   **Consensus in the Community:** The standard is also shaped by community customs. As a result, different communities with a variety of cultural backgrounds and values have different standards. As an example, bartering and dual relationships may be an inescapable part of rural living (Barnett, 2017b).

How Group Therapists Demonstrate Compliance with Standard of Care

Determining compliance with the standard of care is established predominantly with clinical records. Leaders should be able to explain their techniques and approach, and provide rationales that are tied to a theoretical perspective. Any complex clinical, legal, and ethical cases will require additional documentation. For example, cases of emergencies, violence, mandated reporting, boundary-crossing, and dual relationships will need careful documentation; also, any non-mainstream interventions need to be explained (Zur, n.d.). When therapists choose not to use standard treatment interventions, they must articulate a solid rationale for their preferred treatment. The clinical notes will also need to identify settings and situations where dual or multiple relationships are unavoidable (e.g., prisons) or common occurrences, such as those in rural recovery communities or colleges. Tele-mental health has also introduced newer means of delivering group therapy; hence, the standard of care is evolving together with tele-mental health. If the clinician has used the services of a consultant, that factor should also be documented. The clinician's rationale for a particular decision may or may not be accepted. However, if that rationale is documented carefully, it demonstrates the conscientiousness the leader demonstrated in arriving at, and implementing the decision (Knapp et al., 2013).

Being Informed by Research and Using Appropriate Treatments

As the standard of care evolves with new treatments and modalities, group leaders should also be aware that keeping abreast of new techniques and theoretical developments is also important. We now have strong support for the notion that therapists informed about contemporary research findings are better able to apply this information to increase the effectiveness of groups. Greene (2012) emphasizes that group therapists are scientists who must assess and track what is working and why on an ongoing basis.

Modern best practice approaches to group therapy include using clinical experience, flexible techniques, practical skills, practice guidelines, practiced-based evidence, and empirically supported treatments (Barlow, 2013; Barlow et al., 2015; Greene et al., 2019; Leszcz, 2018; Miles & Paquin, 2014). Some authors use an approach guided by clinical practice guidelines that integrate scientific literature and consensus to assist therapists regarding the *implementation of effective treatment in ways that augment their clinical judgment* (Bernard et al., 2008; Burlingame et al., 2013; Leszcz, 2018). Leszcz (2018) helpfully notes that being guided by an understanding of the scientific literature includes (a) being aware of the research that identifies factors that contribute to increased therapist effectiveness, (b) reviewing complex and difficult cases, (c) reflecting on past sessions, and (d) considering interventions in future sessions—all blended with accrued clinical wisdom.

Clinical practice combined with research knowledge can also improve the group climate or cohesiveness. For example, leaders can benefit from knowing that allowing intense conflict or strong expression of affect *too early in a group before strong relationships are developed* can be detrimental (Yalom & Leszcz, 2020). Ideally, current research findings can inform leaders, who can then test out the information with intuitive probing, leading to a deeper understanding of the therapeutic forces for members. This evidence-based practice builds upon the common principles and models that contemporary group therapists recognize, appreciate, and aim to use: Developing strongly cohesive groups by intentionally working with a *self-reflective and empathic manner* (Leszcz, 2018). Even the contemporary administration of documented manualized treatments is further improved with a solid clinical foundation based on an understanding of group dynamics and processes that are therapeutic (Paquin, 2017).

Evaluating Progress and Outcome Related to Standard of Care

We know that for group leaders to make complex clinical decisions and interventions, we need to incorporate reliable and accurate information. For example, shy Beatriz may have become more depressed and withdrawn lately, so letting her group leader know she has had suicidal urges is less likely when other members are more dominant. For less verbal and more complex clients, it can be difficult in a group modality to monitor each member's symptoms and risk of deterioration. Many have argued that we have an ethical obligation to evaluate the services we provide, although the majority of therapists in North America do not regularly assess client progress or outcome (Muir et al., 2019; Pinner & Kivlighan, 2018; Tasca et al., 2019; Yalom & Leszcz, 2020). There is solid evidence finding that giving feedback about progress to group members can lead to increased treatment gains and better attendance rates than groups not using such measures (Slone et al., 2015). The consensus is that the use of measures to take the pulse of the group and its members should supplement, not replace, clinical judgment (Greene et al., 2019). So, therapists must not only document client progress but also must be accountable for our treatments (Leszcz, 2018). The use of measures can support that accountability.

Continuous assessment by the therapist at regular time intervals may be referred to as *progress monitoring* and can be added to any intake and termination measures that offer pretreatment and posttreatment information (sometimes termed *outcome monitoring*; Tasca et al., 2019). Other authors use the combined term, *routine outcome monitoring* (ROM), to make the case for ethical treatment through ongoing assessments. When leaders include ROM, they can combine the data with clinical judgment with the goal of better intervening or shifting the therapy promptly as needed (Muir et al., 2019). This process is also more recently referred to as measurement-based care (MBC) or practice-based evidence, emphasizing routine assessments throughout the group that can occur at weekly or spaced intervals (Marmarosh, 2018, 2021; Tasca et al., 2016). Feedback and information can be brought to the whole group to engage in discussions with varying degrees of explicitness, based on the informed consent process and agreements about disclosing individuals' results (Greene et al., 2019).

MBC feedback has been found in research to not only lead to better outcomes in clients but to reduce client deterioration significantly (Lambert et al., 2018). These findings supporting ROM fit perfectly with our ethical aspirations of Beneficence and Non-maleficence. Perhaps that is why psychologists in Canada have a codified ethical obligation to evaluate treatment (Tasca et al., 2019). Along those lines, *The Joint Commission on the Accreditation of Healthcare Organizations* (n.d.), put out a statement noting that measurement-based care has become a high-profile issue in the behavioral health care field and that this standard will help accredited practitioners increase the quality of the care, treatment, and services they provide. MBC feedback also relates to the principle of Autonomy in that the member is getting ongoing information that could feed into their decision-making about whether progress on goals is sufficient to influence the duration of group participation.

An Ethical Approach to Providing Competent Care

Some therapists consistently have good outcomes, some consistently have poor outcomes, and some have mixed outcomes depending on the client presentation (Baldwin & Imel, 2013; Barkham et al., 2017; Norcross & Wampold, 2011). We have also established that therapists may not be accurate in estimating their effectiveness with certain types of therapy groups or client problems. The recommendation to track group member progress would help overcome the demonstrated tendency of therapists to overestimate client improvement and underestimate deterioration; thus, there should be an ethical demand to *remedy the quality gap* in competence by engaging in ROM or MBC (Boswell et al., 2015; Jorm et al., 2017; Lambert et al., 2018; Leszcz, 2018; Pinner & Kivlighan, 2018).

Lambert et al. (2018) and other researchers have therefore developed a strong case for intervening during the process of treatment by using measures *as an ethical imperative.*

MBC can bring an ethical focus to assessing therapist competence and the need for further training and supervision in specific practice areas (Muir et al., 2019; Pinner & Kivlighan, 2018). By assessing outcomes over time, therapists can identify competency issues and clinical skills that may be beneficial. With better awareness of our strengths and weaknesses, we also better fulfill our ethical requirements to use scientific knowledge in our profession (Muir et al., 2019; Pinner & Kivlighan, 2018).

Pinner and Kivlighan (2018) also make a strong case that practicing outside of one's *boundaries of competence* can also lead to unfavorable outcomes. These authors note that since ethics codes often refer to competence using elements such as supervised training, education, and work-related experience *which have not consistently held up in research findings to lead to better client outcomes*, competence as currently defined is problematic.

For psychologists, APA's Standard 2.01(a) states, "Psychologists provide services, teach, and conduct research with populations and in areas only within the boundaries of their competence, based on their education, training, supervised experience, consultation, study, or professional experience" (American Psychological Association, 2017, p.7). Pinner and Kivlighan instead propose using ROM with certain client identities or diagnoses to determine if the therapist is competent. For example, one therapist is able to demonstrate competence in helping her sexual minority group members improve on self-compassion scores; another group leader is also able to help a diverse group of religious minorities achieve high attendance in group therapy and feel accepted as demonstrated by strong therapeutic factor and alliance scores on questionnaires. However, a third leader demonstrates less client improvement with racial minorities and transgendered clients; his supervisor decides to engage in more discussion around showing nonverbal empathy and using appropriate terms with future minority group members.

Lambert et al. (2018) remind us that professional bodies have been quick to recommend MBC methods. For example, the American Psychological Association formed a Presidential Task Force on Evidence-Based Practice in 2006 that recommended that MBC be a part of effective psychological services because monitoring has been shown to enhance client outcomes. The Association of State and Provincial Psychology Boards (2019) also recommended that ROM be a part of competency-based supervision. Within the Substance Abuse and Mental Health Administration's National Registry of Evidence-based Programs and Practices (www.nrepp.samhsa.gov/), two ROM systems have been listed and widely studied regarding their impact on an individual client's psychotherapy outcome: the Partners for Change Outcome Management System (PCOMS; www.pcoms.com; Duncan & Miller, 2008; Prescott, et al., 2017) and the Outcome Questionnaire System (OQ-System; www.oqmeasures.com; Lambert et al., 2013).

In 2021, a joint effort between the Association for Specialists in Group Work and the Association for Assessment and Research in Counseling led to the development of the *Standards of Care for Assessment in Group Work* (Bennett et al., 2021) with a particular emphasis on using appropriate and culturally relevant assessments. These standards suggest determining whether norming groups for a measure adequately represent individuals from diverse backgrounds (Hays & Wood, 2017) and understanding the complexities of using measures developed for special populations (Spurgeon, 2017). The standards focus on *process and outcome* measures rather than selection and screening but do note that group therapists should understand the similarities and differences between informal (screening) tools and formal measures and strategies.

Choosing a Focus of the Measures

What can be measured varies by the agreed-upon goals and the approach to the group treatment. Examples include assessments of mood, quality of life, insight, specific behaviors, interpersonal functioning, cognitions, and overall symptom reduction. The Joint Commission, mentioned earlier, has provided a list of outcome measures used in some systems of healthcare (Joint Commission, n.d.). The CORE Battery-Revised also recommends measures for selection, process, and outcome to group therapists (Burlingame et al., 2006); it is currently being updated and revised by an international team of researchers and practitioners through the American Group Psychotherapy Association's Science to Service Task Force. Considerations for assessment by the ethical leader also include important measures of therapist factors such as alliance, cultural attunement, and empathy (Norcross & Lambert, 2018).

Considering Process

Burlingame et al. (2006) remind group therapists that while individual improvement matters, core group processes that can shift the therapeutic progress for all can also be measured. Understanding how members are experiencing the healing aspects of a group can not only provide information about the responses of individual clients but also about the whole-group processes of engagement, safety, and alliance. For example, since we now know that the therapeutic factors (TFs) in a group can resonate with clients differently (Paquin et al 2013), it is helpful to assess various member reactions to the group climate. Yalom and Leszcz (2020) remind us that taking the pulse of the group can be crucial to a deeper understanding of how the group is being perceived and where treatment strategy might need to shift.

Whereas we have been covering process monitoring generally, at times it is necessary to monitor *highly specific* aspects of the group process. One such area in the recent literature has been racism and ethnicity-related stress.

Measures of Racism and Ethnicity-Related Stress

Leaders should also consider several measures of ethnicity-related stress and an adapted measure of ethnic identity to more fully understand group client diversity. Such measures can be quite helpful for both members and the leader.

The Multiculturally Sensitive Mental Health Scale

Particularly for groups designed to treat and support African Americans, specific information regarding how mental health is impacted by racism can be quite beneficial. The Multiculturally Sensitive Mental Health Scale (MSMHS; Chao & Green, 2011) was developed to assess African Americans' mental health, including perceptions of racism. The MSMHS was designed to reflect the belief that if people want to understand African Americans' psychology, they must more fully understand their experiences of racism. Because racism is a unique stressor for African Americans and almost every African American has experienced racism, it is wise to include perceptions of racism in an instrument measuring African Americans' mental health.

The Perception of Ethnic Discrimination Questionnaire (PEDQ)

Over 20 years ago, ethnicity-related stressors were assessed with multiple instruments in a study by Contrada et al. (2001) and included measures of perceived discrimination, stereotype confirmation concerns, and own-group conformity pressure. Analyses demonstrated that ethnicity-related stress and racial identity constructs captured by the various instruments were associated with measures of psychological and physical well-being. The Perception of Ethnic Discrimination Questionnaire has received confirmatory validation numerous times over the years, and there is now a brief version specifically for community-based groups (PEDQ-CVB; Blair et al., 2021; Brondolo et al., 2005). It is available at https://attcnetwork.org/sites/default/files/2020-12/2-PEDQ-CV-B.pdf.

As more group leaders become better trained to tune in to ethnicity-related stress, using an assessment tool can help validate microaggression experiences from both the past and present to help members better understand each other. Measures can also help show members how they may contribute to these dynamics. Other cultural factors to consider assessing include client-perceived therapist multicultural orientation, collectivist versus individualist orientations, and marginalization and oppression group dynamics (Chang-Caffaro & Caffaro, 2018; Kaklauskas & Nettles, 2019; Kivlighan & Chapman, 2018; Kivlighan et al., 2019a, 2019b; Marmarosh et al., 2013; Ribiero, 2020).

Caveats and Challenges for Therapists Using Measurement-based Care

Using practice-based evidence does have its limitations. The majority of MBC systems do not account for a substantial variety of external factors that can influence treatment outcomes over and above the effectiveness of services delivered (Pinner & Kivlighan, 2018). Some authors estimate that almost 70% of the variance in treatment outcomes is attributable to client and extracurricular factors independent of the therapy (Wampold & Imel, 2015). For example, many colleges and university counseling centers use the well-researched and validated Counseling Center Assessment of Psychological Symptoms (CCAPS-34, Center for Collegiate Mental Health; Carney et al., 2021; Locke et al., 2012; Youn et al, 2020) to track the change in symptoms over time. Other external factors such as experiencing a sexual assault or losing a parent during treatment can certainly worsen client symptoms unrelated to therapist effectiveness. It is for this reason that many agencies, as well as the developers of the CCAPS-34, have explicitly argued against using certain symptom measures to evaluate the competence of the therapist. Therapists may rightfully feel unfairly judged without a full explanation for negative changes in outcomes.

Despite this limitation, some do make a strong case for MBC data to be used as an *estimate* of clinical effectiveness (Miller et al., 2015). The MBC approach could be combined with other processes such as supervision with recordings to examine techniques, alliance or empathy-building, and the deliberate practice of therapeutic skills (see Chow et al., 2015). Readers are referred to Pinner and Kivlighan (2018) for a detailed case example of using MBC to establish the boundaries of competence in practice while simultaneously considering ethical issues by applying Knapp et al.'s (2017) five-step ethical decision-making model. Goldberg et al. (2016) similarly found that therapists in a large agency that systematically implemented MBC and the "deliberate practice" of skills showed a statistically significant improvement in clinical effectiveness over time. When MBC is used as a training method to enhance client outcomes, competency can be increased.

Since MBC has such strong evidence of benefit for clients, Ionita and colleagues (2020) have attempted to study why so few therapists and agencies are currently using MBC. They found the top four barriers to using measures were limited knowledge, limitations in training, the burden on clients, and concerns regarding additional work and time. The results suggest that offering training in different formats, over extended periods, and from a peer trainer, may be the most effective approach to overcoming these barriers. As mentioned earlier, group treatment has been recognized by APA as an accredited specialty. Thus, we now have a professional standard for training and the pathways available to acquire the group competencies (Barlow, 2013), which are provided through both AGPA and APA (Burlingame & Strauss, 2021).

In summary, the evidence has never been stronger for practitioners to use an evidence-based treatment, guided by measurement-based practice and multicultural competence for a variety of clinical indications (Burlingame & Strauss, 2021). In the last decade, the empirical support for practice-based assessment has strengthened significantly, and the AGPA CORE Battery-Revised (Burlingame et al., 2006; Strauss et al., 2008) has been in the process of a third revision to meet this need.

In this section, we have discussed how monitoring progress and outcome can represent a means of achieving standard of care. Monitoring progress and outcome is also a means of supporting sound ethical decision-making when quandaries arise. All else being equal, the therapist is able to arrive at an ethically sound decision when information is abundant rather than when it is lacking. Deficiencies in the therapist's informational base require the therapist to make suppositions that might be incorrect. For example, a particular quandary might arise in relation to whether a group member should remain in the group. An element that could critically feed into the decision is the extent to which the member is benefitting from group participation. Having regular data on the member's status with respect to pertinent variables would provide the therapist with a very strong foundation for this appraisal, particularly when added to other data sources such as the observations of the therapists and other group members, as well as any data from collaterals (e.g., individual therapist and family members).

In the next section, we consider how the group psychotherapist proceeds when facing high-stakes ethical and legal situations.

Risk Management

In addition to obtaining and building solid decision-making skills using an advanced model, all group leaders should be trained in risk management. Given the complexities of intense interpersonal dynamics that surface in a therapy group, the risks of harm to members are numerous. Here, we explore a few of the most common risks that the leader needs to manage and steps to mitigate the risk.

Suicide Risk

Of the most frequent and concerning risks in group treatment, suicidal thoughts and intentions can be quite challenging for both the leader and other members. Suicide is not only one of the most shattering and complex of all human actions, but also it is consistently among the leading causes of death worldwide.

Ethical Principles and Risk Decisions

Ethical principles related to the assessment of suicide risk include Autonomy, Beneficence, Non-maleficence, and Justice. Examples of how they apply are as follows:

- Autonomy: When hearing a group member's thoughts about self-harm or suicide, the leader may need to sacrifice a member's autonomy when the individual is hopeless, cognitively clouded, or has a narrowed perspective.
- Beneficence: If a leader shows care and concern with authentic empathy for the member's extreme pain, this can help open the member to new perspectives around staying alive through the difficult time.
- Non-Maleficence: Prevention of harm and death can occur due to the leader's thorough assessment; the leader is obligated to take steps to prevent risky self-harm or a suicide attempt.
- Justice: A group psychotherapist can be most helpful to a member by looking at suicidal ideation through the lens of the client's culture.

Conceptual Issues in Suicide Risk Assessment and Management

It is common knowledge that group members can be hesitant to share their suicidal thoughts and plans, which means the leader must be *intentional* in approaching the topic of safety with all members. The secrecy of suicidal ideation in group members must always be considered by the leader, with explicit aims to have the group climate become a safe and trusting space for vulnerable disclosures to occur.

Cognitive reactivity—such as maladaptive cognitions triggered by sad mood—has been associated with a history of suicide attempts as well as high hopelessness and aggression (Antypa et al., 2010). Clients with high emotional reactivity—the degree to which one experiences strong negative emotion in response to a stressful event—are more likely to have suicidal behaviors, particularly when combined with poor problem-solving or cognitive inflexibility (Dour et al., 2011). Emotional reactivity might be easier to see in the group than maladaptive cognitions, so cognitions might demand careful focus by the group psychotherapist. Sometimes, it might be necessary to perform follow-up after the group if the leader is not getting a clear read within the group.

Further, the literature indicates that the risk factors for suicidal *ideation* may be different from those that predict suicidal *attempts*. In a recent study, one clear finding is that a history of self-injurious thoughts and behaviors (SITBs) differentiates soldiers with a recent suicide attempt from non-attempting soldiers with current/recent suicidal ideation (Naifeh et al., 2020). Thus, the leader should be particularly aware of members having both *difficulty controlling the ideation and engaging in non-suicidal self-injury.*

Minority Identities and Suicide

We must be aware that group members with minority identities may be at increased risk. Suicide rates tend to vary across different segments of the population (age, race, sexual orientation, class, etc.) and thus, the group therapist should have knowledge about the relative risks of their members (Lindsey et al., 2019; Reisner et al., 2014). This awareness is especially important because, at times, members of a group might be sharing very similar feelings. However, these feelings might have different risk implications for members depending upon their identity status. The World Health Organization (WHO) advises clinicians that the strongest risk factor for suicide is a previous suicide attempt; however, suicide rates are also noted to be high among vulnerable groups who experience discrimination, such as refugees and migrants; indigenous peoples; lesbian, gay, bisexual, transgender, and intersex persons; and prisoners (World Health Organization, 2019). Additionally, Chu et al. (2017) expanded knowledge about risk evaluation practices by studying culturally competent suicide-risk assessments (CCSRA) in training and practice. They found that despite holding beliefs that cultural factors do impact the level of risk, doctoral-level participants had only minimal amounts of training and low levels of comfort employing CCSRA into practice. Leaders are encouraged to consider using the 39-item Cultural Assessment of Risk for Suicide (CARS) Measure (Chu et al., 2013).

Practical Recommendations

Based on a combination of recent suicide theories, Sommers-Flanagan and Shaw (2017) propose that the crucial factors that should guide therapists in their empathic efforts and evaluation include the following:

- substantial psychological or emotional pain
- social disconnectedness or thwarted belongingness
- a sense of being burdensome
- hopelessness about the psychological, emotional, or interpersonal angst ever resolving
- problem-solving deficits

- agitation or arousal
- diminished fear of suicide or increased pain tolerance that push individuals toward an accessible lethal means

The group may also provide a better setting for the assessment of some factors over others. For example, social disconnection might be observed more readily than problem-solving deficits. Also, leaders should consider that members who are new might be disinclined to provide evidence of some of these factors for fear of rejection or disapproval. The clinical interview for the assessment of risk should also include (Sommers-Flanagan & Sommers-Flanagan, 2017): (a) exploration and analysis of pertinent risk and protective factors (but with an emphasis on empathizing with and evaluating psychological pain, social connection, and hope or hopelessness); (b) using clinical strategies to ask directly about current and past suicide ideation; (c) evaluating, as needed, the nature of current and past suicide plans, including previous attempts; (d) assessment of patient self-control and agitation; (e) habituation to pain, fear, and/or death; (f) assessment of suicide intent and reasons for living; and (g) implementation (as needed) of a collaborative safety plan or alternative suicide intervention strategy that assists clients with concrete problem-solving and addresses unique client issues, including lethal means restriction.

PRIOR TO THE GROUP

Setting the norms for safety should begin in the first contact with a potential group member. First, the leader must emphasize that members *do not contact each other* with safety concerns. As an example, the leader might tell a new member to imagine how an established group member, Trey, might feel if a fellow group member Becky reached out when suicidal, but the phone call was not enough to prevent her from later taking her own life. Instead, Becky is advised during a pre-group meeting that all safety issues should be brought to the leader or on-call counselors; reaching out to a group member outside of the group would thus go against agreed-upon norms. The leader should also plan to review these norms in the first session of the group as a reminder.

Chen and Rybak (2017) recommend helping members set an agenda for the group session by *directly addressing* safety and vulnerability disclosures. Members can be explicitly informed that the group *will be building a secure atmosphere for regular discussions around safety issues.* Providing resources for suicide hotlines and after-hours emergency supports through a variety of methods (e.g., handouts, verbal messages, online, or electronic tools) can also be beneficial prior to the group.

Progress has also recently been made with using new assessment instruments and structured interviews that can be processed before starting group therapy. Ballester et al. (2019) studied first-year Spanish students (18–24 years old) as a part of the WHO World Mental Health-International College Student (WMH-ICS) initiative. Psychologists administered the Mini-International Neuropsychiatric Interview (MINI) by telephone. The WMS-ICS survey showed reasonable concordance with the MINI telephone interviews performed by mental health professionals when using cut-off scores. The WMS-ICS survey, thus, might be useful for screening purposes. Though logistics associated with administering such instruments before or after a group are often cited as barriers to more thorough means of assessing risk (Woods & Ruzek, 2018), quick screening assessments can provide valuable information to the leader and potentially save lives. When used as a way to track risk, a consistent measuring tool increases knowledge about member safety. Even simple checklists of several risk items taken just before the group session can provide valuable information. Regular assessments for suicide risk can also be implemented at the pre-group meeting, at regular treatment intervals, and at the end of group members' participation.

ASSESSMENT AND RESPONSE TO SUICIDAL IDEATION WITHIN A GROUP

In addition to objective measures and structured interviews given before the session, the group leader should observe and respond to changes in mental status. Woods and Ruzek (2018) suggest that if the leader notices a deterioration in functioning or observes unusual behaviors, it is important to ask group members about these changes. Conducting a risk assessment and connecting members with additional resources while in group therapy can be a valuable way to both support group cohesion and manage risk. By attending to risk, the leader demonstrates the value of ensuring safety as well as demonstrating that risk can be attenuated through interpersonal relationships. For example, it can be healing for member Becky, who has revealed suicidal thoughts, *to see other members crying at the potential of losing her to suicide.* It can serve as a reminder to Becky that she has established significant relationships with caring and concerned peers, as well as a recognition of the personal value she offers others. Furthermore, the group can be a solid source of emotional regulation for the member at risk (Badenoch & Cox, 2010).

Given that social connection protects against suicide, clinicians should make efforts to establish an authentic, empathic, and supportive interpersonal connection with clients who report suicide-related thoughts and behaviors (Sommers-Flanagan & Sommers-Flanagan, 2017). Imagine Becky starts the group with, "I just want to end it all." The following steps are examples of how the leader can respond:

- verbally appreciate the risk disclosure as a sign of trust in the group *and frame it as a "brave step" by Becky*
- demonstrate the intention to listen to Becky with compassion
- assess Becky's risk using the recommended prompts discussed earlier
- suggest that it would be helpful for other members to relate to Becky by sharing their experiences with suicidal ideation (i.e., "you are not alone")
- elicit more specific feedback from the group about what Becky offers to others in the group such as strengths or supportive qualities
- reflect on the supportive responses of the group to illuminate that the other members seem to value Becky and are displaying caring and concern
- engage in safety planning in front of the group, which can include sharing the risk information with a responsible family member or other supportive adults, using emergency resources, or arranging transport for a hospital evaluation
- process the interactions and any remaining concerns of members, while also praising and reinforcing the demonstrated bonds and caring in the group

The compassionate listening and peer feedback cycle can have quite an impact in helping to *broaden the client's thinking.* If Becky can hear how trusted others *actually* view her, she may gradually shift her self-perception and improve her feelings of self-worth.

Many agencies and settings also suggest therapists use mood ratings with a floor reflecting suicidality to better indicate the level of client risk. It can be helpful to insert a suicide assessment within a mood-based scaling procedure (Sommers-Flanagan & Shaw, 2017) for all group members. This process involves evaluating mood like an extended mental status examination. The procedure involves using scaling questions to assess the current mood, worst mood, and best mood. Such questions and numeric ratings of mood can thus lead to a deeper understanding of the member's distinctive state of mind, which can be quite relieving for the client. It is also important that the use of any form or structure be flexible to maintain the therapeutic alliance. When settings do use forms to guide the information-gathering process, protocols can include cautions that it should not obstruct rapport and therapeutic alliance. Instead of rigidly sticking with an interview protocol, it is important to (1) pause after hearing the member's response to each question, (2) use paraphrasing and feeling reflections to communicate empathic understanding, and (3) ask additional questions that pursue or track the client's unique experience (Simon, 2011).

The leader, however, may need to consider alternatives if other less helpful dynamics surface during such a process or it is not productive. The leader can consider asking the member to remain after the group to assess and manage the risk. In this case, it can be helpful to reassure all members that steps will be taken to engage in an agreed-upon safety plan or that other emergency resources may be considered to keep the member safe.

CONSIDERING ASSESSMENT AND RESPONSE OUTSIDE OF THE GROUP

Reasons for having risk assessment and interventions outside of the group can include:

- a member frequently dominates with safety concerns, which creates disrupts group goals
- a member is less forthcoming in the group or is unable to engage in the process
- other members do not have suicidal ideation or do not seem able to support or relate
- the at-risk member is inconsistent in attendance or does not have good relations with other members
- the leader believes the topic would be overly time-consuming

When a suicide risk assessment is deemed best handled outside of the group, a group member may stay after the group or leave with one of two co-leaders during a group session (Woods & Ruzek, 2018). When extra staffing or a co-therapist team is available, it can be helpful to have one leader complete the risk assessment while another leader attends to any resulting reactions triggered in other group members. For groups that disallow communications outside of the group except for attendance or management-type issues, leaders may want to consider that such policies might disadvantage the therapists in making a suicide assessment.

TRAINING THE LEADER TO RESPOND WITH CALMNESS

As many highly distressed individuals with suicidal impulses suffer from problem-solving deficits, and client arousal or agitation is linked to suicidal behavior (Ribeiro et al., 2015), *it is crucial to calmly broaden the group member's thinking*. The leader needs to *model calmness* at the same time that a careful risk assessment and associated interventions are implemented. Training and experience are crucial for clinicians to become *comfortable and thorough* in group therapy with suicidal members. Graduate students and new practitioners should be taught to normalize suicidal thinking with the assumption that given the current levels of pain, it is natural for such thoughts to surface. Leaders should be thoroughly trained in advanced suicide assessment approaches, recognizing that a comprehensive approach and empathic responding are essential to developing a cohesive group.

Group co-leaders in training may also differ from each other regarding the extent to which they are emotionally triggered by at-risk members, with influences from their own personal and professional encounters with suicide. Furthermore, it is important to stay current on the science around suicide assessment and the risk factors for suicidality and to learn to document carefully. Many practitioners are not using the most updated, reliable, and accurate measures for suicidality; many group therapists are also not documenting the assessment for suicidality adequately (Novotney, 2020). For example, it is helpful to use the client's exact words in notes when they state that they agree to contact emergency resources before taking any self-harm actions.

WHEN A MEMBER ATTEMPTS SUICIDE OR COMPLETES A SUICIDE

A group client's suicide or attempt can be overwhelming and devastating for trainees and seasoned group leaders alike. A leader may experience the following:

- rumination about what might have been done differently
- grief about the loss of a meaningful therapeutic relationship
- loss of confidence and increased self-doubt
- questioning whether to remain in the role of therapist
- a perceived burden of responsibility for keeping clients alive
- worry about other reactions, such as contagion effects or blame from the other group members

Most centers also have policies that mandate a retrospective analysis of actions taken before the death to glean if anything can be learned, and this process can also add to the stress of a trainee or supervisor. An important early study examined prelicensure doctoral supervisees who experienced a client's suicide (Knox et al., 2006). Findings suggested that although these supervisees received minimal training about suicide, support and normalization from supervisors and others helped them to cope with the death.

When a member suicide occurs, the leader also has an obligation to the surviving group members to help them process reactions to the loss. Given each member came to the group to get help with distress, the trauma of losing a peer may instead exacerbate their own symptoms. Additionally, each member may have individual personal histories with suicidal ideation and actions that may affect how they process the loss of a fellow member. The leader will need to consult with other professionals to consider how to assess the impact of the loss and help the members process the death.

In summary, an ethical approach to suicide assessment can be implemented within an empathic pre-group intervention, in which listening includes gentle explorations of unique risk factors, emotional pain, social connectedness, hopelessness or fearlessness, agitation, and access to lethal means. Brief screening measures used throughout the group and a practice of bringing up safety issues regularly can enhance the group climate by normalizing that suicidal ideation is a common response to pain. Whether within or outside of a group, supervisors should assess the capacity of the leader to directly and calmly inquire about suicidal thoughts and plans and engage in the problem-solving phase with the aim to decrease psychological distress, increase connectedness, and promote safety.

Violence

Legal and ethical standards delineate the responsibility of the leader to take action when a client expresses violent intent (Murrie & Kelley, 2017). Again, all risk assessments are a complex and continuous process that must be addressed with relative calm by the leader and be attended to throughout the group's life. When it comes to preparing for such crises, Novotney (2020) suggests practitioners consult with professionals who have expertise in working with volatile patients. Educating oneself on when the duty to warn applies and what the state statute requires in terms of the next steps is crucial. For instance, some states indicate that the duty to warn only arises when there are identifiable victims and the intended violence is imminent, while other states have broader parameters such as a more general threat not limited to a specific person. The National Conference of State Legislatures provides guidance on the duty-to-warn statute in each state, https://www.ncsl.org/research/health/mental-health-professionals-duty-to-warn.aspx. Databases of Tarasoff laws on state websites can also be used to gather more information (Edwards, 2014).

Even after the therapist assesses the risk of potential violence before admission to a group, it is not uncommon for members to deteriorate into higher-risk phases of mental health during treatment. The leader should pay particular attention to:

- romantic relationship endings
- workplace anger
- a history of domestic violence
- thoughts or fantasies related to revenge

As with suicide assessment, ascertaining the intensity of the violent intention and predicting future actions can be challenging for the leader. The leader can consider using ratings with a floor to estimate the likelihood the member will act violently (e.g., numbers between one and ten); asking about access to means and the specifics of what might need to happen for the member to respond with violence is crucial. Exploring alternative actions to violence with coping techniques such as mindfulness, a time out by leaving the situation, or physical or emotional distraction can occur in the group, with other members weighing in around how they calm themselves when anger is escalating. Consideration of outside of group session interventions due to time constraints or lack of progress may also be important.

The leader should also keep in mind that other members may have anxious reactions when hearing threats and yet remain silent or paralyzed in groups. For example, one member may be considering ending the life of a terminally ill spouse. Members may hold values or religious views that disagree with such actions or may respond with heightened worry or conflict. Nonetheless, it may be important for group members to engage with the leader's comprehensive assessments to address their responses and concerns for the volatile member, as well as any concerns for the potential target of harm.

Appropriate training can facilitate leader confidence in risk assessment. Murrie and Kelley (2017) note that by integrating basic knowledge and practices from forensic psychology and psychiatry, clinicians can more comfortably incorporate violence risk assessment and management into their routine care. Therapists with such knowledge incorporate risk assessment into the start of treatment, monitor risk throughout treatment, and respond appropriately to any threats of violence that emerge. For more details regarding the foundational knowledge and techniques useful in behavioral emergencies and crises, and a review of the legal and ethical parameters that guide clinician appraisals of violence risk, see Murrie and Kelly.

Child and Elder Abuse Reporting

Child maltreatment, encompassing emotional, physical, or sexual abuse, and neglect, is a significant public health problem (Centers for Disease Control and Prevention, 2020). Parental characteristics such as psychiatric problems and substance abuse have proven to be the strongest predictors for child neglect (Barth, 2009; Mulder et al., 2018). A leader needs to also have a keen awareness of signs of elder abuse, particularly during an isolating time such as a pandemic or contagious illness. Safe and nurturing caregiving relationships, as well as current social support, can have a buffering effect on those who have suffered abuse (Jaffee et al., 2017).

Ethical principles related to abuse reporting include Autonomy, Beneficence, Justice, and Non-maleficence. For example, it is recommended that all group members are given information about state guidelines for child and elder abuse reporting during a pre-group meeting, providing the client the autonomy to decide what to reveal. Should a member disclose information suggesting evidence that abuse is currently ongoing, states will have specific directives for making a report to social services to investigate to provide protection for a family member (i.e., actions reflecting Beneficence and Non-maleficence). Helping vulnerable populations get assistance in a fair and timely manner can mean the Justice principle is followed.

The leader will need to make decisions about how to further gather more information to determine the extent of the risk, similar to the assessments of suicide or homicide risk. For example, the leader must balance (1) allowing other members to witness or even participate in such discussions with considerations of triggering other members, (2) encouraging the expression of relief by members should the inquiries lead to less risk than initially believed, and (3) reporting quickly to ensure the safety of those at risk (i.e., Non-maleficence) and reassuring members. For instance, other members may express feeling relieved that the leader takes safety seriously by protecting others to the degree that they are able. For a detailed review of interventions and services related to elder abuse, see O'Donnell et al. (2015).

In the pre-group meeting, addressing family history can illuminate patterns that can be shifted through corrective or healing experiences by the leader who demonstrates empathy like that of a "good parent." Treatment groups in the form of family therapy, multisystem treatments, and other interventions can also have an impact on the cycle of violence and patterns of intergenerational transmission of risk (Wu & Slesnick, 2020). When hearing about the potential risk of current or future abuse or neglect, the leader must inquire right away to assess the level of danger. The group members need to see therapeutic actions to protect the potential victim or hear that after the group, a plan will be made for reporting or further problem-solving. Clinicians must realize that they have a moral imperative to intervene appropriately to protect the potentially *vulnerable* populations, children, and the elderly.

Final Note

In this chapter, we reviewed the range of factors that can enter into a group psychotherapist's decision-making about ethical situations. Whereas in Chapter 1 we emphasized the more rational, deliberative factors, this chapter considered the more intuitive, emotional, and motivational elements. Both types of processes are necessary for ethical decision-making. Without a knowledge of the sequence of steps, the group psychotherapist would be prone to proceeding in a chaotic fashion (e.g., implementing a solution before all options had been considered). Without the integration of affect, e.g., the group psychotherapist would lack the empathy that could help in forging solutions reflecting emotional sensitivity to all parties. Without intuition, the group leader fails to draw upon the backlog of clinical experience that could be useful in understanding the present.

This chapter also addressed the product of ethical decision-making, that is, the decision itself and how it can be implemented. Standard of care is a duty to provide treatment that a typical, reasonable, caring, and careful practitioner would have implemented under similar conditions. We have noted that achieving the standard of care is different from achieving perfection. Still, from a virtue ethics perspective, group leaders should strive to do the best they possibly can. To meet and surpass the standard of care, the group leader should incorporate ROM into their practice and use this source of feedback as a means of continually improving the members' group experiences. When evidence exists that members are not progressing adequately, the leader should bring all resources to bear in altering this circumstance, including ROM and the use of supervision and consultation. Challenges to meeting the standard of care can occur when ethical problems arise. Recognizing errors rooted in bias and use of heuristics, knowing one's strengths and weaknesses as a problem-solver and compensating for the latter, being aware of jurisdictional regulations and relevant disciplinary codes of ethics, making use of supervision and consultation, and documenting the rationale for decisions made can serve the group leader well in meeting the standard of care. Risk management approaches with an ethical lens also include knowledge of suicide and violence risk factors and a willingness to explore them directly and thoroughly while considering the group dynamics and reactions.

CEU Questions

1. Stress can lead a decision-maker to generate fewer solutions to a problem. (T/F)
2. Stress decreases as the number of ethical decisions a professional must make increases. (T/F)
3. The use of intuition leads to poor decisions. (T/F)
4. System 2 is highly involved in routine clinical decisions. (T/F)
5. Reamer identified the following principles to assess the standard of care:

   a. Reasonable, practical, and prudent
   b. Reasonable, typical, and prudent
   c. Virtuous, reasonable, and practical
   d. Legal, prudent, and practical

6. To meet the standard of care, group psychotherapists must be aware of the state and federal laws that regulate their practices. (T/F)
7. Licensing boards will sanction a practitioner only when that practitioner has harmed a client. (T/F)
8. In North America, most therapists have adopted a routine outcome monitoring system. (T/F)
9. A therapist who wants to continue to conduct a group despite not being able to maintain a healthy census is likely affected by loss aversion. (T/F)
10. Difficulty controlling suicidal ideation and engaging in non-suicidal self-injury are important to consider in evaluating an individual's suicide potential. (T/F)

Answer Key: 1. T; 2. F; 3. F; 4. F; 5. b.; 6. T; 7. F; 8. F; 9. T; 10. T

Discussion Questions

1. In this chapter, we explored the topic of cognitive biases and in Chapter 3 that of microaggressions. What are the ways in which these two concepts are related?
2. Identify your self-care strategies. Are these strategies sufficient when the stress of group leadership or other work responsibilities becomes intense? What modifications might you make if you regard your current strategies inadequate to help you cope with a high-stress load?
3. If a therapist is conducting a psychotherapy group while pursuing difficult medical treatment such as chemotherapy, what resources might be mobilized to support the therapist?

4. How might the affect bias shape a therapist's decision as to whether to accept a particular candidate in a group?
5. A group psychotherapist claims that members attend group more consistently when they pay for each session whether they are present or not. If this observation is correct, would it be consistent or inconsistent with the loss aversion effect? Why?
6. What are the advantages of instituting a routine outcome monitoring system? Given these advantages, why might the therapist not institute such a system?
7. Think about a group you led in the past in which you did not implement a routine outcome monitoring system. How would group members have reacted to this system? If you identified any member resistances, how might you have surmounted them?
8. Think about past sticky situations you faced in a group. In what situations did you proceed with more intuitive thinking when deliberative thinking might have been in order? What factors led you to emphasize deliberative thinking?

Vignettes/Role Plays

1. Dr. Hote is four months pregnant, but her pregnancy is not evident to many people. She interviews a candidate for a long-term therapy group and does not reveal her pregnancy. Dr. Hote intends to take a three-month sabbatical from the group during which time she will have a substitute therapist. Her rationale for not divulging the pregnancy to the entering member is that she has not yet announced it to the group. Does Dr. Hote have an ethical obligation to reveal her pregnancy to the new member? If so, why? If not, why not? Might any of the factors described in this chapter bear upon Dr. Hote's decision?
2. You are interviewing a prospective employer and attempting to discern the extent to which self-care is valued within the organization. What questions might you pose during the interview? What might help you to know if the organization is committed to self-care in name only? What policies might you ask about that would provide clues to the organization's value of self-care?
3. In Chapter 2, we presented the following situation in a vignette:
   Terrence reported to his group that after his terminally ill wife had months of pain and no quality of life left, he ended her life at her request by giving her more morphine than allowed. Another member wants the leader to report this to the police because it violates her religious values.
   The therapist must formulate a response. One individual should role play deliberate processing and another individual automatic processing. How might this conversation proceed? What contribution does each system make to ethical decision-making?

References

American Psychological Association. (2010). Amending the ethics code. *American Psychological Association, 41*(4), 64. https://www.apa.org/monitor/2010/04/ethics

American Psychological Association. (2017). *Ethical principles of psychologists and code of conduct.* American Psychological Association. https://www.apa.org/ethics/code

American Psychological Association, Presidential Task Force on Evidence-Based Practice. (2006). Evidence-based practice in psychology. *American Psychologist, 61*(4), 271–285. 10.1037/0003-066X.61.4.271

Antypa, N., Van der Does, A. W., & Penninx, B. W. (2010). Cognitive reactivity: Investigation of a potentially treatable marker of suicide risk in depression. *Journal of Affective Disorders*, *122*(1–2), 46–52. 10.1016/j.jad.2009.06.013

Association of State and Provincial Psychology Boards. (2019). Supervision guidelines for education and training leading to licensure as a general applied provider. Retrieved on January 19, 2021 from https://cdn.ymaws.com/www.asppb.net/resource/resmgr/guidelines/supervision_guidelines_for_g.pdf

Badenoch, B., & Cox, P. (2010). Integrating interpersonal neurobiology with group psychotherapy. *International Journal of Group Psychotherapy*, *60*(4), 462–481. 10.1521/ijgp.2010.60.4.462

Baldwin, S. A., & Imel, Z. E. (2013). Therapist effects: Findings and methods. In M. J. Lambert (Ed.), *Bergin and Garfield's handbook of psychotherapy and behavior change*, 6, (pp. 258–297). New York: Wiley.

Ballester, L., Alayo, I., Vilagut, G., Almenara, J., Cebrià, A. I., Echeburúa, E., Gabilondo, A., Gili, M., Lagares, C., Piqueras, J. A., Roca, M., Soto-Sanz, V., Blasco, M. J., Castellví, P., Forero, C. G., Bruffaerts, R., Mortier, P., Auerbach, R. P., Nock, M. K., … UNIVERSAL study group. (2019). Accuracy of online survey assessment of mental disorders and suicidal thoughts and behaviors in Spanish university students. Results of the WHO World Mental Health- International College Student initiative. *PLoS One*, *14*(9), e0221529. 10.1371/journal.pone.0221529

Bargh, J. A., Schwader, K. L., Hailey, S. E., Dyer, R. L., & Boothby, E. J. (2012). Automaticity in social-cognitive processes. *Trends in Cognitive Sciences*, *16*(12), 593–605. 10.1016/j.tics.2012.10.002

Barkham, M., Lutz, W., Lambert, M. J., & Saxon, D. (2017). *Therapist effects, effective therapists, and the law of variability*. In L. G. Castonguay & C. E. Hill (Eds.), *How and why are some therapists better than others?: Understanding therapist effects* (pp. 13–36). American Psychological Association. 10.1037/0000034-002

Barlow, S. H. (2013). *Group specialty practice*. Oxford, UK: Oxford University Press.

Barlow, S., Burlingame, G. M., Greene, L. R., Joyce, A., Kaklauskas, F., Kinley, J., Klein, R. H., Kobos, J. C., Leszcz, M., MacNair-Semands, R., Paquin, J. D., Tasca, G. A., Whittingham, M., & Feirman, D. (2015). *Evidence-based practice in group psychotherapy*. American Group Psychotherapy. http://www.agpa.org/home/practice-resources/evidence-based-practice-in-group-psychotherapy

Barnett, J. E., Baker, E. K., Elman, N. S., & Schoener, G. R. (2007). In pursuit of wellness: The self-care imperative. *Professional Psychology: Research and Practice*, *38*(6), 603–612. 10.1037/0735-7028.38.6.603

Barnett, J. (2017a). An introduction to boundaries and multiple relationships for psychotherapists: Issues, challenges, and recommendations. In O. Zur (Ed.), *Multiple relationships in psychotherapy and counseling: Unavoidable, common and mandatory dual relations in therapy* (pp. 17–29). Routledge.

Barnett, J. (2017b). Unavoidable incidental contacts and multiple relationships in rural practice. In O. Zur (Ed.), *Multiple relationships in psychotherapy and counseling: Unavoidable, common and mandatory dual relations in therapy* (pp. 97–107). Routledge.

Barnett, J. E., Johnston, L. C., & Hillard, D. (2006). Psychotherapist wellness as an ethical imperative. In L. VandeCreek & J. B. Allen (Eds.), *Innovations in clinical practice: Focus on health and wellness* (pp. 257–271). Professional Resources Press.

Baron, J. (2000). *Thinking and deciding* (3rd ed.). Cambridge University Press.

Barth, R. P. (2009). Preventing child abuse and neglect with parent training: Evidence and opportunities. *The Future of Children*, *19*(2), 95–118. 10.1353/foc.0.0031

Bennett, C., Blount, A., Gerlach, J., Schroeder, K., Ausloos, C. D., Bloom, Z., Goodrich, K. M., Hunnicutt Hollenbaugh, K. M., & Taylor, J. (2021). Standards of care for assessment in group work. *The Journal for Specialists in Group Work*, *46*(3), 238–243. 10.1080/01933922.2021.1942346

Bernard, H., Burlingame, G., Flores, P., Greene, L., Joyce, A., Kobos, J. C., Leszcz, M., MacNair-Semands, R. R., Piper, W. E., McEneaney, A. M., & Feirman, D. (2008). Clinical practice guidelines for group psychotherapy. *International Journal of Group Psychotherapy*, *58*(4), 455–542. 10.1521/ijgp.2008.58.4.455

Blair, I. V., Danyluck, C., Judd, C. M., Manson, S. M., Laudenslager, M. L., Daugherty, S. L., Ratliff, E. L., Gardner, J. A., & Brondolo, E. (2021). Validation of the brief perceived ethnic discrimination questionnaire–Community Version in American Indians. *Cultural Diversity and Ethnic Minority Psychology, 27*(1), 47–59. 10.1037/cdp0000419

Boswell, J. F., Kraus, D. R., Castonguay, L. G., & Youn, S. J. (2015). Treatment outcome package: Measuring and facilitating multidimensional change. *Psychotherapy, 52*(4), 422–431. 10.1037/pst0000028

Brabender, V. (2021). Identifying and resolving ethical dilemmas in group psychotherapy. In M. Trachsel, J. Gaab, N. Biller-Andorno, Ş. Tekin, & J. Z. Sadler (Eds.), *The Oxford handbook of psychotherapy ethics* (pp. 625–641). Oxford University Press.

Bricklin, P. (2001). Being ethical: More than obeying the law and avoiding harm. *Journal of Personality Assessment, 77*(2), 195–202. 10.1207/S15327752JPA7702_03

Brondolo, E., Kelly, K. P., Coakley, V., Gordon, T., Thompson, S., Levy, E., & Contrada, R. J. (2005). The perceived ethnic discrimination questionnaire: Development and preliminary validation of a community version. *Journal of Applied Social Psychology, 35*, 335–365. 10.1111/j.1559-1816.2005.tb02124.x

Brown, K. W., & Ryan, R. M. (2003). The benefits of being present: Mindfulness and its role in psychological well-being. *Journal of Personality and Social Psychology 84*(4), 822–848. 10.1037/0022-3514.84.4.822

Burlingame, G. M. & Strauss, B. (2021). Efficacy of small group treatments: Foundation for evidence-based practice. In M. Barkham, W. Lutz, & L. G. Castonguay (Eds.), *Bergin & Garfield's handbook of psychotherapy and behavior change* (7th ed.). Wiley. https://www.wiley.com/en-us/Bergin+and+Garfield%27s+Handbook+of+Psychotherapy+and+Behavior+Change%2C+7th+Edition-p-9781119536581

Burlingame, G. M., Strauss, B., & Joyce, A. (2013). Change mechanisms and effectiveness of small group treatments. In M. J. Lambert (Ed.), *Bergin and Garfield's handbook of psychotherapy and behavior change, 6,* (pp. 640–689). Wiley.

Burlingame, G. M., Strauss, B., Joyce, A., MacNair-Semands, R., MacKenzie, K. R., Ogrodniczuk, J., & Taylor, S. (2006). *CORE Battery—revised: An assessment tool kit for promoting optimal group selection, process and outcome.* Available through the AGPA store.

Carney, D. M., Castonguay, L. G., Janis, R. A., Scofield, B. E., Hayes, J. A., & Locke, B. D. (2021). Center effects: Counseling center variables as predictors of psychotherapy outcomes. *The Counseling Psychologist, 97*(7), 1013–1037. 10.1177/00110000211029271

Centers for Disease Control and Prevention. (2020). *Violence prevention: Child abuse & neglect.* https://www.cdc.gov/violenceprevention/childabuseandneglect/index.html

Chang-Caffaro, S., & Caffaro, J. (2018). Differences that make a difference: Diversity and the process group leader. *International Journal of Group Psychotherapy, 68*(4), 483–497. 10.1080/00207284.2018.1469958

Chao, R. C. L., & Green, K. E. (2011). Multiculturally Sensitive Mental Health Scale (MSMHS): Development, factor analysis, reliability, and validity. *Psychological Assessment, 23*, 876–887. 10.1037/a0023710

Chen, M. W., & Rybak, C. J. (2017). *Group leadership skills: Interpersonal process in group counseling and therapy* (2nd ed.). SAGE Publications. https://us.sagepub.com/en-us/nam/group-leadership-skills/book251766

Chow, D. L., Miller, S. D., Seidel, J. A., Kane, R. T., Thornton, J. A., & Andrews, W. P. (2015). The role of deliberate practice in the development of highly effective psychotherapists. *Psychotherapy, 52*, 337–345. 10.1037/pst0000015

Chu, J., Floyd, R., Diep, H., Pardo, S., Goldblum, P., & Bongar, B. (2013). A tool for the culturally competent assessment of suicide: The Cultural Assessment of Risk for Suicide (CARS) measure. *Psychological Assessment, 25*(2), 424–434. 10.1037/a0031264

Chu, J. P., Poon, G., Kwok, K. K., Leino, A. E., Goldblum, P., & Bongar, B. (2017). An assessment of training in and practice of culturally competent suicide assessment. *Training and Education in Professional Psychology, 11*(2), 69–77. 10.1037/tep0000147

Contrada, R. J., Ashmore, R. D., Gary, M. L., Coups, E., Egeth, J. D., Sewell, A., Ewell, K., Goyal, T. M., & Chasse, V. (2001). Measures of ethnicity-related stress: Psychometric properties, ethnic group differences, and associations with well-being. *Journal of Applied Social Psychology*, *31*(9), 1775–1820. 10.1111/j.1559-1816.2001.tb00205.x

Coombs v. Beede. (1896). https://www.ravellaw.com/opinions/0199f29f379343a7a3a78ba906298aba

Croskerry, P. (2003). The importance of cognitive errors in diagnosis and strategies to minimize them. *Academic Medicine*, *78*(8), 775–780. 10.1097/00001888-200308000-00003

Daw, B., & Joseph, S. (2007). Qualified therapists' experience of personal therapy. *Counselling and Psychotherapy Research*, *7*(4), 227–232. 10.1080/14733140701709064

Dour, H. J., Cha, C. B., & Nock, M. K. (2011). Evidence for an emotion–cognition interaction in the statistical prediction of suicide attempts. *Behaviour Research and Therapy*, *49*(4), 294–298. 10.1016/j.brat.2011.01.010

Duncan, B. L., Miller, S. D. (2008). *The Outcome and Session Rating Scales: The revised administration and scoring manual, including the Child Outcome Rating Scale.* Chicago, IL: Institute for the Study of Therapeutic Change.

Edwards, G. (2014). Doing their duty: An empirical analysis of the unintended effect of Tarasoff v. Regents on homicidal activity. *The Journal of Law and Economics*, *57*(2), 321–348. 10.2139/ssrn.1544574

Forsyth, D. R. (2020). Group-level resistance to health mandates during the COVID-19 pandemic: A groupthink approach. *Group Dynamics: Theory, Research, and Practice*, *24*(3), 139–152. 10.1037/gdn0000132

Franklin, J. C., Ribeiro, J. D., Fox, K. R., Bentley, K. H., Kleiman, E. M., Huang, X., Musacchio, K. M., Jaroszewski, A. C., Chang, B. P., & Nock, M. K. (2017). Risk factors for suicidal thoughts and behaviors: A meta-analysis of 50 years of research. *Psychological Bulletin*, *143*(2), 187–232. 10.1037/bul0000084

Freudenberger, H. J. (1990). Hazards of psychotherapeutic practice. *Psychotherapy in Private Practice*, *8*, 31–34. 10.1300/J294v01n01_14

Gal, D. & Rucker, D. D. (2018). The loss of loss aversion: Will it loom larger than its gain? *Journal of Consumer Psychology*, *28*, 497–516. 10.1002/jcpy.1047

Goldberg, S. B., Babins-Wagner, R., Rousmaniere, T., Berzins, S., Hoyt, W. T., Whipple, J. L., Miller, S. D., Wampold, B. E. (2016). Creating a climate for therapist improvement: A case study of an agency focused on outcomes and deliberate practice. *Psychotherapy*, *53*, 367–375. 10.1037/pst0000060

Graber, M. L., Kissam, S., Payne, V. L., Meyer, A. N., Sorensen, A., Lenfestey, N., Tant, E., Henriksen, K., LaBresh, K. , & Singh, H. (2012). Cognitive interventions to reduce diagnostic error: A narrative review. *BMJ Quality & Safety*, *21*(7), 535–557. 10.1136/bmjqs-2011-000149

Greene, L. R. (2012). Group therapist as social scientist, with special reference to the psychodynamically oriented psychotherapist. *American Psychologist*, *67*(6), 477–489. 10.1037/a0029147

Greene, L. S., Kaklauskas, F. J., & Rutan, J. S. (2019). Advanced skills. In F. J. Kaklauskas & L. S. Greene (Eds.), *Core principles of group psychotherapy: A training manual for theory, research, and practice.* New York, NY: Routledge.

Grenon, R., Schwartze, D., Hammond, N., Ivanova, I., Mcquaid, N., Proulx, G., & Tasca, G. A. (2017). Group psychotherapy for eating disorders: A meta-analysis. *International Journal of Eating Disorders*, *50*, 997–1013. 10.1002/eat.22744

Hampton, H. P. (1984). Malpractice in psychotherapy: Is there a relevant standard of care? *35 Case Western Reserve Law Review*, 35, 251–281. https://scholarlycommons.law.case.edu/cgi/viewcontent.cgi?article=2435&context=caselrev

Hayes, S. C., Strosahl, K. D., & Wilson, K. G. (2012). *Acceptance and commitment therapy: An experiential approach to behavioral changes* (2nd ed.). Guilford Press.

Hays, D. G., & Wood, C. (2017). Stepping outside the normed sample: Implications for validity. *Measurement and Evaluation in Counseling and Development*, *50*(4), 282–288. 10.1080/07481756.2017.1339565

Ionita, G., Ciquier, G., & Fitzpatrick, M. (2020). Barriers and facilitators to the use of progress-monitoring measures in psychotherapy. *Canadian Psychology/Psychologie canadienne, 61*(3), 245–256. 10.1037/cap0000205

Jaffee, S. R., Takizawa, R., & Arseneault, L. (2017). Buffering effects of safe, supportive, and nurturing relationships among women with childhood histories of maltreatment. *Psychological Medicine, 47*(15), 2628–2639. 10.1017/S0033291717001027

Johnson, W. B. & Johnson, S. J., (2017). Unavoidable and mandated multiple relationships in military settings. In O. Zur (Ed.), *Multiple Relationships in Psychotherapy and Counseling: Unavoidable, Common and Mandatory Dual Relations in Therapy* (pp. 49–60). Routledge.

Joint Commission (n.d.) https://manual.jointcommission.org/BHCInstruments/WebHome?_ga=2.268348040.768402592.1609957597-1468227570.1609352814

Jorm, A. F., Patten, S. B., Brugha, T. S., & Mojtabai, R. (2017). Has increased provision of treatment reduced the prevalence of common mental disorders? Review of the evidence from four countries. *World Psychiatry, 16*(1), 90–99. 10.1002/wps.20388

Joyce, A. S., MacNair-Semands, R., Tasca, G. A., & Ogrodniczuk, J. S. (2011). Factor structure and validity of the therapeutic factors inventory-short form. *Group Dynamics: Theory, Research, and Practice, 15*(3), 201. 10.1037/a0024677

Jurist, E. (2021). Mentalizing heath: Newsletter #4. https://elliot4cc.substack.com/p/mentalizing-health-30f?token=eyJ1c2VyX2lkIjoyNjAyODgyOSwicG9zdF9pZCI6MzI1NzMwOTEsIl8iOiJxVmZvdCIsImlhdCI6MTYxMzQ0OMjgzNSwiZXhwIjoxNjEzNDQ2NDM1LCJpc3MiOiJwdWItMjcwMjgyIiwic3ViIjoicG9zdC1yZWFjdGlvbiJ9.dw_syxKEtp4bRx1uM3XqB-pWuUq3ZLlOwJ9LBC7uk3Y&utm_source=substack&utm_medium=email&utm_content=share

Kahneman, D. (2011). *Thinking, fast and slow.* Farrar, Strauss, and Giroux.

Kahneman, D., & Tversky, A. (1982). The psychology of preferences. *Scientific American, 246*(1), 160–173. https://www.jstor.org/stable/24966506

Kaklauskas, F. J., & Nettles, R. (2019). Towards multicultural and diversity proficiency as a group psychotherapist. In F. J. Kaklauskas & L. S. Greene (Eds.), *Core principles of group psychotherapy: A training manual for theory, research, and practice* (pp. 25–45). Routledge.

Kälvemark, S., Höglund, A. T., Hansson, M. G., Westerholm, P., and Arnetz, B. (2004). Living with conflicts-ethical dilemmas and moral distress in the health care system. *Social Science and Medicine, 58*, 1075–1084. doi: 10.1016/S0277-9536(03)00279-X

Kivlighan III, D. M., Adams, M. C., Drinane, J. M., Tao, K. W., & Owen, J. (2019a). Construction and validation of the Multicultural Orientation Inventory—Group Version. *Journal of Counseling Psychology, 66* (1), 45. 10.1037/cou0000294

Kivlighan III, D. M., & Chapman, N. A. (2018). Extending the multicultural orientation (MCO) framework to group psychotherapy: A clinical illustration. *Psychotherapy, 55*(1), 39. 10.1037/pst0000142

Kivlighan III, D. M., Drinane, J. M., Tao, K. W., Owen, J., & Liu, W. M. (2019b). The detrimental effect of fragile groups: Examining the role of cultural comfort for group therapy members of color. *Journal of Counseling Psychology, 66* (6), 763. 10.1037/cou0000352

Knapp, S., & VandeCreek, L. (2007). Balancing respect for autonomy with competing values with the use of principle-based ethics. *Psychotherapy: Theory, Research, Practice, Training, 44*(4), 397–404. 10.1037/0000036-003

Knapp, S., Handelsman, M. M., Gottlieb, M. C., & VandeCreek, L. D. (2013). The dark side of professional ethics. *Professional Psychology: Research and Practice, 44*(6), 371–377. 10.1037/a0035110

Knapp, S. J., VandeCreek, L. D., & Fingerhut, R. (2017). Ethical decision making. In S. J. Knapp, L. D. VandeCreek, & R. Fingerhut (Eds.), *Practical ethics for psychologists: A positive approach,* (pp. 39–50). American Psychological Association. 10.1037/0000036-003.

Knox, S., Burkard, A. W., Jackson, J. A., Schaack, A. M., & Hess, S. A. (2006). Therapists-in-training who experience a client suicide: Implications for supervision. *Professional Psychology: Research & Practice, 37*(5), 547–557. 10.1037/0735-7028.37.5.547

Lambert, M. J., Kahler, M., Harmon, C., Burlingame, G. M., Shimokawa, K., White, M. M. (2013). *Administration and scoring manual: Outcome questionnaire OQ®-45.2.* Salt Lake City, UT: OQMeasures.

Lambert, M. J., Whipple, J. L., & Kleinstäuber, M. (2018). Collecting and delivering progress feedback: A meta-analysis of routine outcome monitoring. *Psychotherapy*, *55*(4), 520–537. 10.1037/pst0000167

Leszcz, M. (2018). The evidence-based group psychotherapist. *Psychoanalytic Inquiry*, *38*, 285–298. 10.1080/07351690.2018.1444853

Leszcz, M., & Kobos, J. C. (2008). Evidence-based group psychotherapy: Using AGPA's practice guidelines to enhance clinical effectiveness. *Journal of Clinical Psychology*, *64*: 1238–1260. 10.1002/jclp.20531

Lichner, V., Halachová, M., & Lovaš, L. (2018). The concept of self-care, work engagement, and burnout syndrome among slovak social workers. *Czech and Slovak Social Work*, *18*(4), 62–75.

Lindsey, M. A., Sheftall, A. H., Xiao, Y., & Joe, S. (2019). Trends of suicidal behaviors among high school students in the United States: 1991–2017. *Pediatrics*, *144*(5). 10.1542/peds.2019-1187

Locke, B. D., McAleavey, A. A., Zhao, Y., Lei, P. W., Hayes, J. A., Castonguay, L. G., Li, H., Tate, R., & Lin, Y. C. (2012). Development and initial validation of the Counseling Center Assessment of Psychological Symptoms–34. *Measurement and Evaluation in Counseling and Development*, *45*(3), 151–169. 10.1177/0748175611432642

MacKenzie, K. R. (1981). Measurement of group climate. *International Journal of Group Psychotherapy*, *31*(3), 287–295. 10.1080/00207284.1981.11491708

Maltzman, S. (2011). An organizational self-care model: Practical suggestions for development and implementation. *The Counseling Psychologist*, *39*(2), 303–319. 10.1177/0011000010381790

Marmarosh, C. L. (2018). Introduction to special issue: Feedback in group psychotherapy. *Psychotherapy*, *55*, 101–104. 10.1037/ pst0000178

Marmarosh, C. L. (2021). Ruptures and repairs in group psychotherapy: From theory to practice. *International Journal of Group Psychotherapy*, *71*(2), 205–223. 10.1080/00207284.2020.1855893

Marmarosh, C. L., Markin, R. D., & Spiegel, E. B. (2013). *Attachment theory and group psychotherapy*. American Psychological Association. 10.1037/14186-000

McCutchen, J. L. (2017). Multiple relationships in police psychology: Common, unavoidable, and navigable occurrences. In O. Zur (Ed.), *Multiple relationships in psychotherapy and counseling: Unavoidable, common and mandatory dual relations in therapy* (pp. 61–71). Routledge.

Merriam-Webster. (n.d.). Standard of care. *Merriam-Webster.com legal dictionary*. Retrieved December 7, 2020, from https://www.merriam-webster.com/legal/standard%20of%20care

Miles, J. R., & Paquin, J. D. (2014). Best practices in group counseling and psychotherapy research. In J. L. DeLucia-Waack, C. R. Kalodner, & M. T. Riva (Eds.), *The handbook of group counseling and psychotherapy* (2nd ed., pp. 178–192). Sage Publications.

Miller, S. D., Duncan, B. L., Brown, J., Sparks, J. A., & Claud, D. A. (2003). The outcome rating scale: A preliminary study of the reliability, validity, and feasibility of a brief visual analog measure. *Journal of Brief Therapy*, *2*(2), 91–100.

Miller, S. D., Hubble, M. A., Chow, D., & Seidel, J. (2015). Beyond measures and monitoring: Realizing the potential of feedback-informed treatment. *Psychotherapy*, *52*, 449–457. 10.1037/pst0000031

Mortier, P., Auerbach, R. P., Alonso, J., Bantjes, J., Benjet, C., Cuijpers, P., Ebert, D. D., Green, J. G., Hasking, P., Nock, M. K., O'Neill, S., Pinder-Amaker, S., Sampson, N. A., Vilagut, G., Zaslavsky, A. M., Bruffaerts, R., & Kessler, R. C. (2018). Suicidal thoughts and behaviors among first-year college students: Results from the WMH-ICS project. *Journal of the American Academy of Child and Adolescent Psychiatry*, *57*(4), 263–273. 10.1016/j.jaac.2018.01.018

Muir, H. J., Coyne, A. E., Morrison, N. R., Boswell, J. F., & Constantino, M. J. (2019). Ethical implications of routine outcomes monitoring for patients, psychotherapists, and mental health care systems. *Psychotherapy*, *56*(4), 459–469. 10.1037/pst0000246

Mulder, T. M., Kuiper, K. C., van der Put, C. E., Stams, G. J. J., & Assink, M. (2018). Risk factors for child neglect: A meta-analytic review. *Child Abuse & Neglect*, *77*, 198–210. 10.1016/j.chiabu.2018.01.006

Mullen, P. R., Morris, C., & Lord, M. (2017). The experience of ethical dilemmas, burnout, and stress among practicing counselors. *Counseling and Values*, *62*(1), 37–56. 10.1002/cvj.12048

Mumford, M. D., Devenport, L. D., Brown, R. P., Connelly, S., Murphy, S. T., Hill, J. H., & Antes, A. L. (2006). Validation of ethical decision making measures: Evidence for a new set of measures. *Ethics & Behavior, 16*(4), 319–345. 10.1207/s15327019eb1604_4

Mumford, M. D., Murphy, S. T., Connelly, J. H., Hill, A. L., Antes, R. P., Brown, R. P., & Devenport, L. D. (2007). Environmental influences on ethical decision-making: Climate and environmental predictors of research integrity. *Ethics and Behavior, 17*, 337–366. 10.1080/10508420802487815

Murrie, D. C., & Kelley, S. (2017). Evaluating and managing the risk of violence in clinical practice with adults. In P. M. Kleespies (Ed.), *The Oxford handbook of behavioral emergencies and crises* (pp. 126–145). Oxford University Press. 10.1093/oxfordhb/9780199352722.013.11

Naifeh, J. A., Nock, M. K., Dempsey, C. L., Georg, M. W., Bartolanzo, D., Ng, T. H. H., Aliaga, P. A., Dinh, H. M., Fullerton, C. S., Mash, H. B. H., Kao, T. C., Sampson, N. A., Wynn, G. H., Zaslavsky, A. M., Stein, M. B., Kessler, R. C., & Ursano, R. J. (2020). Self-injurious thoughts and behaviors that differentiate soldiers who attempt suicide from those with recent suicide ideation. *Depression and Anxiety, 37*(8), 738–746. 10.1002/da.23016

Nock, M. K., Kessler, R. C., & Franklin, J. C. (2016). Risk factors for suicide ideation differ from those for the transition to suicide attempt: The importance of creativity, rigor, and urgency in suicide research. *Clinical Psychology: Science and Practice, 23*(1), 31–34. 10.1111/cpsp.12133

Norcross, J. C. (2000). Psychotherapist self-care: Practitioner-tested, research-informed strategies. *Professional Psychology: Research and Practice, 31*(6), 710–713. 10.1037/0735-7028.31.6.710

Norcross, J. C., & Lambert, M. J. (2018). Psychotherapy relationships that work III. *Psychotherapy, 55*(4), 303–315. 10.1037/pst0000193

Norcross, J. C., & Wampold, B. E. (2011). Evidence-based therapy relationships: Research conclusions and clinical practices. *Psychotherapy, 48*, 98–102. 10.1037/a0022161

Norman, G. R., Monteiro, S. D., Sherbino, J., Ilgen, J. S., Schmidt, H. G., & Mamede, S. (2017). The causes of errors in clinical reasoning: Cognitive biases, knowledge deficits, and dual process thinking. *Academic Medicine, 92*(1), 23–30. 10.1097/ACM.0000000000001421

Novemsky, N., & Kahneman, D. (2005). The boundaries of loss aversion. *Journal of Marketing research, 42*(2), 119–128. 10.1509/jmkr.42.2.119.62292

Novotney, A. (2020). Common ethical principles and how to avoid them. *Monitor on Psychology, 51*(2), 36–40. https://www.apa.org/monitor/2020/03/ce-corner-missteps

O'Donnell, P., Farrar, A., BrintzenhofeSzoc, K., Conrad, A. P., Danis, M., Grady, C., Taylor, C., & Ulrich, C. M. (2008). Predictors of ethical stress, moral action and job satisfaction in health care social workers. *Social Work in Health Care, 46*(3), 29–51. 10.1300/J010v46n03_02

O'Donnell, D., Phelan, A., & Fealy, G. (2015). *Interventions and services which address elder abuse: An integrated review.* NCPOP. https://docplayer.net/20248210-Interventions-and-services-which-address-elder-abuse-an-integrated-review-deirdre-o-donnell-amanda-phelan-gerard-fealy.html

Paquin, J. D. (2017). Delivering the treatment so that the therapy occurs: Enhancing the effectiveness of time-limited, manualized group treatments. *International Journal of Group Psychotherapy, 67*(1), S141–S153. 10.1080/00207284.2016.1218771

Paquin, J. D., Kivlighan, D. M., Jr., & Drogosz, L. M. (2013). Person–group fit, group climate, and outcomes in a sample of incarcerated women participating in trauma recovery groups. *Group Dynamics: Theory, Research, and Practice, 17*(2), 95–109. 10.1037/a0032702

Pinner, D. H., & Kivlighan, D. M. III. (2018). The ethical implications and utility of routine outcome monitoring in determining boundaries of competence in practice. *Professional Psychology: Research and Practice, 49*(4), 247–254. 10.1037/pro0000203

Prescott, D. S., Maeschalck, C. L., & Miller, S. D. (Eds.). (2017). Feedback-informed treatment in clinical practice: Reaching for excellence. American Psychological Association. 10.1037/0000039-000

Quirk, K., Miller, S., Duncan, B., & Owen, J. (2013). Group Session Rating Scale: Preliminary psychometrics in substance abuse group interventions. *Counselling and Psychotherapy Research, 13*(3), 194–200. 10.1080/14733145.2012.744425

Raines, M. L. (2000). Ethical decision making in nurses. Relationships among moral reasoning, coping style, and ethics stress. *JONA'S Healthcare Law, Ethics and Regulation, 2*(1), 29–41.

Reamer, F. G. (2014). The Concept of Standard of Care. Social Work Today (May). https://www.socialworktoday.com/news/eoe_051314.shtml

Reid, W. H. (1998). Standard of care and patient need. *The Journal of Psychiatric Practice*, http://www.reidpsychiatry.com/columns/Reid05-98.pdf

Reisner, S. L., Biello, K., Perry, N. S., Gamarel, K. E., & Mimiaga, M. J. (2014). A compensatory model of risk and resilience applied to adolescent sexual orientation disparities in nonsuicidal self-injury and suicide attempts. *American Journal of Orthopsychiatry*, *84*(5), 545–556. 10.1037/ort0000008

Ribeiro, M. D. (Ed.). (2020). *Examining social identities and diversity issues in group therapy: Knocking at the boundaries*. Routledge. 10.4324/9780429022364

Ribeiro, J. D., Bender, T. W., Buchman, J. M., Nock, M. K., Rudd, M. D., Bryan, C. J., Lim, I. C., Baker, M. T., Knight, C., Gutierrez, P. M., & Joiner, T. E., Jr. (2015). An investigation of the interactive effects of the capability for suicide and acute agitation on suicidality in a military sample. *Depression and Anxiety*, *32*(1), 25–31. 10.1002/da.22240

Rogerson, M. D., Gottlieb, M. C., Handelsman, M. M., Knapp, S., & Younggren, J. (2011). Nonrational processes in ethical decision making. *American Psychologist*, *66*(7), 614–623. 10.1037/a0025215

Ruedy, N. E., & Schweitzer, M. E. (2010). In the moment: The effect of mindfulness on ethical decision-making. *Journal of Business Ethics*, *95*, 73–87. 10.1007/s10551-011-0796-y

Rupert, P. A., & Dorociak, K. E. (2019). Self-care, stress, and well-being among practicing psychologists. *Professional Psychology: Research and Practice*, *50*(5), 343–350. 10.1037/pro0000251

Shapiro, F. (2002). EMDR and the role of the clinician in psychotherapy evaluation: Towards a more comprehensive integration of science and practice. *Journal of Clinical Psychology*, *58*(12), 1453–1463. 10.1002/jclp.10104

Simon, R. I. (2011). Improving suicide risk assessment: Avoiding common pitfalls. *Psychiatric Times*, *28*(11). https://www.psychiatrictimes.com/view/improving-suicide-risk-assessment

Slone, N., Reese, R. Mathews-Duval, S., & Kodet, J. (2015). Evaluating the efficacy of client feedback in group psychotherapy. *Group Dynamics*, *19*, 122–136. 10.1037/gdn0000026

Sommers-Flanagan, J., & Shaw, S. L. (2017). Suicide risk assessment: What psychologists should know. *Professional Psychology: Research and Practice*, *48*(2), 96–106. 10.1037/pro0000106

Sommers-Flanagan, J., & Sommers-Flanagan, R. (2017). *Clinical interviewing* (6th ed.). Wiley. https://www.wiley.com/en-gu/Clinical+Interviewing,+6th+Edition-p-9781119215585

Spurgeon, S. L. (2017). Evaluating the unintended consequences of assessment practices: Construct irrelevance and construct underrepresentation. *Measurement and Evaluation in Counseling and Development*, *50*(4), 275–281. 10.1080/07481756.2017.1339563

Stenmark, C. K., & Mumford, M. D. (2011). Situational impacts on leader ethical decision-making. *The Leadership Quarterly*, *22*(5), 942–955. 10.1016/j.leaqua.2011.07.013

Strauss, B., Burlingame, G. M., & Bormann, B. (2008). Using the CORE-R battery in group psychotherapy. *Journal of Clinical Psychology*, *11*, 1225–1237. 10.1002/jclp.20535

Tasca, G. A., Angus, L., Bonli, R., Drapeau, M., Fitzpatrick, M., Hunsley, J., & Knoll, M. (2019). Outcome and progress monitoring in psychotherapy: Report of a Canadian Psychological Association Task Force. *Canadian Psychology/Psychologie Canadienne*, *60*(3), 165. 10.1037/cap0000181

Tasca, G. A., Cabrera, C., Kristjansson, E., MacNair-Semands, R., Joyce, A. S., & Ogrodniczuk, J. S. (2016). The Therapeutic Factors Inventory-8: Using item response theory to create a brief scale for continuous process monitoring for group psychotherapy. *Psychotherapy Research*, *26*, 131–145. 10.1080/10503307.2014.963729

Wampold, B. E., & Imel, Z. E. (2015). *The great psychotherapy debate: The evidence for what makes psychotherapy work*. Routledge. 10.4324/9780203582015

Weinberg, M. (2014). The ideological dilemma of subordination of self versus self-care: Identity construction of the 'ethical social worker.' *Discourse & Society*, *25*(1), 84–99. 10.1177/0957926513508855

Wise, E. H., Hersh, M. A., & Gibson, C. M. (2012). Ethics, self-care and well-being for psychologists: Re-envisioning the stress-distress continuum. *Professional Psychology: Research and Practice*, *43*, 487–494. 10.1037/a0029446

Woods, J. D., & Ruzek, N. A. (2018). Ethics in group psychotherapy. In M. D. Ribeiro, J. M. Gross, & M. M. Turner (Eds.), *The college counselor's guide to group psychotherapy* (pp. 83–100). Routledge. 10.4324/9781315545455

World Health Organization. (2019). *Suicide.* https://www.who.int/news-room/fact-sheets/detail/suicide

Wu, Q., & Slesnick, N. (2020). Substance abusing mothers with a history of childhood abuse and their children's depressive symptoms: the efficacy of family therapy. *Journal of Marital and Family Therapy*, *46*(1), 81–94. 10.1111/jmft.12364

Yalof, J., & Brabender, V. (2001). Ethical dilemmas in personality assessment courses: Using the classroom for in vivo training. *Journal of Personality Assessment*, *77*(2), 203–213. 10.1207/S1532 7752JPA7702_04

Yalom, I., & Leszcz, M. (2020). *The theory and practice of group psychotherapy* (6th ed.). Basic Books. https://www.basicbooks.com/titles/irvin-d-yalom/the-theory-and-practice-of-group-psychotherapy/ 9781541617575/

Yechiam, E. (2019). Acceptable losses: The debatable origins of loss aversion. *Psychological Research*, *83*(7), 1327–1339. 10.1207/S15327752JPA7702_04

Youn, S. J., Castonguay, L. G., McAleavey, A. A., Nordberg, S. S., Hayes, J. A., & Locke, B. D. (2020). Sensitivity to change of the Counseling Center Assessment of Psychological Symptoms-34. *Measurement and Evaluation in Counseling and Development*, *53*(2), 75–88. 10.1080/07481756.2019. 1691459

Younggren, J., & Gottlieb, M. (2017). Mandated multiple relationships and ethical decision-making. In O. Zur (Ed.), *Multiple relationships in psychotherapy and counseling: Unavoidable, common and mandatory dual relations in therapy* (pp. 30–44). Routledge.

Youssef, F. F., Dookeeram, K., Basdeo, V., Francis, E., Doman, M., Mamed, D., Maloo, S., Degannes, J., Dobo, L., Ditshotlo, P. , & Legall, G. (2012). Stress alters personal moral decision making. *Psychoneuroendocrinology*, *37*(4), 491–498. 10.1016/j.psyneuen.2011.07.017

Zeni, T. A., Buckley, M. R., Mumford, M. D., & Griffith, J. A. (2016). Making "sense" of ethical decision making. *The Leadership Quarterly*, *27*(6), 838–855. 10.1016/j.leaqua.2016.09.002

Zur, O. (Ed.) (2017). *Multiple relationships in psychotherapy and counseling: Unavoidable, common and mandatory dual relations in therapy.* Routledge.

Zur, O. (n.d.). *The standard of care in psychotherapy and counseling.* Zur Institute. https://www. zurinstitute.com/standard-of-care-therapy/

Afterword

We have presented many vignettes in this text, but we would like to offer our readers one more:

The mid-career group leader left her session feeling unsettled. She believed the session had been helpful to most of the members. But, overall, the session had a dull quality that troubled her. Moreover, she recalled that, recently, the sessions had generally had a bland quality. She asked herself if she herself had been disengaged but that did not seem to be the case. She wondered if the fact that the membership had remained unusually constant over a longer period of time (nearly 18 months) was creating a feeling of staleness. She also contemplated whether particular issues were likely to be threatening to her, leading her to discourage any further emergence or contemplation.

She contacted a supervisor who had been very helpful to her in her early work as a group leader. Her former supervisor would now function as a consultant. She shared with the supervisor process notes on several sessions and obtained the members' permission to share an audio recording with her. The consultation sessions yielded three insights. The consultant noted – in addition to members' occasional self-reports about their progress – the group leader's heavy reliance upon her own impressions as to how they were benefitting from the group. The supervisor suggested that repeated outcome management could supplement the therapist's evaluation of the group.

The review of process notes from earlier sessions revealed that two events in the group had received what seemed at the time adequate attention but, in retrospect, might have been resolved incompletely. One issue pertained to the racial composition of the group, i.e., that a single Black man was present in an otherwise all-White group. In fact, he had been in the group for a lengthy period, and occasionally brought up experiences of being a Black man in the world. The leader had somewhat tentatively asked him if he had similar experiences within the session but he had always responded in the negative. The consultant helped the leader to appreciate how difficult it might be for that member to acknowledge any parallels between his experiences in the room and outside. The group therapist admitted that the idea of having a deep, thoroughgoing exploration of race was frightening to her. She was afraid of making a misstep. It also aroused her guilt in that she had always had doubt about whether it was appropriate to have a single Black individual in the group. She consoled herself with the fact that other racial minorities were present, and she wondered why they never connected around the themes of discrimination and oppression.

Another issue was the fact that four members of the group were seeing her in individual psychotherapy. The others were either seeing another individual therapist or pursuing group psychotherapy as their sole therapeutic experience. Reference had been made to this variation at different points in the life of the group. Recently, however, an event occurred in which members perceived that she had softened a piece of feedback they were delivering to a member. They speculated that her individual therapy relationship led her to feel unduly protective of the member. The three other members who were also her individual therapy clients disputed that perspective, saying that on a number of occasions, they had wished she would have come to their aid. Another member said she remembered the leader framing members' feedback to her in more palatable terms even though she was not her individual client.

The consultant observed that privilege inside and outside of the group might have been an issue the therapist evaded—the privilege of being White, the privilege of having other members of the group share one's identity status, the privilege of being the group leader's individual therapy client. Whether it was the avoidance of a thorough exploration of issues related to privilege that was responsible for the group's flatness could not be known absolutely, but it was plausible to believe that this was a factor. In any case, the leader was able to acknowledge insecurity and lack of skill in regard to exploring issues of race and privilege. Collaboratively, the consultant and leader fashioned a set of experiences that would better equip the leader to work with the group in this area. This collection included participation in a weekend racial awareness group, completion of a set of readings on race and white privilege, and involvement in a peer supervision group that met bi-weekly. The consultant and leader put in place a routine outcome management system so that the leader could better ascertain members' progress. The consultant also indicated that she would continue to be available to the leader as needed.

Many aspects of this vignette could be explored further, such as how race and privilege are addressed in the psychotherapy group. We invite the reader to do so independently, applying the concepts presented in these chapters. However, what we want to comment upon as our final word to the reader is this leader's willingness to recognize when the group experiences being offered to members might not be optimal for their development. Moreover, the leader in our vignette took decisive action to remediate likely deficiencies in her approach to the group. Notice that nothing had occurred in the group that would constitute an emergency. Rather, the therapist's initiation of a course of action resulted from her continuing monitoring of the group's progress and yearning to offer treatment that would be as beneficial as possible to her members. In doing so, she took the risks that she might learn about her own weaknesses and might experience discomfort. She accepted these risks.

In 2001, Patricia Bricklin wrote an article entitled "Being ethical is more than obeying the law and avoiding harm." What she meant by this statement is that ethical mindedness is not something that the leader should bring out for special occasions such as, for example, when some troubling situation emerges. It's a state of mind that the therapist achieves in an abiding way. The presence of this state of mind leads the leader to reflect with consistency on the work, recognize the potential for achieving even greater good, and pursue the steps for realizing that potential.

Reference

Bricklin, P. (2001). Being ethical: More than obeying the law and avoiding harm. *Journal of Personality Assessment, 77*(2), 195–202. 10.1207/S15327752JPA7702_03

Index

Locators in **bold** refer to tables.

ableness **52**, **54**
abuse 57, 113, 159–160
accountability 148–149
acculturation: Ethics Acculturation model
    122–123, 144; organizational guidelines **54**;
    resources for multicultural competence **52**
adequate containers 73
administrative supervision 127
adolescents: decision-making processes 133;
    informed consent 110–112
advertising 111–112
affect heuristic 136
age **52**, **54**
alcohol 17, 18, 59, 107
alliance, between group leaders and prospective
    members 67; with personality traits 72;
    preparing members 81
alternative treatments 109–110
American Board for Group Psychology
    (ABPP) 10
American Counseling Association (ACA)
    10, **120**
American Group Psychotherapy Association
    (AGPA) 10, 59, 89, 152
American Psychiatric Association (APA) 11
American Psychological Association (APA) 10,
    11, **120**, 150, 152
American Telemedicine Association 11
anchoring-and-adjustment strategy 136
anxious attachment style 70
Aristotle 6–7
assimilist strategy 123
attachment styles 70, 78–80
attendance 71, 76, 78, 106–107
automatic processing 134–135
autonomy in decision-making 134
autonomy, respect for 2, **3**, 3; attachment styles
    and personality traits 78–79; decision-making
    processes 143; sharing norms 87; information
    about leader credentials 87; social relations
    with other members 87; extra-group contact

90; informed consent 111; pre-group selection
    67–68, 73–74; suicide risk 153
availability heuristic 135–136
avoidant attachment style 70

Beauchamp, T. L. 2–3
beneficence 2, 3, **3**; excluding a group member
    87; informed consent 99; multicultural
    competence 50; pre-group selection 73;
    relational style 79; suicide risk 153
Bernard, H. 10, 69–71, 73, 76, 80–82, 88–89, **90**
biases: decision-making 134–135, 139–144;
    optimism/pessimism 74; prejudice from group
    members 56–57, 82–85, 89
Black Identity theory 51
boundaries: addressing rupture and repair 58;
    extra-group contact 47–49; feminist ethics 6;
    multicultural competence 51–56; therapist's
    role in managing 43–45
boundaries of competence 149–150
boundary crossing 6, 43–45, 137
boundary violation 43
Brabender, V. 2, 29, 30–32, **33**, 36, 42, 46, 84, 88,
    101, 104, 106, 120–122, 127, 133
brainstorming 16–17
Bricklin, P. 12, 172
Brown, L. 6
bullying xi

care, ethics of 6
case law 146
character of the professional 8
child abuse reporting 159–160
children, informed consent 110–112
Childress, J. F. 2–3
clinical supervision 127; *see also* supervision
Clinically-Oriented Research Evaluation
    (CORE) Battery-R 104
codes of ethics 9–11, **120**, 146–147
coercion xi, 7, 57, 60, 67–68, 105, 125
cognitive interferences (therapist) 42
cognitive processing 135, 140

cognitive reactivity 154
Commission for the Recognition of Specialties and Proficiencies in Professional Psychology (CRSPPP) 10
communication, privileged 26–28, 35–37
community consensus 147
competences of supervisors 119–120, 124
competences of therapist 43; ethical decision-making 149–150; influencing factors 42; pre-group preparation 91–92; scope of responsibility 59
competent care 149–150
confidentiality 26–27; challenges of 28–37; consequences of breaches in 29–30, 32–34; decision-making processes 133; fostering 30–31; informed consent 100; risk of confidentiality breaches 103–104
consultation: decision-making processes 16; versus supervision 127; value of 171
contextual analysis 18
contextual capability 42
contextual challenges in decision-making 132–134
continuing education 42
continuous assessment 149
Cottone, R. R. 18–19
Counseling Center Assessment of Psychological Symptoms (CCAPS-34) 152
court orders 36–37
Covid-19 pandemic 100, 107, 108–109
Cultural Assessment of Risk for Suicide (CARS) 154
cultural humility 50, **52–55**
cultural influences: addressing rupture and repair 58–59; assessments for 89–90; community consensus 147; gifts and gift-giving 46–47; and identity 49; interpersonal distress 79; Koocher and Keith-Spiegel Model 15–16; marginalized identities 51, **52–55**; multicultural competence 49–50, **52–55**; preparing for diversity and difference 82–85
cultural oppression 56
culturally competent suicide-risk assessments (CCSRA) 154

decision-making biases 134–135
decision-making processes: approaches, techniques, and tips 138–144; challenges to ethical decision-making 132–138; ethical paradigms 13–19; pre-group selection 70–71; risk management 153–160; Standard of Care 144–153; supervisor's role 121–122, 141–142
deliberate thinking 135, 140
disabilities: ableness **52**, **54**; informed consent 112–113
discrimination 57, 83–84, 151–152, 154; *see also* multicultural competence
diversity: differences within the microcosm 56–57; group composition 73–74, 171;

interpersonal distress 79; managing differences among members 49–56; managing member-to-member relations 57–58; multicultural competence and humility 49–56, **52–55**; Multiculturally Sensitive Mental Health Scale 151; Perception of Ethnic Discrimination Questionnaire (PEDQ) 151–152; pre-group meetings 68; preparing for diversity and difference 82–85
documentation, for supervision 126
dropout: exclusion criteria 71–72, 80–81; lack of progress 104; progress monitoring 149; selection instruments 76–77; *see also* pre-group selection

elder abuse reporting 159–160
emotional interferences (therapist) 42
emotional load 138–139
emotions: affect heuristic 136; decision-making processes 15; ethics of care 7; interpersonal skills 72; supervisor's role 120
ethical judgment: approaches, techniques, and tips 138–144; challenges to ethical decision-making 132–138; risk management 153–160; Standard of Care 144–153; supervisor's role 122, 141–142
ethical paradigms 1–2; codes of ethics and standards of practice 9–11; comment on ethical models 8–9; decision-making processes 13–19; ethics of care 7; feminist ethics 4–7, 121; principlism 2–4, 7, 99; regulatory bodies and the law 12–13; virtue ethics 6–7
ethical practitioners 122–123
Ethics Acculturation model 122–123, 144
ethics of care 7
ethnicity: organizational guidelines **55**; preparing for diversity and difference 84–85; resources for multicultural competence **53**
evidence-based treatment 148–153
exclusion criteria 71–72; *see also* pre-group selection
experiential training groups 125–126
external factors in decision-making 132–134
extra-group contact 47–49, 90–91
Eye Movement Desensitization and Reprocessing (EMDR) 147

feedback: measurement-based care systems (MBC) 58–59, 149, 150–152; member questionnaires 58–59; progress monitoring 149; supervisor's role 121–122
fees 105–106
feminist ethics 4–7, 121
fidelity 2–3, **3**
financial responsibilities 105–106
floor approach to ethics 9
Focused on the Needs of Others scale 79
framing the problem 140–141
functional subgrouping 57

Gabbard, G. O. 108
gatekeeping 124, 126
gender: organizational guidelines **54**; resources for multicultural competence **52**
gender identity **53**, **54**, 84
gift-giving 46–47
Greene, L. 42, 57, 71, 78, 89–90, 148–149
group composition 73–74, 171
group dynamics: addressing rupture and repair 58–59; consultation vignette 171–173; dropout 71–72, 76–77; excluding a group member 80–81, 87; extra-group contact 47–49, 90–91; fears and myths 87–88; feedback and questionnaires 58–59; identity differences within the microcosm 56–57; managing differences among members 49–56; managing member-to-member relations 57–58; Standard of Care 148; violent intent 158–159; *see also* pre-group selection
group norms 67, 85–87
group participation sessions 31–34
group psychodynamic-interpersonal psychotherapy (GPIP) model 89–90
Group Questionnaire (GQ) 58–59
Group Readiness Questionnaire (GRQ) 76–77
group screening 67; *see also* pre-group meetings
Group Sessions Rating Scale (GSRS) 58–59
group termination: confidentiality awareness 34; excluding a group member 80–81, 87; progress monitoring 149
Group Therapy Questionnaire (GTQ) 77–78
Group Therapy Questionnaire-Short Version (GTQ-S) 68, 77–78

Haas, L. J. 14, 18, 27
Hampton, H. P. 146
Health Insurance Portability and Accountability Act 12
heterogeneous groups 69
heuristics 135–136, 137–138, 139–144
HIPAA regulations 146
homogeneous groups 69
humility *see* cultural humility

identity: differences within the microcosm 56–57; group composition 73–74; interpersonal distress 79; managing differences among members 49–56; managing member-to-member relations 57–58; multicultural competence and humility 49–56, **52–55**; Multiculturally Sensitive Mental Health Scale 151; Perception of Ethnic Discrimination Questionnaire (PEDQ) 151–152; pre-group meetings 68; preparing for diversity and difference 82–85; suicide risk 154
immigration **52**, **54**
impaired adults 112–113
impulsivity 18, 29, 143

inclusion criteria 69–71; *see also* pre-group selection
indigenous people 53, **54–55**
information gathering 141
informed consent 99; considerations for special populations 110–114; elements 101–110; formats 101; member responsibilities 105–107; as process, not event 99–101; risks of group treatment 102–105; use of technology 107–109
insight 69
integrationist strategy 123
internal factors in decision-making 134–135
interpersonal attachments 89–90
interpersonal distress 79
interpersonal goals 85–86
interpersonal problems inventories 70, 79
interpersonal skills: pre-group selection 69–70, 72; relational style 78–80
Inventory of Interpersonal Problems (IIP) 70

justice 2, **3**; multicultural competence 49; pre-group selection 70–71, 73; preparing for diversity and difference 82–85; suicide risk 153

Kahneman, D. 135–136
Kaklauskas, F. 57, 68, 84, 89–90
Keith-Spiegel, P. 13–18
Knapp, S. 9, 142
Koocher, G. P. 13–18

leader's role *see* therapist's role
leaving a group *see* dropout; group termination
Lefforge, N. L. 58
legal context: confidentiality 103–104; decision-making processes 15; ethical paradigms 12–13; Standard of Care 146; violent intent 158–159
Leszcz, M. 11, 56, 58, 66–74, 69–71, 76–77, 79–82, 84–85, 87–89, **90**, 147–149
licensing boards 12, 146
loss, avoidance of 136–138, 140–141
loyalty 2–3, **3**

MacNair-Semands, R. 11, 49, 68–72, 74, 76–78, 82–83, 84–85, 106
Malat, J. 120–121
Malouf, J. L. 14, 18, 27
mandated treatment 113–114
marginalized identities 51, **52–55**; Multiculturally Sensitive Mental Health Scale 151; Perception of Ethnic Discrimination Questionnaire (PEDQ) 151–152; pre-group selection 70–71; suicide risk 154
marginalizing strategy 123
Marmarosh, C. L. 34, 58, 70, 73, 103, 105, 149, 152
materiality standard 103
measurement-based care systems (MBC) 58–59, 149, 150–152

measures for selection and screening 74–80; *see also* pre-group selection
measures of racism and ethnicity-related stress 151–152
member goals 85–86, 102
member outcomes 148–149
member responsibilities 105–107
member suicide attempt or completion 158
member-to-member relations: addressing rupture and repair 58–59; extra-group contact 47–49, 90–91; fears and myths 87–88; identity differences within the microcosm 56–57; managing differences among members 49–56; managing member-to-member relations 57–58; risk of discomfort 103; risks of group treatment 102–103; *see also* group norms; pre-group selection
microaggressions 56–57, 58–59, 68, 84, 86, 89–90
Mini-International Neuropsychiatric Interview (MINI) 155
minorities *see* marginalized identities
multicultural competence 49–56, **52–55**
Multiculturally Sensitive Mental Health Scale 151

National Association of Social Workers (NASW) 10–11, **120**
non-maleficence 2, **3**; excluding a group member 71; pre-group selection 70–71, 73; preparing for diversity and difference 82–85; expectations for termination 87; suicide risk 153
Norcross, J. C. 138, 139

online group meetings 100, 107, 108–109
optimistic bias 74
oral substances 107
organizational influences 133–134
Outcome Rating Scale 59
outcomes: cultural humility 50; lack of progress 104; measurement-based care systems (MBC) 58–59, 149, 150–152; personality traits 71–72, 79–80; pre-group selection 69, 70, 76, 102; progress monitoring 149, 152–153; risks of group treatment 102–105; self-care (therapist) 139; Standard of Care 148–149; suicide risk 153–158
outside contact *see* extra-group contact

payment 105–106
Perception of Ethnic Discrimination Questionnaire (PEDQ) 151–152
performance pressure 134
personal growth/changes 104–105
Personal Health Information (PHI) 12, 26
personality traits 15–16, 71–72, 78–80
pessimistic bias 74
positive approach to ethics 9

power asymmetries: feminist ethics 4, 7; identity and microaggressions 56–57
practical wisdom 8
practice-based evidence 149, 152; *see also* routine outcome monitoring; measurement-based care
practitioners: character of the professional 8; ethical paradigms 1–2, 19; standards of practice 9–11; training in ethics 122–123; *see also* decision-making processes; standards of practice; therapist's role
pre-group meetings: attachment styles and personality traits 70, 71–72, 78–80; describing the work of group 88–89; fears and myths 87–88; fostering confidentiality 30–31; goals and norms 85–87; Group Therapy Questionnaire (GTQ) 68, 77–78; Group Readiness Questionnaire 76–77; preparing for diversity and difference 82–85; purposes of 67–68
pre-group preparation 81–82, 90; assessments for interpersonal attachments and culture 89–90; competences of therapist 91–92; describing the work of group 88–89; diversity and difference 82–85; extra-group contact 90–91; fears and myths 87–88; goals and norms 85–87; informed consent 99–100; safety norms 155–156; working alliance 81
pre-group selection: appropriate fit 67–68; criteria and procedures 68–76; exclusion criteria 71–72, 80–81; group composition 73–74, 171; Group Readiness Questionnaire (GRQ) 76–77; Group Therapy Questionnaire (GTQ) 68, 77–78; heterogeneous and homogeneous groups 69; inclusion criteria 69–71; screening out 67, 71–72, 80–81; suicide risk 155–156
prejudice: identity and microaggressions 56–57; preparing members 82–85, 89
principlism 2–4, 7, 99
privacy 26; *see also* confidentiality
privilege: group dynamics 172; identity and microaggressions 56–57, 58; preparing for diversity and difference 84–85
privileged communication 26–28, 35–37
process-oriented psychotherapy groups 56, 69
professional associations 9–11, 146–147
professional consensus 147
professional development 119; *see also* supervision
professional self-awareness 143–144
professional standards *see* standards of practice
progress, lack of 104
progress monitoring 149, 152–153
prospect theory 136–138
psychotherapist-patient privilege 27–28
psychotherapy, versus supervision 127
punctuality 106–107

quality gap 149–150
quality of object relations (QOR) 74

race: group composition 171; organizational guidelines **55**; preparing for diversity and difference 84–85; resources for multicultural competence **53**
racial identity theory 51
Rapin, L. S. 11
regulatory bodies 12–13; *see also* legal context
rejection, fear of 87
relational style 70, 78–80
religion: organizational guidelines **55**; resources for multicultural competence **53**
research, informing practice 148–153
respect for autonomy *see* autonomy, respect for
respected minority principle 147
rigid boundaries 43
risk, approaches to decision-making 136–138
risk management 145, 153–161
risks of group treatment 102–105
routine outcome monitoring (ROM) 149, 150; *see also* measurement-based care (MBC)
Rutan, J. S. 58, 75, 91, 105–106

safety norms 155–156
scapegoating 57, 80
selecting members *see* pre-group selection
self-awareness 143–144
self-care (therapist) 42, 138–139
self-disclosure of group members 43–44, 57, 73, 100
self-disclosure of therapist 45–46, 125–126
self-efficacy 134
self-understanding 69
separatist strategy 123
sexual orientation: organizational guidelines **55**; preparing for diversity and difference 84–85; resources for multicultural competence **53**
Shaw, S. L. 154–155
social justice 10, 34, 49, 56, 82, 84, 106
social networking 108
social skills 69–70, 72
social workers, National Association of Social Workers (NASW) 10–11, **120**
socio-economic status: organizational guidelines **55**; resources for multicultural competence **53**
sociocultural dimensions: differences within the microcosm 56–57; group composition 73–74; interpersonal distress 79; managing differences among members 49–56; managing member-to-member relations 57–58; multicultural competence and humility 49–56, **52–55**; Multiculturally Sensitive Mental Health Scale 151; Perception of Ethnic Discrimination Questionnaire (PEDQ) 151–152; pre-group meetings 68; preparing for diversity and difference 82–85; suicide risk 154
Sommers-Flanagan, J. 154–155

spirituality: organizational guidelines **55**; resources for multicultural competence **53**
stakeholders: decision-making processes 16; multiple stakeholders in ethical decisions 132–133
Standard of Care 144–153; legal considerations 146; elements 146–147
standards of practice 9–11; decision-making processes 15; organizational influences on decision-making 133–134; risks of group treatment 103; supervision **120**
state licensing 12, 146
status *see* socio-economic status
stress management 138–139, 151–152
subpoena 36
substances use 107
suicide risk 153–158
supervision 119; clinical versus administrative 127; competences 119–120, 124; versus consultation 127; contracts and documentation 126; duties 120–124; ethical decision-making 122, 141–142; group settings 124–126; organizational guidelines **120**; versus psychotherapy 127
the supervisory alliance 121

Tasca, G. A. 79, 89–90
technology use 107–109
telepsychology 11
termination of group sessions *see* group termination
testimonials 111–112
therapeutic factors (TFs) 151
therapist credentials 102
therapist's role 59–60; addressing rupture and repair 58–59; competences 42–43, 59; ethical practice 42; excluding a group member 80–81, 87; extra-group contact 47–49; gifts and gift-giving 46–47; identity differences within the microcosm 56–57; managing boundaries 43–45; managing differences among members 49–56; managing member-to-member relations 57–58; multicultural competence and humility 49–50, **52–55**; pre-group preparation 81–90; scope of responsibility 59; self-disclosure 45–46; *see also* decision-making processes
therapy services, regulation of 12–13
training: ethical practitioners 122–123; experiential training groups 125–126; suicide risk 154, 157–158; supervisor's role 119, 121–122; violent intent 159
transgender 84
transparency 34

values, pre-group meetings 83–84; *see also* group norms
verbal informed consent 101
Vergés, A. 18

veterans **54**, **55**
violence 158–159
virtual meetings *see* online group meetings
virtue ethics 7–8, 59
vulnerability 155–156, 159–160

White Identity theory 51
Whittingham, M. 68, 77–78, 79, 83, 85, 89

World Mental Health-International College
    Student (WMH-ICS) 155
written informed consent 101

Yalom, I. D. 11, 56, 58, 66–74, 69–71, 76–77,
    79–82, 84–85, 87–89, **90**, 147–149

.

For Product Safety Concerns and Information please contact our EU
representative GPSR@taylorandfrancis.com
Taylor & Francis Verlag GmbH, Kaufingerstraße 24, 80331 München, Germany

www.ingramcontent.com/pod-product-compliance
Ingram Content Group UK Ltd.
Pitfield, Milton Keynes, MK11 3LW, UK
UKHW030828080625
459435UK00014B/589